Recent Advancements in Neuromuscular Medicine

Guest Editor

GREGORY T. CARTER, MD, MS

PHYSICAL MEDICINE AND REHABILITATION CLINICS OF NORTH AMERICA

www.pmr.theclinics.com

Consulting Editor
GREGORY T. CARTER, MD, MS

February 2012 • Volume 23 • Number 1

SAUNDERS an imprint of ELSEVIER, Inc.

W.B. SAUNDERS COMPANY
A Division of Elsevier Inc.

1600 John F. Kennedy Boulevard • Suite 1800 • Philadelphia, Pennsylvania 19103

http://www.theclinics.com

PHYSICAL MEDICINE AND REHABILITATION CLINICS OF NORTH AMERICA Volume 23, Number 1
February 2012 ISSN 1047-9651, ISBN-13: 978-1-4557-3917-2

Editor: David Parsons
Developmental Editor: Teia Stone

Reprints. For copies of 100 or more of articles in this publication, please contact the Commercial Reprints Department, Elsevier Inc., 360 Park Avenue South, New York, NY 10010-1710. Tel.: 212-633-3812; Fax: 212-462-1935; E-mail: reprints@elsevier.com.

Physical Medicine and Rehabilitation Clinics of North America (ISSN 1047-9651) is published quarterly by Elsevier Inc., 360 Park Avenue South, New York, NY 10010-1710. Months of issue are February, May, August, and November. Business and Editorial Offices: 1600 John F. Kennedy Blvd., Suite 1800, Philadelphia, PA 19103-2899. Customer Service Office: 3251 Riverport Lane, Maryland Heights, MO 63043. Periodicals postage paid at New York, NY and additional mailing offices. Subscription price per year is $248.00 (US individuals), $441.00 (US institutions), $132.00 (US students), $302.00 (Canadian individuals), $575.00 (Canadian institutions), $189.00 (Canadian students), $373.00 (foreign individuals), $575.00 (foreign institutions), and $189.00 (foreign students). Foreign air speed delivery is included in all *Clinics* subscription prices. All prices are subject to change without notice. **POSTMASTER:** Send address changes to *Physical Medicine and Rehabilitation Clinics of North America,* Customer Service Office: Elsevier Health Sciences Division, Subscription Customer Service, 3251 Riverport Lane, Maryland Heights, MO 63043. **Customer Service: 1-800-654-2452 (US). From outside of the United States, call 314-447-8871. Fax: 314-447-8029. E-mail: JournalsCustomer Service-usa@elsevier.com (for print support); JournalsOnlineSupport-usa@elsevier.com (for online support).**

Physical Medicine and Rehabilitation Clinics of North America is indexed in *Excerpta Medica, MEDLINE/ PubMed (Index Medicus), Cinahl, and Cumulative Index to Nursing and Allied Health Literature.*

Printed and bound by CPI Group (UK) Ltd, Croydon, CR0 4YY

Transferred to Digital Print 2012

Contributors

CONSULTING EDITOR

GREGORY T. CARTER, MD, MS
Medical Director, Muscular Dystrophy Association Regional Neuromuscular Center, Providence Medical Group, Clinical Neurosciences Division, Olympia, Washington

GUEST EDITOR

GREGORY T. CARTER, MD, MS
Medical Director, Muscular Dystrophy Association Regional Neuromuscular Center, Providence Medical Group, Clinical Neurosciences Division, Olympia, Washington

AUTHORS

RICHARD T. ABRESCH, MS
Department of Physical Medicine and Rehabilitation, University of California Davis, Sacramento, California

DANIEL J. BOGAN, BA
Department of Pathology and Laboratory Medicine, The Gene Therapy Center, School of Medicine; Senator Paul D. Wellstone Muscular Dystrophy Cooperative Research Center, University of North Carolina-Chapel Hill, Chapel Hill, North Carolina

JANET R. BOGAN, BS
Department of Pathology and Laboratory Medicine, The Gene Therapy Center, School of Medicine; Senator Paul D. Wellstone Muscular Dystrophy Cooperative Research Center, University of North Carolina-Chapel Hill, Chapel Hill, North Carolina

GREGORY T. CARTER, MD, MS
Medical Director, Muscular Dystrophy Association Regional Neuromuscular Center, Providence Medical Group, Clinical Neurosciences Division, Olympia, Washington

MICHAEL S. CARTWRIGHT, MD
Assistant Professor, Department of Neurology, Wake Forest School of Medicine, Winston-Salem, North Carolina

MARTIN K. CHILDERS, DO, PhD
Professor, Section of PM&R, Department of Neurology, School of Medicine; Wake Forest Institute for Regenerative Medicine, Wake Forest University, Winston-Salem, North Carolina

JARED W. COBURN, PhD
Department of Kinesiology, California State University, Fullerton, Fullerton, California

CLARK E. CULLEN, MD
Principal Investigator and Research Director, Sunstone Medical Research, Medford, Oregon

J. DAVOODI, PhD
Assistant Professor, Institute of Biochemistry and Biophysics, University of Tehran, Iran; Human Nutrition, Foods and Exercise, Virginia Tech, Blacksburg, Virginia

JENNIFER L. DOW, BS
Department of Pathology and Laboratory Medicine, and The Gene Therapy Center, School of Medicine; Senator Paul D. Wellstone Muscular Dystrophy Cooperative Research Center, University of North Carolina-Chapel Hill, Chapel Hill, North Carolina

ZHENG FAN, MD
Department of Neurology, School of Medicine; Senator Paul D. Wellstone Muscular Dystrophy Cooperative Research Center, University of North Carolina-Chapel Hill, Chapel Hill, North Carolina

MARK R. FERGUSON, MD
Assistant Professor, Department of Radiology, Seattle Children's Hospital, Seattle, Washington

ERIKA L. FINANGER, MD, MS
Assistant Professor, Departments of Pediatrics and Neurology, Oregon Health and Science University; Shriners Hospital, Portland, Oregon

SEAN C. FORBES, PhD
Research Assistant Professor, Department of Physical Therapy, University of Florida, Gainesville, Florida

LAWRENCE FRANK, PhD
Department of Radiology, University of California San Diego; Research Service, VA San Diego Healthcare System, San Diego, California

JAN FRIDÉN, MD, PhD
Professor of Hand Surgery, Department of Hand Surgery, Institute of Clinical Sciences, Sahlgrenska University Hospital, Göteborg, Sweden; Swiss Paraplegic Centre, Nottwil, Switzerland

SETH D. FRIEDMAN, PhD
Department of Radiology, Center for Clinical and Translational Research, Seattle Children's Hospital, Seattle, Washington

WALTER R. FRONTERA, MD, PhD
Professor, Department of Physical Medicine and Rehabilitation; Professor, Department of Physiology, University of Puerto Rico School of Medicine, San Juan, Puerto Rico

MELISSA A. GODDARD, BSc
Wake Forest Institute for Regenerative Medicine, Wake Forest University, Winston-Salem, North Carolina

ANDREAS GOHRITZ, MD
Department of Plastic, Hand and Reconstructive Surgery, Hannover Medical School, Hannover, Germany

ROBERT W. GRANGE, PhD
Associate Professor and Assistant Department Head, Department of Human Nutrition, Foods, and Exercise, Virginia Tech University, Blacksburg, Virginia

PETER A. GRANT, MD
Electrodiagnostic Medicine, Medford, Oregon

JAY J. HAN, MD
Associate Professor, Department of Physical Medicine and Rehabilitation, University of California Davis, Sacramento, California

ERIC P. HOFFMAN, PhD
Department of Integrative Systems Biology, George Washington University School of Medicine; Research Center for Genetic Medicine, Children's National Medical Center, Washington, DC

JAMES F. HOWARD Jr, MD
Department of Neurology, School of Medicine; Senator Paul D. Wellstone Muscular Dystrophy Cooperative Research Center, University of North Carolina-Chapel Hill, Chapel Hill, North Carolina

S.M. HUTSON, PhD
Department of Human Nutrition, Foods and Exercise, Virginia Tech, Blacksburg, Virginia

JOE N. KORNEGAY, DVM, PhD
Departments of Pathology and Laboratory Medicine and Neurology, and The Gene Therapy Center, School of Medicine; Senator Paul D. Wellstone Muscular Dystrophy Cooperative Research Center, University of North Carolina-Chapel Hill, Chapel Hill, North Carolina

RICHARD LIEBER, PhD
Departments of Orthopaedic Surgery and Bioengineering, University of California San Diego La Jolla; Research Service, VA San Diego Healthcare System, San Diego, California

JAU-SHIN LOU, MD, PhD
Director, Neuromuscular Center of Oregon; Director, EMG Laboratory, Department of Neurology, Oregon Health & Science University, Portland, Oregon

MOH H. MALEK, PhD
Integrative Physiology of Exercise Laboratory, Eugene Applebaum College of Pharmacy & Health Sciences, Wayne State University, Detroit, Michigan

C.D. MARKERT, PhD
Wake Forest Institute for Regenerative Medicine, Winston-Salem, North Carolina

DAVID MAYANS, MD
Department of Neurology, Wake Forest School of Medicine, Winston-Salem, North Carolina

CRAIG M. MCDONALD, MD
Professor and Chair, Department of Physical Medicine and Rehabilitation, University of California Davis, Sacramento, California

ERIN MITCHELL, DVM
Department of Physical Therapy, University of Florida, Gainesville, Florida

PETER NGHIEM, DVM
Department of Integrative Systems Biology, George Washington University School of Medicine; Research Center for Genetic Medicine, Children's National Medical Center, Washington, DC

RANDOLPH K. OTTO, MD
Assistant Professor, Department of Radiology, Seattle Children's Hospital, Seattle, Washington

SHAWN E. PARNELL, MD
Assistant Professor of Radiology, Department of Radiology; Seattle Children's Center for Clinical and Translational Research, Seattle Children's Hospital, Seattle, Washington

SANDRA L. POLIACHIK, PhD
Department of Radiology; Seattle Children's Center for Clinical and Translational Research, Seattle Children's Hospital, Seattle, Washington

DANNY A. RILEY, PhD
Professor, Department of Cell Biology, Neurobiology & Anatomy, Medical College of Wisconsin, Milwaukee, Wisconsin

NATIVIDAD RODRIGUEZ, MT
Department of Physiology, University of Puerto Rico School of Medicine, San Juan, Puerto Rico

ANA RODRIGUEZ ZAYAS, PhD
Post-doctoral Fellow, Professor, Department of Physiology, University of Puerto Rico School of Medicine, San Juan, Puerto Rico

WILLIAM D. ROONEY, PhD
Advanced Imaging Research Center, Oregon Health and Science University, Portland, Oregon

BARRY RUSSMAN, MD
Professor, Departments of Pediatrics and Neurology, Oregon Health and Science University; Shriners Hospital, Portland, Oregon

DAVID SCOTT SAPERSTEIN, MD
Phoenix Neurological Associates Ltd, Phoenix, Arizona

SCOTT J. SCHATZBERG, DVM, PhD
Veterinary Emergency and Specialty Center of New Mexico, Albuquerque, New Mexico

SIMON SCHENK, PhD
Department of Orthopaedic Surgery, University of California San Diego, La Jolla, California

DENNIS W. SHAW, MD
Professor of Radiology and Division Chief, Magnetic Resonance Imaging, Division Chief, Vascular/Interventional Imaging, Department of Radiology, Seattle Children's Hospital; Seattle Children's Center for Clinical and Translational Research, Seattle, Washington

ANDREW J. SKALSKY, MD
Assistant Professor, Department of Pediatrics, University of California San Diego, Rady Children's Hospital and Health Center, San Diego, California

BARBARA K. SMITH, PhD, PT
Animal Resources Program, Wake Forest University, Winston-Salem, North Carolina

MARTIN A. STYNER, PhD
Departments of Computer Science and Psychiatry, University of North Carolina-Chapel Hill, Chapel Hill, North Carolina

MARK TARNOPOLSKY, MD, PhD, FRCPC
Professor, Departments of Pediatrics; Department of Medicine, McMaster University, Hamilton, Ontario, Canada

KRISTA VANDENBORNE, PT, PhD
Professor and Chair, Department of Physical Therapy, University of Florida, Gainesville, Florida

J.M. VAN DYKE, PhD
Department of Cell Biology, Neurobiology & Anatomy, Medical College of Wisconsin, Milwaukee, Wisconsin

K.A. VOELKER, PhD
Department of Human Nutrition, Foods and Exercise, Virginia Tech, Blacksburg, Virginia

KATHRYN R. WAGNER, MD, PhD
Director, Center for Genetic Muscle Disorders, Kennedy Krieger Institute; Departments of Neurology and Neuroscience, The Johns Hopkins School of Medicine, Baltimore, Maryland

FRANCIS O. WALKER, MD
Professor of Neurology, Department of Neurology, Wake Forest School of Medicine, Winston-Salem, North Carolina

GLENN A. WALTER, PhD
Associate Professor, Department of Physiology and Functional Genomics, University of Florida, Gainesville, Florida

JIAHUI WANG, PhD
Department of Psychiatry, University of North Carolina-Chapel Hill, Chapel Hill, North Carolina

SAMUEL WARD, PT, PhD
Departments of Radiology and Orthopaedic Surgery, La Jolla; Department of Bioengineering, University of California San Diego, San Diego, California

MICHAEL D. WEISS, MD
Associate Professor of Neurology and Director of the Neuromuscular Diseases Division and Electrodiagnostic Laboratory, Department of Neurology, University of Washington Medical Center, Seattle, Washington

Contents

Preface: Advancing Neuromuscular Medicine Through Integration, Translation, and Collaboration   xv

Gregory T. Carter

Use of Skeletal Muscle MRI in Diagnosis and Monitoring Disease Progression in Duchenne Muscular Dystrophy   1

Erika L. Finanger, Barry Russman, Sean C. Forbes, William D. Rooney, Glenn A. Walter, and Krista Vandenborne

> Studies have shown promise in using various approaches of magnetic resonance imaging (MRI) and magnetic resonance spectroscopy to evaluate skeletal muscle involvement in Duchenne muscular dystrophy. However, these studies have mainly been performed using a cross-sectional design, and the correlation of these MRI changes with disease progression and disease severity has not been fully elucidated. Overall, skeletal muscle MRI is a powerful and sensitive technique in the evaluation of muscle disease, and its use as a biomarker for disease progression or therapeutic response in clinical trials deserves further study.

Techniques in Assessing Fatigue in Neuromuscular Diseases   11

Jau-Shin Lou

> Fatigue is common in neuromuscular disease and it may affect quality of life; however, it has not been adequately studied. We can approach fatigue in neuromuscular diseases systematically. Questionnaires are used to assess subjective or experienced fatigue, and with the wide availability of the Internet, many patients can fill out questionnaires through Web-based surveys. Researchers can use force-generation protocols to evaluate physical fatigability and attention protocols to evaluate mental fatigability. Using these techniques to further understand the mechanisms of subjective and physiologic fatigue will help physicians to develop more effective treatments for fatigue and improve patients' quality of life.

The Utility of Electromyography and Mechanomyography for Assessing Neuromuscular Function: A Noninvasive Approach   23

Moh H. Malek and Jared W. Coburn

> This article introduces the utility of electromyography (EMG) and mechanomyography (MMG) for the assessment of neuromuscular function, and discusses the interpretation of the EMG and MMG signals for various exercise perturbations. The results of these studies suggest that the use of EMG and MMG to determine muscle fatigue is robust. Future studies with clinical populations are needed, however, to determine the optimal use of EMG and/or MMG for assessing muscle function in rehabilitative settings.

Novel Concepts Integrated in Neuromuscular Assessments for Surgical Restoration of Arm and Hand Function in Tetraplegia   33

Jan Fridén and Andreas Gohritz

> Surgical restoration of key functions of the upper extremity has tremendous potential to increase autonomy, mobility, and self-esteem by

resuming critical abilities in patients with tetraplegia. New strategies of surgical reconstruction and postoperative rehabilitation of upper extremity function in tetraplegic patients have been developed, based on basic science and clinical studies. In contrast to traditional hand reconstruction with separate flexors and extensors phases, combining 7 individual procedures provides key pinch and finger flexion together with passive opening of hand in one stage. Further research should aim at combining traditional algorithms with new approaches, such as immediate postoperative activation, combined procedures and nerve transfers.

The Effects of Active and Passive Stretching on Muscle Length   51

Danny A. Riley and J.M. Van Dyke

Active stretch is necessary for regulating muscle fiber length (ie, the number of series sarcomeres). Elevated cytoplasmic calcium is the proposed component of contractile activity required to activate signaling pathways for sarcomere number regulation. Passive stretch reduces muscle tissue stiffness, most likely by signaling connective tissue remodeling via fibroblasts. Passive stretch may induce sarcomere addition if the muscle fibers are lengthened sufficiently to raise cytoplasmic calcium through stretch-activated calcium channels. The magnitude of stretch in vivo is limited by the physiologic range of movement and stretch pain tolerance. The greatest effect of stretching muscle fibers is expected when the lengthening exceeds the optimum fiber length (Lo).

Hypohomocysteinemia: A Potentially Treatable Cause of Peripheral Neuropathology?   59

Clark E. Cullen, Gregory T. Carter, Michael D. Weiss, Peter A. Grant, and David Scott Saperstein

Perturbations of homocysteine metabolism are associated with increased risk for cardiovascular disease, stroke, dementia, and depression, among other major diseases. To assess the relationship between hypohomocysteinemia (HH) and idiopathic peripheral neuropathy (IPN), a retrospective review of 37,442 patients from a tertiary medical clinic was performed. Of patients with HH, 5.9% had IPN versus 0.6% of patients without IPN. Overall, 41% of patients with HH had IPN. These observations indicate that although HH is uncommon in the general population, there is a striking relationship between HH and the incidence of IPN. This article discusses the clinical ramifications of these findings.

Regional and Whole-Body Dual-Energy X-Ray Absorptiometry to Guide Treatment and Monitor Disease Progression in Neuromuscular Disease   67

Andrew J. Skalsky, Jay J. Han, Richard T. Abresch, and Craig M. McDonald

Dual-energy x-ray absorptiometry (DEXA) is a safe, noninvasive, inexpensive tool for managing patients with neuromuscular diseases. Regional and whole-body DEXA can be used to guide clinical treatments, such as determining body composition to guide nutritional recommendations, as well as to monitor disease progression by assessing regional and whole-body lean tissue mass. DEXA can also be used as an outcome measure for clinical trials.

Establishing Clinical End Points of Respiratory Function in Large Animals for Clinical Translation   75

Melissa A. Goddard, Erin L. Mitchell, Barbara K. Smith, and Martin K. Childers

Respiratory dysfunction due progressive weakness of the respiratory muscles, particularly the diaphragm, is a major cause of death in the neuromuscular disease (NMD) X-linked myotubular myopathy (XLMTM). Methods of respiratory assessment in patients are often difficult, especially in those who are mechanically ventilated. The naturally occuring XLMTM dog model exhibits a phenotype similar to that in patients and can be used to determine quantitative descriptions of dysfunction as clinical endpoints for treatment and the development of new therapies. In experiments using respiratory impedance plethysmography (RIP), XLMTM dogs challenged with the respiratory stimulant doxapram displayed significant changes indicative of diaphragmatic weakness.

New Opportunities and Novel Paradigms to Support Neuromuscular Research   95

Richard Lieber, Samuel Ward, Lawrence Frank, and Simon Schenk

This article provides an overview of the structure and function of the National Skeletal Muscle Research Center (NSMRC) at the University of California, San Diego, which is one of the 7 research centers of the Medical Rehabilitation Research Infrastructure Network, created to facilitate access for physicians to experts, technology, and resources from scientific fields related to medical rehabilitation. The 4 cores of the NSMRC are described as a resource for rehabilitation medicine practitioners to use for clinically relevant muscle research.

Skeletal Muscle Edema in Muscular Dystrophy: Clinical and Diagnostic Implications   107

Sandra L. Poliachik, Seth D. Friedman, Gregory T. Carter, Shawn E. Parnell, and Dennis W. Shaw

Muscle degeneration in muscular dystrophies often includes a period of edema before fatty replacement of muscle tissue. Magnetic resonance imaging (MRI) has been used successfully to characterize muscle and fat patterns in several types of muscular dystrophies. Recent MRI techniques enable characterization of edema in tissues. This article reviews the advantages of using MRI assessment of edema and fat in muscle tissue to evaluate disease progression, and discusses inflammation and sarcolemma compromise as sources of edema in muscular dystrophy. Lastly, refining current techniques and adapting other MRI capabilities may enhance detection and assessment of edema for better evaluation of disease progression and treatment outcomes.

Cardiac MRI in Muscular Dystrophy: An Overview and Future Directions   123

Randolph K. Otto, Mark R. Ferguson, and Seth D. Friedman

Cardiac complications are a common feature of many muscular dystrophies. Although many modalities (eg, ultrasound) provide exceptional efficacy for early diagnosis, repeated monitoring, and therapeutic management, MRI has become the gold standard for anatomic and functional characterization. An increasing number of studies, especially in the dystrophinopathies, use strain imaging to evaluate function. This article summarizes these studies and attempts to integrate an understanding of other relevant cardiac features (eg, fibrosis) into interpreting this work. Finally, a general roadmap forward is provided as these tools are increasingly used for treatment assessment and tactical patient management in the future.

Neuromuscular Ultrasonography: Quantifying Muscle and Nerve Measurements   133

David Mayans, Michael S. Cartwright, and Francis O. Walker

Neuromuscular ultrasonography can be used both descriptively and quantitatively in the evaluation of patients with neuromuscular disorders. This article reviews the quantitative use of this technology, particularly measurements of the size and echogenicity of nerve and muscle, as a tool for assessing the severity, progression, and response of these tissues to therapeutic interventions. Neuromuscular ultrasonography has several features, including portability and noninvasiveness, that make it an attractive research tool for advancing the diagnosis and treatment of neuromuscular disorders.

The Paradox of Muscle Hypertrophy in Muscular Dystrophy   149

Joe N. Kornegay, Martin K. Childers, Daniel J. Bogan, Janet R. Bogan, Peter Nghiem, Jiahui Wang, Zheng Fan, James F. Howard Jr, Scott J. Schatzberg, Jennifer L. Dow, Robert W. Grange, Martin A. Styner, Eric P. Hoffman, and Kathryn R. Wagner

Mutations in the dystrophin gene cause Duchenne and Becker muscular dystrophy in humans and syndromes in mice, dogs, and cats. Affected humans and dogs have progressive disease that leads primarily to muscle atrophy. Mdx mice progress through an initial phase of muscle hypertrophy followed by atrophy. Cats have persistent muscle hypertrophy. Hypertrophy in humans has been attributed to deposition of fat and connective tissue (pseudohypertrophy). Increased muscle mass (true hypertrophy) has been documented in animal models. Muscle hypertrophy can exaggerate postural instability and joint contractures. Deleterious consequences of muscle hypertrophy should be considered when developing treatments for muscular dystrophy.

Exercise Testing in Metabolic Myopathies   173

Mark Tarnopolsky

Metabolic myopathies are a group of genetic disorders specifically affecting glucose/glycogen, lipid, and mitochondrial metabolism. The main metabolic myopathies that are evaluated in this article are the mitochondrial myopathies, fatty acid oxidation defects, and glycogen storage disease. This article focuses on the usefulness of exercise in the evaluation of genetic metabolic myopathies.

Nutrition Strategies to Improve Physical Capabilities in Duchenne Muscular Dystrophy   187

J. Davoodi, C.D. Markert, K.A. Voelker, S.M. Hutson, and Robert W. Grange

There is no current cure for Duchenne muscular dystrophy (DMD), and palliative and prophylactic interventions to improve the quality of life of patients remain limited, with the exception of corticosteroids. This article describes 2 potential nutritional interventions for the treatment of DMD, green tea extract (GTE) and the branched-chain amino acid leucine, and their positive effects on physical activity. Both GTE and leucine are suitable for human consumption, are easily tolerated with no side effects, and, with appropriate preclinical data, could be brought forward to clinical trials rapidly.

Aging of Human Muscle: Understanding Sarcopenia at the Single Muscle Cell Level 201

Walter R. Frontera, Ana Rodriguez Zayas, and Natividad Rodriguez

The loss of muscle mass with age, also known as sarcopenia, is a major scientific and public health problem. Muscle atrophy is associated with the loss of functional capacity and poor health outcomes in elderly men and women. A detailed understanding of this problem in humans can be enhanced by the use of experiments with single muscle fibers. It is likely that both muscle atrophy and a decrease in muscle-fiber quality contribute to muscle dysfunction among the elderly. A better understanding of sarcopenia at the single-fiber level may lead to the design of more effective rehabilitative interventions.

Index 209

FORTHCOMING ISSUES

May 2012
**Patient Safety in the Practice
of Rehabilitation Medicine**
Adrian Cristian, MD, *Guest Editor*

August 2012
Neuromuscular Disease Rehabilitation
Craig McDonald, MD, Jay Han, MD,
and Nanette Joyce, DO, *Guest Editors*

November 2012
**Electrodiagnosis of Neuromuscular
Disorders**
Michael Weiss, MD, *Guest Editor*

RECENT ISSUES

November 2011
Youth Sports Concussions
Kathleen Bell, MD and
Stan Herring, MD, *Guest Editors*

August 2011
Management of Neck Pain
Allen Sinclair Chen, MD, MPH,
Guest Editor

May 2011
Burn Rehabilitation
Peter C. Esselman, MD and
Karen Kowalske, MD,
Guest Editors

February 2011
Radiculopathy
David J. Kennedy, MD,
Guest Editor

THE CLINICS ARE NOW AVAILABLE ONLINE!
Access your subscription at:
www.theclinics.com

Preface

Advancing Neuromuscular Medicine Through Integration, Translation, and Collaboration

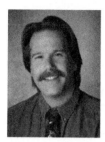

Gregory T. Carter, MD, MS
Guest Editor

I was quite honored a few years back when I was invited by my friend and colleague, Dr Rick Lieber, to become a member of the external advisory board for his National Institutes of Health investigator-initiated grant entitled "Medical Rehabilitation Research Infrastructure Program in Muscle (MRRPM)" based at the University of California, San Diego. This is part of the Medical Rehabilitation Research Infrastructure Network. These grants were designed to facilitate integration and collaboration among physicians and basic science researchers with expertise in specific areas of biomedical research. The goals are to allow cross-collaboration and access to the latest technology and resources from all across the spectrum of scientific, in order to foster translational research. While I have been a part of many program project grants in my career, this new opportunity sounded very appealing to me.

After visiting Dr Lieber's center this past summer, I came away thinking that this is the way rehabilitation research should be done. Physiatrists understand that the clinical problems confronting us in rehabilitation medicine are complex, involving virtually every aspect of the neuromuscular system. Our disabled neuromuscular patients encounter problems that will require the brightest and the best researchers pushing themselves to the limit to solve. Yet, no one single person or persons will be able to conquer disorders like muscular dystrophy or peripheral neuropathy working by themselves. Even when ideas are exchanged openly at meetings there are still missed opportunities. Why not have the brightest and the best muscle histologists working directly with the brightest and the best clinicians from all over America? With everyone working at the top of their game on specific aspects of a complex, multifaceted problem, there suddenly becomes a fighting chance that we can come up with truly effective treatment paradigms.

Phys Med Rehabil Clin N Am 23 (2012) xv–xvii
doi:10.1016/j.pmr.2011.11.018
1047-9651/12/$ – see front matter © 2012 Elsevier Inc. All rights reserved.

pmr.theclinics.com

After the site visit, I was treated to a wonderful lunch near the beach in La Jolla, a place known for stimulating good ideas. As I sat there and listened to brilliant minds discussing their research in an open, collaborative fashion, the idea for this volume of *Physical Medicine and Rehabilitation Clinics of North America* was born. Now the important thing to understand here is that these centers exist for all of us, including clinicians who are not necessarily affiliated with a major academic center. Physiatrists should be comfortable with multidisciplinary, cross-collaboration and open sharing of information, as well a willingness to confront complex problems. The mission statement of rehabilitation professionals should also include both an academic and a clinical perspective. I am very excited about the opportunity to help introduce physiatrists and other rehabilitation clinicians to these research concepts.

My primary goal with this volume of *Physical Medicine and Rehabilitation Clinics of North America* is to provide you with an overview of the University of California, San Diego center followed by a series of cutting-edge articles that were born of this cross-collaborative methodology and offer the latest information on a myriad of clinical problems encountered in neuromuscular medicine. A secondary goal is to stimulate you to consider tapping in to this rich source of readily available help that will enhance your capability of doing medical rehabilitation research and clinical investigation. The third and ultimate goal is, of course, to improve the quality of life for people with neuromuscular disabilities but that cycles back in to my first two goals.

Finally, I want to personally thank all of the contributing authors for all their time and hard work invested here to provide you with an amazing wealth of cutting-edge information that can be directly applied to your clinical practice.

Gregory T. Carter, MD, MS
Muscular Dystrophy Association, Regional Neuromuscular Center
410 Providence Lane, Building 2
Olympia, WA 98506, USA

E-mail address:
gtcarter@uw.edu

Dedication

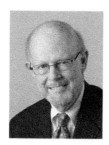

George H. Kraft, MD, MS

This volume is dedicated to Dr George H. Kraft, consulting editor of the *Physical Medicine and Rehabilitation (PM&R) Clinics of North America* for over 20 years. Under George's leadership, the Clinics are now the preeminent clinical reviews, with all papers cited on PubMed (National Library of Medicine). George has decided to step down and I am deeply honored to assume his position.

George is the consummate academician, leading by example and our field is deeply indebted to him. His career is hallmarked by novel, insightful research which profoundly improved quality of life for people battling multiple sclerosis (MS). For this, George received the coveted lifetime achievement award from the National MS Society. He is a past recipient of the Krusen award, our PM&R Academy's highest honor, and many other awards for groundbreaking work in MS and Electrodiagnosis. George accomplished this all while training countless medical students, residents, and fellows.

Yet George remains humble and caring, focused on things dearest to his heart: family, friends, mentees, and research. He is a role model for us all, with amazing zest for life, and tireless pursuit of excellence.

I close with a quote from naturalist John Burroughs, reminding me of George:

"I still find each day too short for all the thoughts I want to think, all the walks I want to take, all the books I want to read, and all the friends I want to see."

With sincere gratitude,
Gregory T. Carter, MD, MS

Use of Skeletal Muscle MRI in Diagnosis and Monitoring Disease Progression in Duchenne Muscular Dystrophy

Erika L. Finanger, MD, MS[a,b,c],*, Barry Russman, MD[a,b,c],
Sean C. Forbes, PhD[d], William D. Rooney, PhD[e],
Glenn A. Walter, PhD[f], Krista Vandenborne, PT, PhD[d]

KEYWORDS

• MRI • Duchenne muscular dystrophy • Skeletal muscle

In clinical practice, diseases of the neuromuscular system, particularly those that are of primary muscle origin, are evaluated with history and examination; electrodiagnostic testing (nerve conduction testing and electromyography); genetic testing; and muscle biopsy. Recently, there has been increasing interest in noninvasive imaging modalities, particularly muscle magnetic resonance imaging (MRI), for the diagnosis and assessment of disease progression for various neuromuscular diseases, including Duchenne muscular dystrophy (DMD).

[a] Department of Pediatrics, Oregon Health and Science University, 707 SW Gaines Street, CDRC-P, Portland, OR 97239, USA
[b] Department of Neurology, Oregon Health and Science University, 707 SW Gaines Street, CDRC-P, Portland, OR 97239, USA
[c] Shriners Hospital for Children Portland, 3101 SW Sam Jackson Park Road, Portland, OR 97239, USA
[d] Department of Physical Therapy, University of Florida, Gainesville, FL 32610, USA
[e] Advanced Imaging Research Center, Oregon Health and Science University, 3181 SW Sam Jackson Park Road, Portland, OR 97239, USA
[f] Department of Physiology and Functional Genomics, University of Florida, Gainesville, FL 32610, USA
* Corresponding author. Oregon Health and Science University, Pediatric Neurology, 707 SW Gaines Street, CDRC-P, Portland, OR 97239.
E-mail address: hedderic@ohsu.edu

Phys Med Rehabil Clin N Am 23 (2012) 1–10
doi:10.1016/j.pmr.2011.11.004
1047-9651/12/$ – see front matter © 2012 Published by Elsevier Inc.

MUSCLE IMAGING

Muscle Ultrasound

The use of muscle ultrasound in the assessment of muscle disease began to gain interest in the 1980s.[1,2] This technique is still used clinically to identify muscle involvement[3] and to aid in the selection of muscles for biopsy. However, the use of muscle ultrasound is limited because this technique is operator-dependent and not all muscles can be adequately assessed.

Muscle MRI and Magnetic Resonance Spectroscopy

MRI is a noninvasive imaging method without ionizing radiation, which has the ability to resolve muscle, fat, connective tissue, and bone. MRI has several advantages over muscle ultrasound, including that MRI has minimal operator-dependence and allows for excellent visualization of all muscles. Magnetic resonance spectroscopy (MRS) is a related noninvasive biochemical sampling technique that has been used in conjunction with MRI to quantify lipid fraction and metabolic products within muscle.[4]

DUCHENNE MUSCULAR DYSTROPHY

DMD is the most common muscular dystrophy affecting children. It is an X-linked recessive disorder with an incidence of 1 in 3300 live male births.[5] The disease is caused by mutations in the gene coding for the dystrophin protein.[6] The dystrophin protein is a member of the dystrophin glycoprotein complex, an essential component of the muscle membrane[7] that provides a link to the extracellular matrix. Mutations in the gene leading to abnormal or absent dystrophin protein lead to absence of localization of dystrophin to the dystrophin-associated glycoprotein complex as seen in muscle biopsy specimens. Disruption of the dystrophin glycoprotein complex and its linkage to the extracellular matrix leads to muscle membrane fragility[8] and renders the myofiber more susceptible to contraction-induced injury. Repeated cycles of myofiber degeneration and necrosis ultimately lead to fatty and connective tissue replacement.[9]

Clinical Course

Boys with DMD typically come to clinical attention before age 5, presenting with delayed motor milestone acquisition, abnormal gait, and difficulty rising from the floor or ascending stairs. Patients experience progressive weakness, beginning in the proximal hip and shoulder girdle muscles, and later progressing to involve more distal muscles. Loss of ambulatory function is usually observed between the age of 10 and 15 years, and by the late teenage years or early twenties most patients die of cardiopulmonary complications.

Diagnosis

The diagnosis of dystrophin-related muscular dystrophy is made by history, physical examination, and markedly elevated serum creatine kinase level, and confirmed by genetic analysis of the dystrophin gene looking for deletions, duplications, or sequence variations.

Current Treatment

Glucocorticoids, a class of corticosteroids, are the only current pharmaceutical agent found to be beneficial in slowing disease progression in boys with DMD and are recommended as standard of care after boys enter the plateau or decline phases of the disease.[10] Steroid therapy has been shown to benefit boys with DMD, with improved muscle strength, prolonged ambulation, stabilized pulmonary and cardiac function, and a reduced incidence of scoliosis.[10–13] Despite known clinical benefit, the cellular mechanism by which steroid agent stabilizes muscle function has not been clearly elucidated. Although glucocorticoids have been shown to reduce the number of cytotoxic T cells,[14] the immunosuppressant action of this drug is likely not the only mechanism protecting muscle in boys with DMD.[15]

POTENTIAL USES OF MRI IN DMD
MRI Findings in DMD

Numerous studies have shown the ability of MRI to detect alterations in skeletal muscle structure and composition in patients with muscular dystrophy.[16–19] Initial studies used T1-weighted images and postcontrast imaging to document structural alterations in patients with muscular dystrophy and provide a qualitative assessment of skeletal muscle.[18–21] Mercuri and colleagues[22,23] developed a four-point grading system to categorize disease severity, based on visual inspection of fatty tissue infiltration. This strategy was recently used to screen DMD subjects in a clinical trial involving injection with antisense oligonucleotides.[24] However, there is considerable interest in using quantitative imaging to monitor disease progression and efficacy of treatment strategies, which is the focus of the remainder of this article.

T1-Weighted Imaging

Quantitative evaluation with T1 imaging has been used to evaluate MRI changes in DMD. T1 values in DMD subjects are high early in the course of disease and fall with increasing clinical severity, associated with increasing fatty replacement of muscle.[20] More recently, Garrood and colleagues[25] showed that in eight of nine muscles analyzed, there was a statistically significant difference in the median muscle signal intensities on T1-weighted imaging between DMD subjects treated with steroids and control subjects.

T1-weighted imaging and gadolinium enhancement
Gadolinium contrast is used in MRI to better visualize vascular structures. In animal models of muscular dystrophy, gadolinium, which in normal muscle remains extracellular, is taken up into muscle fibers with damaged membranes.[26,27] Given that membrane damage is present since birth, some hypothesize that this technique may be more appropriate for evaluating DMD patients early in the course of disease, before fatty infiltration is significant. In a recent study, Garrood and colleagues[25] showed a significant increase in gadolinium uptake in the tibialis anterior muscles after stepping exercise in subjects with DMD, but not in the six other muscles studied and no change in the T2 value.

Muscle cross-sectional area
Some studies have used various MRI approaches to measure muscle size in DMD. Muscle cross-sectional area is a quantitative measure, typically calculated from manually tracing individual muscles in axial slices from T1-weighted images (**Fig. 1**). Recently, Mathur and colleagues[28] used muscle cross-sectional area to compare boys with DMD with age-matched control subjects. They found that muscle cross-sectional area of the posterior calf muscles (soleus, medial, and lateral gastrocnemius) was approximately 60% greater in boys with DMD compared with control subjects, but this finding was not found in the two other muscles tested (tibialis anterior and quadriceps). Furthermore, they showed that there was an age-dependent relationship between the muscle cross-sectional area of the quadriceps muscle, with larger cross-sectional area in boys with DMD compared with control subjects less than

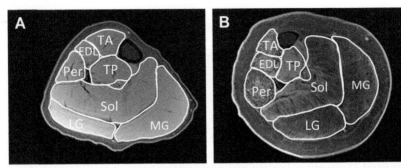

Fig. 1. Representative T1-weighted fat-suppressed images of the lower leg of a boy with DMD that seems to have relatively little involvement (*A*) and of a boy in whom the disease is more progressed (*B*). This MRI sequence can be used to determine maximal cross-sectional area in various lower leg muscles, including the tibialis anterior (TA), extensor digitorum longus (EDL), tibialis posterior (TP), peroneaus (Per), soleus (Sol), lateral gastrocnemius (LG), and medial gastrocnemius (MG).

the age of 10 years with a reversal of this association in boys aged 11 years and older. Therefore, the rate of progression of disease depends on muscle group, and an advantage of MRI is that numerous muscles can be evaluated at the same time.

Although the calculation of muscle cross-sectional area is valuable, it does not discriminate between muscle tissue and fatty tissue/edema. These two components can be separated to calculate the muscle contractile and noncontractile tissue within an individual muscle. A recent study used this technique to compare 28 boys with DMD with 10 control subjects.[29] It was shown that boys with DMD had a significantly greater proportion of noncontractile tissue compared with control subjects and that the proportion of noncontractile tissue increased significantly with age. Further, the proportion of noncontractile tissue correlated with a number of functional tests, including time to walk 30 ft; rise from the floor (supine up); and ascend four steps.[29]

T2-Weighted Imaging

Other investigators have used T2-weighted imaging to reflect muscle composition, including damage, inflammation, and lipid composition. T2-weighted imaging has been used to visualize dystrophic lesions in animals, and T2 mapping enables a quantifiable measure that enables more direct comparisons over time and at different sites. Kim and colleagues[30] recently used a T2 mapping strategy to correlate mean T2 values with the nonquantitative MRI grading scale developed by Mercuri and colleagues[3] and with clinical measures of disease severity. They found that the mean T2 of the gluteus maximus muscle showed significant correlation with the nonquantitative MRI score for fatty infiltration. Furthermore, they showed a significant positive correlation between the mean T2 value for the gluteus maximus muscle and several clinical measures, including patient age, clinical function scale, timed Gower score, and time to run 30 ft.[30] In addition, distribution of T2 values in a region-of-interest has been examined on a pixel-by-pixel basis to provide information about muscle heterogeneity.[16] An example of how this may be used to monitor progression of disease is shown in **Fig. 2**.

Fat-Suppression Sequences

Implementing a fat-suppression procedure during a spin echo sequence (eg, short-tau inversion recovery imaging) suppresses the signal from adipose tissue, and thus the

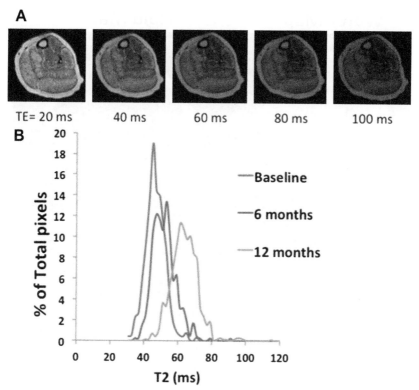

Fig. 2. (A) Representative T2-weighted images acquired with a TE of 20, 40, 60, 80, and 100 ms. (B) Using these images a T2 map can be created, then the pixels plotted within a region of interest to create a histogram. Note the rightward shift of the histogram indicating progression of disease in the soleus over a 1-year period in this subject.

resulting signal is more sensitive to increased extracellular or unbound water content, consistent with edema or inflammation. This may be a particularly useful technique in younger boys with DMD in whom inflammatory changes with edema may be better markers than fatty infiltration because the latter change occurs later in the disease process. This is supported by a study by Marden and colleagues,[18] using short-tau inversion recovery imaging, which found regions of increased signal intensity or muscle inflammation in dystrophic muscles of young boys with DMD in the absence of fatty tissue infiltration.

Three-Point Dixon Technique

In standard MRI sequences, the signal intensity for each voxel (the unit of measurement) is determined based on the fat and water signal intensities within that voxel. The three-point Dixon technique allows separation of MRI signal intensity into separate values for the individual contributions of fat and water in each voxel of tissue.[31] This results in high-resolution water and fat maps (**Fig. 3**), and enables quantifying fat fractions of individual muscles. In addition, this sequence has the advantage of correcting for MRI inhomogeneities.[32] Recently, Wren and colleagues[33] implemented a three-point Dixon MRI technique to quantify the amount of lipid infiltration in the thigh

Water Map   Lipid Map

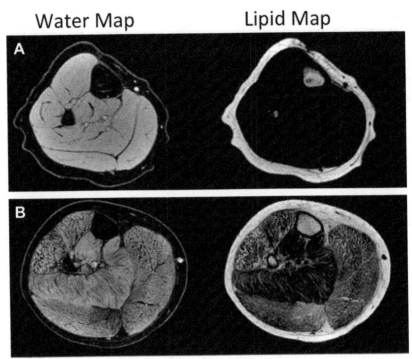

Fig. 3. Example water and lipid maps of the lower leg of a control subject (*A*) and a boy with DMD (*B*) using three-point Dixon technique.

muscles of nine boys with DMD and showed that quantitative measures of muscle adiposity correlate better with disease severity than strength measures.

Similarly, preliminary data from our multisite study of the use of MRI in boys with DMD quantified the intramuscular lipid accumulation in the soleus muscle of 24 ambulatory boys with DMD. A strong correlation was found between the amount of intramuscular lipid assessed by volume localized 1H spectroscopy and measures of functional ability, including the Brooke lower extremity score ($R^2 = 0.78$) and the time to walk 30 ft ($R^2 = 0.80$) (Vandenborne, ImagingDMD, unpublished data, 2011).

Spectroscopy

In addition to MRI, various approaches of MRS have been used to study muscle involvement in muscular dystrophy, including proton spectroscopy (^{1}H-MRS) and ^{31}phosphorus MRS (^{31}P-MRS).[34,35] Although spectroscopy provides limited spatial information, it has proved to accurately quantify muscle metabolites and does not suffer from partial volume filling.[16] One approach is to acquire a spectrum from a single voxel that is maximized in size within an individual muscle to obtain a large representation of the relative lipid concentration (**Fig. 4**). Recently, Torriani and colleagues (in press) used a similar approach to evaluate lipid composition in children with DMD in the soleus and tibialis anterior. In that study relationships between lipid fraction and functional measures were observed. Alternatively, Hsieh and colleagues[36] used MRS to show that the trimethylamines-to-muscle total creatine ratio is significantly reduced in boys with DMD and correlates negatively with function. Therefore, there are a variety of MRS measures that show promise in measuring disease progression in DMD.

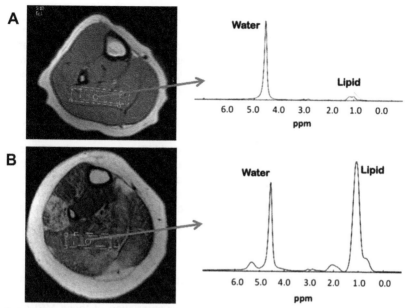

Fig. 4. Example spectrum acquired from the soleus of a control subject (*A*) and a boy with DMD (*B*). Lipid peak includes a composite of intramyocellular and extramyocelluar lipid.

MRI AS A BIOMARKER FOR CLINICAL TRIALS

With a number of potential therapeutic interventions for DMD under development, and some in phase I and II clinical trials, there is an immediate need for such a noninvasive biomarker and MRI seems to be an enticing option. However, few MRI studies have presented a robust quantitative approach to monitor disease progression in DMD. Therefore, although MRI is a promising noninvasive method, further longitudinal studies are required to validate the sensitivity of the measures to monitor disease progression and treatment.

MRI Compared with Muscle Biopsy

Muscle biopsy, used to document the restoration of the dystrophin protein to the muscle membrane, is the gold standard for assessing benefit of potential therapeutic interventions for DMD. The value of muscle biopsy is based on its use in the diagnosis of DMD and its use for drug development and preclinical studies in model systems of DMD. In addition, a recent study by Kinali and colleagues[37] showed a correlation between MRI changes (based on subjective scoring system) and histopathologic changes on muscle biopsy. They showed that there was a good correlation between MRI severity score and a categorical assessment of muscle involvement on standard histologic staining.

There are several concerns, however, with the use of muscle biopsy in clinical trials. First, it is an invasive procedure that involves taking repeated samples from individuals who may already have limited muscle mass. Second, it is susceptible to considerable human error, particularly with specimen processing. Furthermore, recent studies have suggested considerable variability of muscle involvement in DMD, even within a single muscle (eg, rectus femoris), and a muscle biopsy may not provide a true representation of the overall disease progression or therapeutic response.

MRI Correlation with Functional Outcome Measures

Functional measures including timed performance tests (6-minute walk, 30-m walk, time to ascend four stairs, and so forth) and quantitative strength measures have also been routinely used as outcome measures in DMD treatment trials. The study by Wren and colleagues[33] and our preliminary data have shown correlation of various MRI modalities with standard functional measures.

Treatment Response

Notably, several recent treatment trials have included MRI as part of the study protocol. For example, a recent study implemented MRI to compare the T2 relaxation times of the myocardium and sternocleidomastoid muscle (accessory respiratory muscle) of boys chronically treated with deflazacort (treatment duration of at least 7 years) with a younger group of untreated boys.[38] In addition, several studies have used MRI to quantify changes in skeletal muscle volume after treatment with either a neutralizing antibody to myostatin[39] or after myoblast transplants.[40]

SUMMARY

Studies have shown promise in using various approaches of MRI and MRS to evaluate skeletal muscle involvement in DMD. However, these studies have mainly been performed using a cross-sectional design, and the correlation of these MRI changes with disease progression and disease severity has not been fully elucidated. Overall, skeletal muscle MRI is a powerful and sensitive technique in the evaluation of muscle disease, and its use as a biomarker for disease progression or therapeutic response in clinical trials deserves further study.

ACKNOWLEDGMENTS

The authors would like to thank the NIH/NIAMS/NINDS for their funding via a multi-center grant (R01 AR056973) which supported this research.

REFERENCES

1. Heckmatt JZ, Dubowitz V, Leeman S. Detection of pathological change in dystrophic muscle with B-scan ultrasound imaging. Lancet 1980;1(8183):1389–90.
2. Heckmatt JZ, Leeman S, Dubowitz V. Ultrasound imaging in the diagnosis of muscle disease. J Pediatr 1982;101(5):656–60.
3. Mercuri E, Pichiecchio A, Allsop J, et al. Muscle MRI in inherited neuromuscular disorders: past, present, and future. J Magn Reson Imaging 2007;25(2):433–40.
4. Prompers JJ, Jeneson JA, Drost MR, et al. Dynamic MRS and MRI of skeletal muscle function and biomechanics. NMR Biomed 2006;19(7):927–53.
5. Emery AE. The muscular dystrophies. Lancet 2002;359(9307):687–95.
6. Hoffman EP, Brown RH Jr, Kunkel LM. Dystrophin: the protein product of the Duchenne muscular dystrophy locus. Cell 1987;51(6):919–28.
7. Watkins SC, Hoffman EP, Slayter HS, et al. Immunoelectron microscopic localization of dystrophin in myofibres. Nature 1988;333(6176):863–6.
8. Petrof BJ, Shrager JB, Stedman HH, et al. Dystrophin protects the sarcolemma from stresses developed during muscle contraction. Proc Natl Acad Sci U S A 1993;90(8):3710–4.
9. Dubowitz V. Muscle disorders in children. 2nd edition. Kidlington (UK): Bailliere Tindall; 1995.

10. Moxley RTIII, Ashwal S, Pandya S, et al. Practice parameter: corticosteroid treatment of Duchenne dystrophy: report of the quality standards subcommittee of the American Academy of Neurology and the practice committee of the Child Neurology Society. Neurology 2005;64(1):13–20.
11. Angelini C. The role of corticosteroids in muscular dystrophy: a critical appraisal. Muscle Nerve 2007;36(4):424–35.
12. Manzur AY, Kuntzer T, Pike M, et al. Glucocorticoid corticosteroids for Duchenne muscular dystrophy. Cochrane Database Syst Rev (Online) 2008;1:CD003725.
13. Markham LW, Spicer RL, Khoury PR, et al. Steroid therapy and cardiac function in Duchenne muscular dystrophy. Pediatr Cardiol 2005;26(6):768–71.
14. Kissel JT, Burrow KL, Rammohan KW, et al. Mononuclear cell analysis of muscle biopsies in prednisone-treated and untreated Duchenne muscular dystrophy. CIDD study group. Neurology 1991;41(5):667–72.
15. Griggs RC, Moxley RTIII, Mendell JR, et al. Duchenne dystrophy: randomized, controlled trial of prednisone (18 months) and azathioprine (12 months). Neurology 1993;43(3 Pt 1):520–7.
16. Huang Y, Majumdar S, Genant HK, et al. Quantitative MR relaxometry study of muscle composition and function in Duchenne muscular dystrophy. J Magn Reson Imaging 1994;4(1):59–64.
17. Kuriyama M, Hayakawa K, Konishi Y, et al. MR imaging of myopathy. Comput Med Imaging Graphv 1989;13(4):329–33.
18. Marden FA, Connolly AM, Siegel MJ, et al. Compositional analysis of muscle in boys with Duchenne muscular dystrophy using MR imaging. Skeletal Radiol 2005;34(3):140–8.
19. Matsumura K, Nakano I, Fukuda N, et al. Duchenne muscular dystrophy carriers. Proton spin-lattice relaxation times of skeletal muscles on magnetic resonance imaging. Neuroradiology 1989;31(5):373–6.
20. Matsumura K, Nakano I, Fukuda N, et al. Proton spin-lattice relaxation time of Duchenne dystrophy skeletal muscle by magnetic resonance imaging. Muscle Nerve 1988;11(2):97–102.
21. Sookhoo S, Mackinnon I, Bushby K, et al. MRI for the demonstration of subclinical muscle involvement in muscular dystrophy. Clin Radiol 2007;62(2):160–5.
22. Mercuri E, Talim B, Moghadaszadeh B, et al. Clinical and imaging findings in six cases of congenital muscular dystrophy with rigid spine syndrome linked to chromosome 1p (RSMD1). Neuromuscul Disord 2002;12(7-8):631–8.
23. Mercuri E, Bushby K, Ricci E, et al. Muscle MRI findings in patients with limb girdle muscular dystrophy with calpain 3 deficiency (LGMD2A) and early contractures. Neuromuscul Disord 2005;15(2):164–71.
24. van Deutekom JC, Janson AA, Ginjaar IB, et al. Local dystrophin restoration with antisense oligonucleotide PRO051. N Engl J Med 2007;357(26):2677–86.
25. Garrood P, Hollingsworth KG, Eagle M, et al. MR imaging in Duchenne muscular dystrophy: quantification of T1-weighted signal, contrast uptake, and the effects of exercise. J Magn Reson Imaging 2009;30(5):1130–8.
26. Amthor H, Egelhof T, McKinnell I, et al. Albumin targeting of damaged muscle fibres in the mdx mouse can be monitored by MRI. Neuromuscul Disord 2004;14(12):791–6.
27. Thibaud JL, Monnet A, Bertoldi D, et al. Characterization of dystrophic muscle in golden retriever muscular dystrophy dogs by nuclear magnetic resonance imaging. Neuromuscul Disord 2007;17(7):575–84.
28. Mathur S, Lott DJ, Senesac C, et al. Age-related differences in lower-limb muscle cross-sectional area and torque production in boys with Duchenne muscular dystrophy. Arch Phys Med Rehabil 2010;91(7):1051–8.

29. Akima H, Lott D, Senesac C, et al. Relationships of thigh muscle contractile and non-contractile tissue with function, strength, and age in boys with Duchenne muscular dystrophy. Neuromuscul Disord 2011. [Epub ahead of print].

30. Kim HK, Laor T, Horn PS, et al. T2 mapping in Duchenne muscular dystrophy: distribution of disease activity and correlation with clinical assessments. Radiology 2010;255(3):899–908.

31. Dixon WT. Simple proton spectroscopic imaging. Radiology 1984;153(1):189–94.

32. Glover GH, Schneider E. Three-point Dixon technique for true water/fat decomposition with B0 inhomogeneity correction. Magn Reson Med 1991;18(2):371–83.

33. Wren TA, Bluml S, Tseng-Ong L, et al. Three-point technique of fat quantification of muscle tissue as a marker of disease progression in Duchenne muscular dystrophy: preliminary study. AJR Am J Roentgenol 2008;190(1):W8–12.

34. Kan HE, Klomp DW, Wong CS, et al. In vivo 31P MRS detection of an alkaline inorganic phosphate pool with short T1 in human resting skeletal muscle. NMR Biomed 2010;23(8):995–1000.

35. Torriani M, Townsend E, Thomas BJ, et al. Lower leg muscle involvement in Duchenne muscular dystrophy: an MR imaging and spectroscopy study. Skeletal Radiol 2011. [Epub ahead of print].

36. Hsieh TJ, Jaw TS, Chuang HY, et al. Muscle metabolism in Duchenne muscular dystrophy assessed by in vivo proton magnetic resonance spectroscopy. J Comput Assist Tomogr 2009;33(1):150–4.

37. Kinali M, Arechavala-Gomeza V, Cirak S, et al. Muscle histology vs MRI in Duchenne muscular dystrophy. Neurology 2011;76(4):346–53.

38. Mavrogeni S, Papavasiliou A, Douskou M, et al. Effect of deflazacort on cardiac and sternocleidomastoid muscles in Duchenne muscular dystrophy: a magnetic resonance imaging study. Eur J Paediatr Neurol 2009;13(1):34–40.

39. Wagner KR, Fleckenstein JL, Amato AA, et al. A phase I/IItrial of MYO-029 in adult subjects with muscular dystrophy. Ann Neurol 2008;63(5):561–71.

40. Miller RG, Sharma KR, Pavlath GK, et al. Myoblast implantation in Duchenne muscular dystrophy: the San Francisco study. Muscle Nerve 1997;20(4):469–78.

Techniques in Assessing Fatigue in Neuromuscular Diseases

Jau-Shin Lou, MD, PhD

KEYWORDS

- Neuromuscular diseases • Fatigue • Fatigue questionnaires
- Subjective and physiologic fatigue • Physical fatigability
- Mental fatigability

Neuromuscular diseases include a group of conditions that involve lower motor neurons (such as amyotrophic lateral sclerosis [ALS]), nerve roots (such as radiculopathy), plexuses (such as brachial plexopathy), peripheral nerves (such as axonal or demyelinating neuropathy), neuromuscular junctions (such as myasthenia gravis), and muscles (such as inflammatory myopathy). Some neuromuscular diseases can also involve upper motor neurons or the brain, however. For example, one of the diagnostic criteria for ALS is involvement of upper motor neurons. Patients with myotonic dystrophy have cognitive dysfunction and the severity of cognitive dysfunction correlates with the size of the CTG repeat.[1]

DEFINITION OF FATIGUE

Fatigue is common in many medical and neurologic conditions. One of the major challenges in studying fatigue is the lack of a commonly accepted definition; both physicians and patients often talk about "fatigue" without explicitly defining the term. *Harrison's Principles of Internal Medicine* describes chronic fatigue syndrome as "a disorder characterized by debilitating fatigue and several associated physical, constitutional, and neuropsychological complaints," yet never defines fatigue.[2] In practice, "fatigue" may have meanings ranging from mental depression to neuromuscular weakness. Establishing a working definition is the first step in assessing fatigue.

One obstacle in defining fatigue is that it is used to describe either a trait or a state. Whereas a trait is more or less chronic, a state is a relatively temporary condition. In the body of fatigue research, the term "subjective fatigue" or "experienced fatigue" usually refers to the general sensation of tiredness or of difficulty in initiating physical

Department of Neurology, Oregon Health & Science University, CR120, 3181 Southwest Sam Jackson Park Road, Portland, OR 97239, USA
E-mail address: Louja@ohsu.edu

Phys Med Rehabil Clin N Am 23 (2012) 11–22
doi:10.1016/j.pmr.2011.11.003
1047-9651/12/$ – see front matter © 2012 Published by Elsevier Inc.

pmr.theclinics.com

or mental activity over several days to weeks. This is often assessed by questionnaires completed by the subject. The term "fatigability" or "physiologic fatigue" refers to difficulty in maintaining the physical or mental activity at a desired level. Physicians are familiar with the fatigability test used to examine a patient who is suspected to have myasthenia gravis. In the fatigability test, the examiner asks the patient to contract a muscle (for example, the deltoid muscle) repetitively and evaluates whether or not the force generated declines after a few repetitions. The muscle tested is judged to be "fatigable" if the examiner detects a decline in the force generated. Fatigability occurs in a short period of time; therefore, it can be measured quantitatively in a laboratory setting. It is important to note that subjective fatigue and fatigability are not necessarily correlated. In other words, even if patients complain that they are "tired all the time," they may perform well on measures of fatigability. Researchers need to be careful to correctly define and interpret findings of subjective fatigue and fatigability.

A second important differentiation is "physical" versus "mental" subjective fatigue and fatigability. Subjective physical fatigue refers to the amount of effort a subject feels he or she needs to complete certain physical activities, such as performing manual labor, walking, jogging, running, or lifting weights, which require skeletal muscles to generate force. Physical fatigability is the type of fatigability that is induced by motor tasks, such as force generation. Subjective mental fatigue refers to the effort subjects feel they must put forth to pay attention to tasks. Mental fatigability is the degree of attention a subject can maintain when required to sustain attention or concentration for a certain period of time. Subjective mental fatigue and physical fatigue are not always correlated with each other.[3] To the best of the author's knowledge, no studies have examined the correlation between mental and physical fatigability.

SYSTEMATIC APPROACH OF FATIGUE IN NEUROMUSCULAR DISEASES

One of the best ways to assess fatigue in neuromuscular diseases is to take a systematic approach (**Fig. 1**). We can assess subjective physical and mental fatigue using 1 dimensional and multidimensional questionnaires while assessing mental and physical fatigability in a laboratory setting. Researchers often use exercise protocols to evaluate physical fatigability and reaction time paradigms to evaluate mental fatigability.

Using Questionnaires to Assess Subjective Physical and Mental Fatigue

Both 1-dimensional and multidimensional questionnaires are valuable in assessing the presence, severity, and prevalence of subjective fatigue. One-dimensional instruments, such as the Visual Analog Scale (VAS)[4] and 9-item Fatigue Severity Scale (FSS),[5] give a single score to indicate the severity of fatigue. Multidimensional fatigue instruments, such as the Multidimensional Fatigue Inventory (MFI)[6] and the Piper Fatigue Scale (PFS),[7] contain several subscales usually based on a factor analysis. These 4 fatigue instruments have been used in other neurologic or neuromuscular diseases, such as multiple sclerosis,[5] Parkinson disease (PD),[3] ALS,[8] and postpolio syndrome.[9]

The Visual Analog Scale of fatigue

The VAS of fatigue is a 100-mm horizontal line representing the severity of fatigue ranging from 0 (right) to 100% (left). The subjects mark a point on the line that best represents the severity of their fatigue. The distance from the right is scored from 0 to 1.0. The scores in the Visual Analog Scale of fatigue correlated significantly with the multi-item

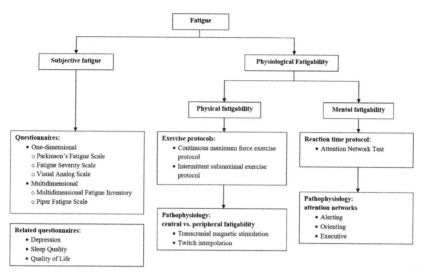

Fig. 1. Systematic approach to fatigue. There are 2 aspects of fatigue: subjective fatigue and physiologic fatigability. We can characterize subjective fatigue (also known as experienced fatigue) using questionnaires. Other symptoms that are related (such as depression, sleep quality, and quality of life) are measured with appropriate questionnaires. We measure physiologic fatigability objectively in the laboratory setting. Physical fatigability is measured by continuous or intermittent exercise paradigms. The pathophysiology of physical fatigability (central vs peripheral) can be explored using transcranial magnetic stimulation or twitch interpolation. Mental fatigability is measured by a reaction time protocol, such as the Attention Network Test (ANT). The information obtained from the ANT allows us to differentiate deficits in alerting, orienting, or executive networks.

fatigue subscale of the Profile of Mood States in subjects receiving chronic hemodialysis.[10]

Not all of these questionnaires are suitable for all neuromuscular diseases. To choose a suitable questionnaire for a particular neuromuscular disease, researchers need to determine the reliability, ease of use, and construct validity of that fatigue questionnaire for measuring fatigue in that particular disease.[11] In addition, scores of a questionnaire should independently predict quality of life when adjusted for severity of associated conditions, such as immobility, depression, sleepiness, pulmonary function, and pain.

The Fatigue Severity Scale

Krupp and colleagues[5] developed this 1-dimensional, 9-item fatigue inventory and validated its internal consistency, sensitivity, and test-retest reliability. The 9-item FSS was selected from a 28-item questionnaire. The investigators administered the 28-item questionnaire to 25 subjects with multiple sclerosis, 29 subjects with systematic lupus erythematosus, and 20 healthy controls. They asked subjects to read each statement of the questionnaire and choose the number between 1 and 7 that best described their degree of agreement with each statement: 1 indicates strongly disagree and 7 strongly agree. Using factor analysis, item analysis, and theoretical considerations, they chose 9 items from this questionnaire to form the FSS. They found that the FSS has good internal consistency (with a Cronbach's alpha of 0.89 for multiple sclerosis, 0.81 for systemic lupus erythromatosus, and 0.88 for healthy controls). They also examined sensitivity of the scale (ie, the ability of the scale to detect clinically appropriate and predicted changes in fatigue) by administering the scale to 6 subjects with Lyme disease before and after antibiotic treatment and 2 subjects with multiple sclerosis before and after treatment with pemoline, a stimulant. In all of these subjects, clinical improvement was associated with reduced scores. In addition, they examined the test-retest reliability of the scale by administering the scale to subjects in whom there was no clinical reason to expect changes in their fatigue state. The subjects were tested at 2 points of time separated by 5 to 33 weeks. As hypothesized, no significant changes in the scores were noted.

The Multidimensional Fatigue Inventory

The MFI is a 20-item self-report instrument designed to measure fatigue.[6] The 20 items cover 5 dimensions of fatigue: general fatigue, physical fatigue, mental fatigue, reduced motivation, and reduced activity. Smets and colleagues[6] tested the psychometric properties of the MFI in 111 cancer subjects receiving radiotherapy, 395 subjects with chronic fatigue syndrome, 481 psychology students, 158 medical students, 46 junior physicians, 160 army recruits during their stay in the barracks, and 156 army recruits in the second week of intensive training. They demonstrated that the MFI was well accepted in both general and clinical populations. Ninety-six percent of the respondents completed the MFI without omitting items. They determined the 5-dimensional structure using confirmatory factor analysis and demonstrated that the 5-factor model fit the data in all samples tested. The instrument had good internal consistency with a Cronbach's alpha of 0.84. They also established the construct validity of the instrument by comparing groups, assuming differences in fatigue based on differences in circumstances or activity level. For example, subjects with chronic fatigue syndrome scored higher than students and army recruits in barracks. Army recruits scored higher during intensive training than when they were in barracks.

Researchers have used the MFI to assess fatigue in subjects with cancer[12,13] and chronic obstructive pulmonary disease (COPD).[14,15] In a study of subjects with COPD, Breslin and colleagues[14] measured pulmonary function, fatigue using the MFI, and depression using the Center for Epidemiologic Studies Depression Scale. They showed that depression correlated with general fatigue and mental fatigue but not with physical fatigue in the MFI. On the contrary, the severity of the pulmonary function impairment correlated with physical fatigue and reduced activity but not with mental fatigue. Other investigators have shown this separation between physical fatigue and mental fatigue as well.[13,15]

A multidimensional fatigue questionnaire, such as the MFI, is useful in characterize fatigue in different diseases. In studies in which the MFI was administered to patients with PD or ALS[4,8] (**Fig. 2**), a stark contrast in the distribution of MFI subscores emerged. Patients with PD or ALS had greater overall MFI scores than controls. The subscores revealed that patients with ALS do not show significantly higher fatigue in the "Reduced Motivation" and "Mental Fatigue" subscores than controls, whereas patients with PD display significantly higher fatigue in these categories than controls.

The Piper Fatigue Scale

The PFS is a multidimensional questionnaire and includes 22 characteristics of fatigue in 4 different dimensions: behavioral/severity, affective meaning, sensory, and cognitive/mood.[16] The validity and reliability of the PFS have been well established in subjects with cancer,[7,17] myocardial infarction,[18] and HIV.[19] The PFS has been validated in postpolio syndrome,[9] a lower motor neuron disease. Strohschein and

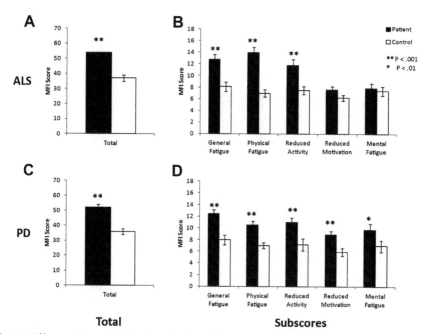

Fig. 2. Different characteristics of subjective fatigue in patients with ALS or PD measured by the Multidimensional Fatigue Inventory (MFI). The total MFI score is higher in patients with PD or ALS than in healthy controls (*A* and *C*). The MFI subscores "General Fatigue," "Physical Fatigue," and "Reduced Activity" are higher in patients with PD or ALS than in healthy controls; however, the MFI subscores "Reduced Motivation" and "Mental Fatigue" are not different from the controls in patients with ALS, but are higher in patients with PD (*B* and *D*).

colleagues[9] administered the PFS to 64 subjects with postpolio syndrome and 25 healthy controls. They demonstrated that the instrument has a high internal consistency with a Cronbach's alpha coefficient of 0.98 and strong test-retest reliability with an intraclass correlation coefficient of 0.98. The convergent validity of the instrument was shown with a strong positive correlation between the PFS and Chalder Fatigue Questionnaire.[20]

Subjects do not need to fill out these questionnaires in the presence of clinicians or researchers. Widely available Internet access is now making it possible for Web-based surveys to replace paper surveys.[21] Many subjects can fill out these questionnaires online with minimum effort.

Measuring Physical Fatigability in a Laboratory Setting

Physical fatigability is the inability to maintain the desired force during sustained or repeated exercise. It can be assessed objectively is a laboratory setting. Two most commonly used exercise protocols are intermittent submaximal exercise protocol and continuous maximum force exercise protocol.

In the submaximal force protocol, the subject generates submaximal (usually 50% of MVC) contraction intermittently (eg, 3 to 5 repetitions per minute) (**Fig.** 3A). The submaximal force protocol mimics activities, such as walking or cycling, and fatigue develops over a longer period (10–30 minutes) than in the maximal force exercise protocol. Submaximal force generation is more common for activities of daily living

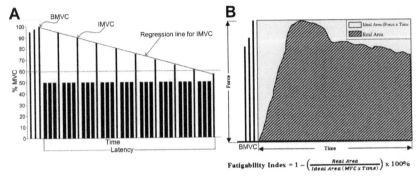

$$\text{Fatigability Index} = 1 - \left(\frac{Real\ Area}{Ideal\ Area\ (MVC\ x\ Time)}\right) \times 100\%$$

Fig. 3. Exercise paradigms used to determine physical fatigability. (*A*) The intermittent submaximal force exercise paradigm, and (*B*) the continuous maximum force exercise paradigm. At the beginning of the trial, the subject is encouraged to generate as much force as possible. The largest force of 3 attempts is the maximal voluntary contraction (MVC) or baseline MVC (BMVC). In the intermittent paradigm (*A*), each subject then performs cycles of exercise lasting for 10 to 7 seconds of muscle contraction at 50% of BMVC and 3 seconds of rest. An interval maximal voluntary contraction (IMVC) is performed after every 3 cycles. This continues until the subject develops fatigue, defined as the inability to generate an IMVC greater than 60% of BMVC.[8] In the continuous maximum force paradigm (*B*), subjects attempt to maintain the muscle contraction at the maximal force for a period of time (for example, 30 seconds). The actual force generated (the curved line) will decline owing to development of physical fatigability. The Fatigability Index is calculated using the equation in the figure. A higher Fatigability Index indicates more physical fatigability.

and therefore is more relevant to study fatigue. In the submaximal exercise protocol, we first measure the baseline maximal voluntary contraction (BMVC) of the muscles of interest as the greatest MVC in 3 trials. We use the BMVC to calculate the 50% MVC to be used in the submaximal force protocol. For a duty cycle of 70%, the subject sustains a contraction of 50% MVC for 7 seconds and rests for 3 seconds repeatedly. After every 3 cycles, the subject attempts to perform an interval MVC (IMVC). This series is repeated until the subject is unable to generate an IMVC above 60% of the MVC. We use the slope of the IMVC to measure the development of physical fatigability.

In the maximum force exercise protocol (see **Fig. 3**B), the subject is instructed to generate sustained maximal voluntary contraction (MVC). The MVC is the force generated with the subject's maximal effort with feedback and encouragement. During a sustained MVC, the force will decline gradually and fatigue will develop over a short period (<60 seconds). The maximal force protocol mimics activities, such as lifting heavy objects.

PHYSICAL FATIGABILITY HAS A CENTRAL OR PERIPHERAL ORIGIN

The generation of force during the maximal or submaximal exercise protocol includes a sequence of events, and fatigability can develop at any site involved.[22] The activation of the upper motor neurons may be influenced by other processes in the central nervous system, such as motivation and integration of sensory inputs. Lower motor neurons in the anterior horn of the spinal cord and the signal transfer across the neuromuscular junction are other potential sites for development of fatigability.[22] In addition, events occurring in the muscle during exercise can also result in fatigability. Central fatigability refers to reduced force generation caused by events at or proximal to the anterior horn cells, including the corticospinal tract, pyramidal cells, and motor cortex. Peripheral fatigability refers to the failure at or beyond the neuromuscular junction (**Fig. 4**).

The development of central or peripheral fatigability depends on the exercise protocol.[22] In the maximum force exercise protocol, the blood supply to the muscle is completely occluded during sustained MVC. As a result, K+ ion and other

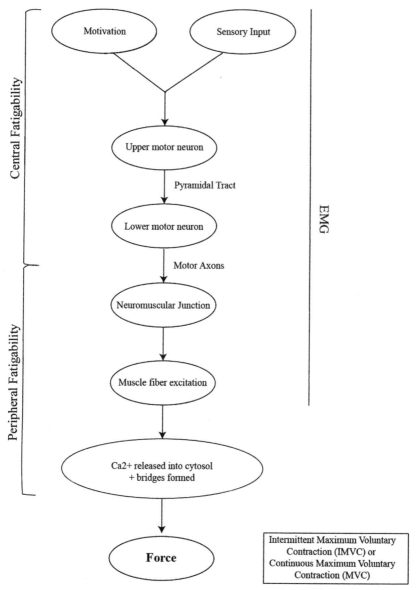

Fig. 4. Central and peripheral fatigability. Physical fatigability can be central or peripheral in origin. Central fatigability is fatigability originating at a site proximal to the neuromuscular junction. Peripheral fatigability is fatigability originating at or distal to the neuromuscular junction. Electromyelogram (EMG), twitch interpolation, and transcranial magnetic stimulation are techniques used to determine if physical fatigability is central or peripheral.

metabolites accumulate in the extracellular muscle space within seconds and cause peripheral fatigability. During the submaximal force exercise protocol, blood supply may be hindered during the contractions; however, hyperemia between contractions may still provide the muscle with enough blood and oxygen to prevent local accumulation of metabolites and causes less peripheral fatigability. The submaximal force exercise model is therefore used widely in studying central fatigability.

Twitch Interpolation and Transcranial Magnetic Stimulation (TMS) are Used to Differentiate Central from Peripheral Fatigability

In twitch interpolation, an electrical stimulus is delivered to the muscle or nerve to induce a maximal evocable force (MEF).[22] The MEF is the force generated by a muscle when additional electrical stimulation does not result in further force increase. Based on this technique, central fatigability can be defined as any exercise-induced reduction in maximal voluntary contraction force that is not accompanied by the same reduction in maximal evocable force. In contrast, there is a parallel decrease in MVC and MEF in peripheral fatigability. The technique of twitch interpolation has been proven to be a useful tool in studying the mechanism of fatigability.

Schillings and colleagues[23] used a modified twitch interpolation method to study the relative contribution of central and peripheral fatigability during a 2-minute maximum sustained muscle contraction. They assessed peripheral fatigability in 2 ways. First, by measuring muscle fiber conduction velocity during maximal voluntary contraction. Muscle fiber conduction velocity was determined with surface electromyography when stimulating the muscle endplate. Second, by comparing force level before and after a period of MVC. They assessed central fatigability by first measuring central activation failure (CAF). CAF was calculated using a formula[23] that evaluated the relative size of the superimposed force (responding to the electrical stimulation) during a 2-minute sustained contraction. The central fatigability was the difference between the CAF at the beginning and the CAF at the end of the sustained muscle contraction.

Central fatigability can also be measured by transcranial magnetic stimulation (TMS). In TMS, a magnetic coil stimulator is placed over the motor cortex area. A changing magnetic field delivered by the stimulator induces an electric field in the motor cortex and excites the cortical motor neurons. The signals travel down the spinal cord and activate the lower motor neurons that in turn activate muscles. The responses from the muscle are recorded as motor-evoked potentials (MEPs). The excitability of the cortical motor neurons can be assessed either by comparing the amplitudes of MEPs at a given stimulus intensity or by calculating the probability of MEPs by stimulation at the threshold levels. Cortical processes, such as motivation and sensory integration, could influence the excitability of cortical motor neurons. A change of the excitability of cortical motor neurons associated with central fatigability would imply that processes proximal to upper motor neurons most likely cause central fatigability.

Samii and colleagues[24] used TMS to investigate the change in cortical excitability associated with physical fatigability in healthy subjects. Subjects performed an intermittent isometric exercise of the extensor carpi radialis muscle for 30-second periods at half maximum force until fatigability (the inability to maintain half maximum force). The MEP amplitudes, measured after each exercise period, were on average 2 times larger than the MEP amplitudes before the exercise, a phenomenon they called postexercise facilitation. The increased MEPs decayed to baseline values over several minutes after the exercise ended. When fatigability developed, the MEP amplitudes were approximately 60% of the values taken before the exercise, a phenomenon they called postexercise depression. These depressed MEPs recovered to preexercise value over several minutes of rest. They hypothesized that postexercise MEP facilitation and depression are caused by intracortical mechanisms. Their findings suggest that TMS is a useful tool to measure and study the mechanism of central fatigability.

Our laboratory has used TMS to investigate the physiologic mechanisms of physical fatigability in Parkinson disease (PD). The increased physical fatigability in PD was associated with increased cortical excitability, and both were normalized by administration of levodopa.[8]

Gandevia and colleagues[25] used TMS and twitch interpolation to investigate the mechanisms of central fatigability. Healthy subjects performed a sustained fatiguing MVC of the biceps muscle for 1.5 to 2.0 minutes. TMS stimuli were delivered before, during, and after MVC. TMS initially produced a small increase in biceps force and larger with the development of fatigability. To examine if peripheral fatigability played a role in fatigability development during this exercise, they induced ischemia in the biceps by using a blood pressure cuff. Neither maximal voluntary force, nor voluntary activation recovered during ischemia; however, the fatigability-induced changes in MEP recovered rapidly, despite maintained ischemia. Therefore, they concluded that reduced output from the motor cortex was associated with fatigability.

Twitch interpolation and TMS techniques allow researchers to measure central and peripheral fatigability, as well as to investigate the mechanisms of physical fatigability in neuromuscular diseases. The advantages and the limitations of twitch interpolation are thoroughly discussed in a recent article.[26] Understanding the mechanisms of physical fatigability is the first step in developing effective treatments.

Peripheral and Central Physical Fatigability in Neuromuscular Diseases

Many patients with different types of neuromuscular diseases suffer from both peripheral and central fatigability. Schillings and colleagues[27] investigated the experienced (or subjective) fatigue and physiologic fatigability in 3 genetically distinct neuromusucular disorders. They studied 65 pateints with facioscapulohumeral dystrophy, 79 patients with classical myotonic dystrophy, 73 patients with hereditary motor and sensory neuropathy type I, and 24 age-matched healthy controls. They used a 4-item fatigue questionnaire to measure experienced fatigue at the current moment just before the physiologic measurement. The subjects made a 2-minute sustained maximal voluntary contraction of the biceps brachii muscle. They used the techniques described in their previous article[23] to measure peripheral and central fatigability. They found that patients had an increased level of experienced fatigue and less peripheral fatigability compared with controls; however, central fatigability was not different between patients and controls. Most interestingly, they found that patients had more than a threefold increase in central activation failure (CAF) than healthy controls (36% to 41% vs 12%). Furthermore, CAF slightly correlated with the level of experienced fatigue immediately before the test. They speculated that the large CAF in patients may be a result of reduced concentration, reduced motivation, or reduced effort.

Subjects with ALS also have more subjective fatigue and physical fatigability. Patients with ALS have been shown to have more pronounced subjective fatigue than healthy controls,[8] and have excessive physical fatigability that has peripheral and central components.[28,29]

Mental Fatigability in Neuromuscular Diseases

No studies have examined mental fatigability in neuromuscular diseases; however, it is likely that patients with neuromuscular diseases may suffer from mental fatigability in addition to physical fatigability. For example, Schilling and colleagues[27] speculated that the marked increase in CAF in patients with neuromuscular diseases may be a result of reduced concentration.

Mental fatigability can be defined as "deterioration in the performance of attention tasks over an extended period of time." We can quantitatively assess mental fatigability by measuring reaction times or error rates over an extended period in a reaction time paradigm, commonly used to assess attention.[30] An increase in reaction time or error rates over time would indicate development of mental fatigability.

Posner and Petersen[31] brought the concept that attention comprises 3 anatomically defined brain networks: the alerting network, the orienting network, and the executive network. Each of these networks has been related to specific cortical sites and neurotransmitters. The alerting network involves the cortical projection of the norepinephrine system from the locus ceruleus to the parietal and frontal cortex,[32] reflecting the ability to maintain alert state. The orienting network involves the cortical projection of the cholinergic system from the nucleus basalis to the temporal parietal junction, superior parietal lobe, and frontal eye fields,[33] performing selection of information from sensory inputs. The executive network involves projection of the dopaminergic system from the substantia nigra to the anterior cingulate cortex and lateral prefrontal cortical regions[34] for self-regulation of cognition and conflict-solving.

Fan and colleagues[35] have developed a computerized attention network test (ANT) that provides a behavioral measure of the efficiency of the 3 attention networks within a single task. The ANT measures reaction times to visual stimuli in 12 different experimental conditions (3 different target types with 4 different cue conditions). The efficiency of the alerting, orienting, and executive networks can be measured by calculating the difference in reaction times between different experimental conditions. This test has been used as a behavioral test to evaluate the performance of healthy children,[36,37] children with chromosome 22q11.2 deletion syndrome,[38,39] children with attention-deficit hyperactivity disorder (ADHD),[40] adults with borderline personality disorder,[41] and patients with schizophrenia.[42]

Mental fatigability has not been investigated in subjects with neuromuscular diseases; however, patients with myotonic dystrophy may suffer from excessive mental fatigability because of their cognitive dysfunction.[1] Patients with Duchenne muscular dystrophy also suffer from higher rates ADHD, autism spectrum disorder, and obsessive-compulsive disorder.[43,44] It is crucial for us to examine if these patients suffer from more mental fatigability that would affect their quality of life.

SUMMARY

Fatigue is common in neuromuscular disease and it may affect quality of life[8,21]; however, it has not been adequately studied. We can approach fatigue in neuromuscular diseases systematically. Questionnaires are used to assess subjective or experienced fatigue. With the wide availability of the Internet, many patients can fill out questionnaires through a Web-based survey. Researchers can use force-generation protocols to evaluate physical fatigability and attention protocols to evaluate mental fatigability. Using these techniques to further understand the mechanisms of subjective and physiologic fatigue will help physicians to develop more effective treatments for fatigue and improve patients' quality of life.

REFERENCES

1. Angeard N, Gargiulo M, Jacquette A, et al. Cognitive profile in childhood myotonic dystrophy type 1: Is there a global impairment? Neuromuscul Disord 2007;17:451–8.
2. Fauci AS, Braunwald E, Kasper DL, et al. Harrison's principles of internal medicine. 17th edition. New York: McGraw-Hill Medical; 2008.

3. Lou JS, Kearns G, Oken B, et al. Exacerbated physical fatigue and mental fatigue in Parkinson's disease. Mov Disord 2001;16:190–6.
4. Krupp LB, Avarez LA, Larocca NG, et al. Fatigue in multiple sclerosis. Arch Neurol 1988;45:435–7.
5. Krupp LB, LaRocca NG, Muir-Nash J, et al. The fatigue severity scale: application to patients with multiple sclerosis and systemic lupus erythematosus. Arch Neurol 1989;46:1121–3.
6. Smets EM, Grassen B, Bonke B, et al. The Multidimensional Fatigue Inventory (MFI) psychometric qualities of an instrument to assess fatigue. J Psychosom Res 1995;39:315–25.
7. Piper PF, Dibble SL, Dodd MJ, et al. The revised Piper Fatigue Scale: psychometric evaluation in women with breast cancer. Oncol Nurs Forum 1998;25:677–84.
8. Lou JS, Reeves A, Benice T, et al. Fatigue and depression are associated with poor quality of life in ALS. Neurology 2003;60:122–3.
9. Strohschein FJ, Kelly CG, Clarke AG, et al. Applicability, validity, and reliability of the Piper Fatigue Scale in postpolio patients. Am J Phys Med Rehabil 2003;82:122–9.
10. Brunier G, Graydon J. A comparison of two methods of measuring fatigue in patients on chronic haemodialysis: visual analogue vs Likert scale. Int J Nurs Stud 1996;33:338–48.
11. Meek PM, Nail LM, Barsevick A, et al. Psychometric testing of fatigue instruments for use with cancer patients. Nurs Res 2000;49:181–90.
12. Smets EM, Garssen B, Schuster-Uitterhoeve AL, et al. Fatigue in cancer patients. Br J Cancer 1993;68:220–4.
13. Schneider RA. Reliability and validity of the Multidimensional Fatigue Inventory (MFI-20) and the Rhoten Fatigue Scale among rural cancer outpatients. Cancer Nurs 1998;21:370–3.
14. Breslin E, van der Schans C, Breukink S, et al. Perception of fatigue and quality of life in patients with COPD. Chest 1998;114:958–64.
15. Breukink SO, Strijbos JH, Koorn M, et al. Relationship between subjective fatigue and physiological variables in patients with chronic obstructive pulmonary disease. Respir Med 1998;92:676–82.
16. Piper PF, Lindsey AM, Dodd MJ, et al. The development of an instrument to measure the subjective dimension of fatigue. In: Funk SG, Tornquist EM, Champagne MT, et al, editors. Key aspects of comfort: management of pain, fatigue, and nausea. New York: Springer; 1989. p. 199–208.
17. Dean GE, Spears L, Ferrell BR, et al. Fatigue in patients with cancer receiving interferon alpha. Cancer Pract 1995;3:164–72.
18. Varvaro FF, Sereika SM, Zullo TG, et al. Fatigue in women with myocardial infarction. Health Care Women Int 1996;17:593–602.
19. Grady C, Anderson R, Chase GA. Fatigue in HIV-infected men receiving investigational interleukin-2. Nurs Res 1998;47:227–34.
20. Chalder T, Berelowitz G, Pawlikowska T, et al. Development of a fatigue scale. J Psychosom Res 1993;37:147–53.
21. Boentert M, Dziewas R, Heidbreder A, et al. Fatigue, reduced sleep quality and restless legs syndrome in Charcot-Marie-Tooth disease: a web-based survey. J Neurol 2010;257:646–52.
22. Vollestad NK. Measurement of human muscle fatigue. J Neurosci Methods 1997;74:219–27.
23. Schillings ML, Hoefsloot W, Stegeman DF, et al. Relative contributions of central and peripheral factors to fatigue during a maximal sustained effort. Eur J Appl Physiol 2003;90:562–8.

24. Samii A, Wassermann EM, Ikoma K, et al. Characterization of postexercise facilitation and depression of motor evoked potentials to transcranial magnetic stimulation. Neurology 1996;46:1376–82.
25. Gandevia SC, Allen GM, Butler JE, et al. Supraspinal factors in human muscle fatigue: evidence for suboptimal output from the motor cortex. J Physiol 1996; 490:529–36.
26. Gandevia SC. Twitch interpolation: a valid measure with misinterpreted meaning. J Appl Physiol 2009;107(1):363–4 [discussion: 367–8].
27. Schillings ML, Kalkman JS, Janssen HM, et al. Experienced and physiological fatigue in neuromuscular diseases. Clin Neurophysiol 2007;118:292–300.
28. Sharma KR, Kent-Braun JA, Majumdar S, et al. Physiology of fatigue in amyotrophic lateral sclerosis. Neurology 1995;45:733–40.
29. Kent-Braun J, Miller RG. Central fatigue during isometric exercise in amyotrophic lateral sclerosis. Muscle Nerve 2000;23:909–14.
30. Oken BS, Salinsky MC, Elsas SM. Vigilance, alertness, or sustained attention: physiological basis and measurement. Clin Neurophysiol 2006;117(9):1885–901.
31. Posner MI, Petersen SE. The attention system of the human brain. Annu Rev Neurosci 1990;13:25–42.
32. Marrocco RT, Davidson MC. Neurochemistry of attention. In: Parasuraman R, editor. The attentive brain. Cambridge (MA): MIT; 1998. p. 35–50.
33. Corbetta M, Shulman GL. Control of goal-directed and stimulus-driven attention in the brain. Nat Rev Neurosci 2002;3(3):201–15.
34. Benes FM. Emerging principles of altered neural circuitry in schizophrenia. Brain Res Brain Res Rev 2000;31(2-3):251–69.
35. Fan J, McCandliss BD, Sommer T, et al. Testing the efficiency and independence of attentional networks. J Cogn Neurosci 2002;14(3):340–7.
36. Mezzacappa E. Alerting, orienting, and executive attention: developmental and socio-demographic properties in an epidemiological sample of young, urban children. Child Dev 2004;75(5):1373–86.
37. Rueda R, Fan J, McCandliss BD, et al. Development of attentional networks in childhood. Neuropsychologia 2004;42(8):1029–40.
38. Bish JP, Ferrante SM, McDonald-McGinn D, et al. Maladaptive conflict monitoring as evidence for executive dysfunction in children with chromosome 22q11.2 deletion syndrome. Dev Sci 2005;8(1):36–43.
39. Sobin C, Kiley-Brabeck K, Daniels, et al. Networks of attention in children with the 22q11 deletion syndrome. Dev Neuropsychol 2004;26(2):611–26.
40. Mullane JC, Corkum PV, Klein RM, et al. Alerting, orienting, and executive attention in children with ADHD. J Atten Disord 2011;15(4):310–20.
41. Posner MI, Rothbart MK, Vizueta N, et al. Attentional mechanisms of borderline personality disorder. Proc Natl Acad Sci U S A 2002;99(25):16366–70.
42. Wang K, Fan J, Dong Y, et al. Selective impairment of attentional networks of orienting and executive control in schizophrenia. Schizophr Res 2005;78(2–3): 235–41.
43. Hendriksen JG, Vles JS. Neuropsychiatric disorders in males with duchenne muscular dystrophy: frequency rate of attention-deficit hyperactivity disorder (ADHD), autism spectrum disorder, and obsessive–compulsive disorder. J Child Neurol 2008;23(5):477–81.
44. Boosman H, Visser-Meily JM, Meijer JW, et al. Evaluation of change in fatigue, self-efficacy and health-related quality of life, after a group educational intervention programme for persons with neuromuscular diseases or multiple sclerosis: a pilot study. Disabil Rehabil 2011;33(8):690–6.

The Utility of Electromyography and Mechanomyography for Assessing Neuromuscular Function: A Noninvasive Approach

Moh H. Malek, PhD[a],*, Jared W. Coburn, PhD[b]

KEYWORDS

• Exercise physiology • Fatigue • Muscle • Rehabilitation

ELECTROMYOGRAPHY

Electromyography (EMG) has been used to study muscle function for decades.[1] During voluntary contraction, action potentials are sent from the brain to the motor unit, ultimately leading to the contraction of muscle fibers.[1] EMG, therefore, allows investigators to measure muscle activation.[1] EMG can be divided into invasive and noninvasive methods. For invasive methods, fine-wire or needle EMG is used, with recording wires directly inserted into the muscle,[1] whereas with noninvasive EMG, electrodes are placed on the skin over the muscle of interest (**Fig. 1**).[1] This latter approach is the focus of the first half of the paper. The second half of the paper introduces a complementary method of examining muscle function called *mechanomyography* (MMG). MMG measures the sound produced by activated muscle, and thus represents the mechanical counterpart to EMG. Therefore, this article introduces and discusses two noninvasive methods of examining muscle function that may be potentially useful in clinical settings (**Fig. 2**).

[a] Integrative Physiology of Exercise Laboratory, Eugene Applebaum College of Pharmacy & Health Sciences, Wayne State University, 259 Mack Avenue, Room 5344, Detroit, MI 48201, USA
[b] Department of Kinesiology, California State University, Fullerton, 800 North State College Boulevard, Fullerton, CA 92834-6870, USA
* Corresponding author.
E-mail address: en7488@wayne.edu

Phys Med Rehabil Clin N Am 23 (2012) 23–32
doi:10.1016/j.pmr.2011.11.005
1047-9651/12/$ – see front matter © 2012 Elsevier Inc. All rights reserved.

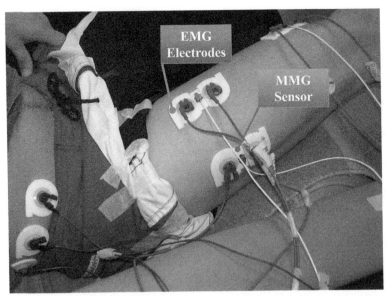

Fig. 1. Placement of the surface EMG electrodes and MMG sensors on the superficial quadriceps muscles. The ground electrodes for EMG are placed on the iliac crest. The MMG sensors are accelerometers.

The EMG signal derived from muscle contraction is characterized into two domains called *time* and *frequency*.[1] The time domain of the EMG signal is a measure of EMG amplitude (voltage) and reflects the number of motor units activated and the frequency of activation. The frequency domain of the EMG signal is a measure of how frequently the waveform crosses the baseline and is measured in hertz (Hz). It is related to the conduction velocity of the action potentials,[1] at least for isometric muscle actions. The EMG time and frequency domains have been examined under various perturbations, such as isometric,[2] isokinetic,[2] eccentric,[3] and dynamic muscle actions.[4–6]

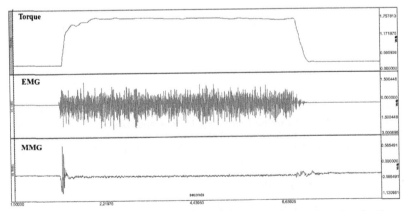

Fig. 2. The raw signal for torque, EMG, and MMG for isometric muscle action for the vastus lateralis muscle.

EMG RESPONSES TO ISOMETRIC AND DYNAMIC SUBMAXIMAL TO MAXIMAL MUSCLE ACTIONS

A variety of muscle action types (concentric, eccentric, and isometric) are typical of activities of daily living. Methodologies such as EMG suggest that the nervous system uses unique strategies to control muscle force production during each of these different types of muscle actions. This concept may have important implications for clinicians who are responsible for assessing muscle function and conducting strength training programs designed to assist with movement tasks that require the use of different muscle actions.

Isometric muscle actions are typically characterized by linear or curvilinear increases in EMG amplitude with force caused by concurrent increases in motor unit recruitment and firing rates to 50% to 80% of maximal voluntary contraction (MVC), and then increases in firing rates only between 50% to 80% and 100% of MVC.[7–11] Investigators have also suggested that a curvilinear EMG amplitude versus isometric torque relationship may be caused by increases in the firing rates of motor units with fused twitches.[12] Theoretically, increases in the firing rates of these motor units (with fused twitches) could cause an increase in EMG amplitude without a corresponding increase in torque production. This response would result in curvilinear EMG amplitude versus isometric torque relationships.[1,12]

During isometric muscle actions, the frequency content of the EMG signal is believed to reflect the average conduction velocity of the action potential.[13] This response is related to the number and type of the activated motor units.[14] Theoretically, the progressive recruitment of fast-twitch motor units, with higher conduction velocities of action potentials, would lead to increases in EMG frequency with increases in torque muscle,[1] although this is a debated concept.

For concentric muscle actions, the amplitude of the EMG signal increases linearly with increases in force. The limited number of studies[3,15–17] that have examined eccentric muscle actions have found that they involve unique motor control strategies compared with isometric or concentric muscle actions. For example, muscle activation is lower during eccentric than concentric or isometric muscle actions,[18,19] and preferential recruitment of fast-twitch motor units may occur during eccentric, as opposed to concentric, muscle actions.[15–17,20]

USING EMG TO IDENTITY FATIGUE THRESHOLD
EMG Amplitude

Although several methods are available to identify fatigue threshold using cardiorespiratory indices, deVries and colleagues[21] introduced the use of EMG to identify neuromuscular fatigue using cycle ergometry (**Fig. 3**). The fatigue threshold or physical

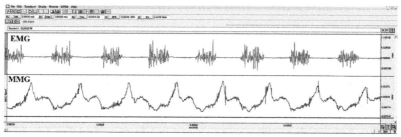

Fig. 3. Screen shot of EMG and MMG raw signal for cycle ergometry for the vastus lateralis muscle.

working capacity (PWC) uses mathematical modeling and physiologic indices such as the EMG amplitude or frequency to identify a workload that an individual can theoretically perform indefinitely.[21] Briefly, the EMG fatigue threshold is identified from a series of visits during which the subject performs constant power output exercise on a cycle ergometer.[21] The power outputs are selected to elicit a continuous increase in muscle activity during the ride.[21] The duration of each ride, therefore, may be until voluntary exhaustion occurs[22] or for a set period, such as 8 minutes (**Fig. 4**).[23] In their original work, deVries and colleagues[21] focused on EMG amplitude, and therefore plotted EMG amplitude versus time for each power output. Thereafter, the investigators used linear regression to determine the slope of the relationship between EMG amplitude and time. Subsequently, the slope coefficients were plotted for each power output and linear regression was performed. The intersection between the regression line and the y-intercept is identified as the fatigue threshold for that individual, and is theoretically the maximal workload that the individual could continue indefinitely.

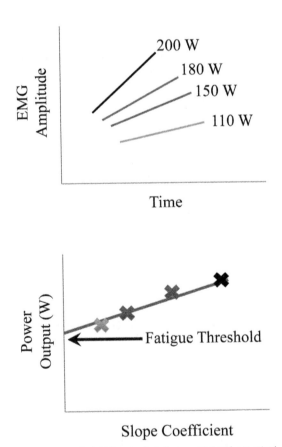

Fig. 4. Theoretical depiction of deVries and colleagues' mathematical model for determining fatigue threshold for cycle ergometry from four separate constant power output rides for a set time. (*From* deVries HA, Tichy MW, Housh TJ, et al. A method for estimating physical working capacity at the fatigue threshold (PWCFT). Ergonomics 1987;30(8): 1195–204; with permission.)

Recently, Camic and colleagues[24] proposed a method of determining EMG fatigue threshold from a single incremental cycle ergometry test. Briefly, the investigators recorded EMG amplitude from the vastus lateralis at each workload. Thereafter, linear regression was performed to determine if the slope of the regression line was significantly different from zero. The investigators then selected the highest workload that had a nonsignificant ($P>.05$) slope and the first workload that had a significant ($P<.05$) slope. These two workloads were then averaged to provide an estimate of the EMG fatigue threshold from a single incremental test to voluntary exhaustion. This new approach may have applications in a clinical setting if future studies validate this method and show that it is sensitive for detecting changes in the muscle with various interventions, such as endurance training.

EMG Frequency

Several studies have examined measures of EMG frequency during various fatiguing exercise tasks,[25,26] including those performed by clinical populations.[27] Typically, these studies have found that fatigue is associated with decreases in EMG frequency measures. During incremental cycle ergometry to exhaustion, however, there is a lack of consistency in the patterns of responses for EMG frequency.[28–30] To determine whether the consistencies in EMG frequency were from the mode of exercise (multijoint vs single-joint), Malek and colleagues[30] had the same subjects perform incremental cycle ergometry and double-legged knee-extensor ergometry. Briefly, the knee-extensor ergometry is a model of isolating the exercise workout to the quadriceps femoris muscles with little to no neuromuscular activity in other lower limb muscles.[31] The investigators found that the patterns of responses for EMG frequency were still inconsistent during incremental exercise regardless of whether the mode was multijoint or single-joint. Several recent studies have successfully attempted to use the EMG frequency domain as an index of neuromuscular fatigue during isometric muscle action of the biceps brachii[32–34] or the vastus lateralis during cycle ergometry.[24,35] Future studies, however, are needed to validate these new methods and determine their application in rehabilitation settings.

MMG

The previous section discussed the use of EMG for examining motor control strategies and determining contributors to neuromuscular fatigue under various perturbations. This section introduces MMG, which can be used in conjunction with EMG to examine neuromuscular function. MMG is the recording and quantification of sounds produced by low-frequency lateral oscillation of muscle fibers.[36,37] Although in more recent years the term *MMG* has been more routinely used, initial studies used various terms such as *vibromyography*, *sound myogram*, or *acoustic myography* to describe this phenomenon of the muscle.[36,37] Regardless of terminology, investigators have suggested that MMG reflects the mechanical counterpart of motor unit activity measured by EMG.[38] In addition, several investigators[37,39] have found that the lateral oscillations reflected in the MMG signal are generated by (1) a gross lateral movement of the muscle at the initiation of a contraction that is generated by nonsimultaneous activation of muscle fibers, (2) smaller sequential lateral oscillations occurring at the resonant frequency of the muscle, and (3) dimensional changes of the active muscle fibers. Similar to the EMG signal, the MMG signal has a time and frequency domain, with the time domain related to motor unit recruitment and the frequency domain being unique in that it provides information regarding motor unit firing rates.[40,41]

MMG RESPONSES TO ISOMETRIC AND DYNAMIC SUBMAXIMAL TO MAXIMAL MUSCLE ACTIONS

As with EMG, MMG has been used to examine the motor control strategies used to vary force production during concentric, eccentric, and isometric contractions of the superficial quadriceps femoris muscles.[3,7–9,11,42–47] Some studies have found linear or curvilinear increases in MMG amplitude to 100% MVC for isometric muscle actions,[8,9,11,43–45,47] whereas others have found increases in MMG amplitude to 75% to 80% of MVC, followed by a plateau or decrease to 100% of MVC. This plateau or decrease in MMG amplitude may be from the fusion of motor unit twitches or the end of motor unit recruitment.

POTENTIAL APPLICATION OF EMG AND MMG WITH CLINICAL POPULATIONS

The simultaneous use of EMG and MMG can provide complementary but unique information to clinicians interested in studying neuromuscular function. For example, one recent study[48] examined MMG and EMG amplitude and frequency values from the biceps brachii and triceps brachii of patients with Parkinson disease and age-matched controls while they performed a submaximal load-holding task. Marusiak and colleagues[48] found that patients with Parkinson disease had higher MMG amplitude values from the biceps brachii but lower MMG frequency from both muscles. In addition, EMG frequency of the triceps brachii was higher for these patients compared with controls. The authors concluded that MMG may be a useful clinical tool for evaluating neuromuscular function in patients with Parkinson disease.[48] Previous studies have used MMG to examine cerebral palsy,[49] myotonic dystrophy,[50,51] and externally powered prostheses.[52] Although more studies are required, the potential application of EMG and MMG for assessing neuromuscular function in various clinical populations is feasible.

USING MMG FOR CONTINUOUS MUSCLE ACTIONS

Studies examining MMG amplitude or frequency responses during dynamic muscle action have used either incremental or constant workload cycle ergometry.[53,54] For example, Stout and colleagues[55] and Shinohara and colleagues[56] initially used MMG to determine the relationship between MMG amplitude versus power output for the vastus lateralis muscle. Stout and colleagues[55] reported a linear relationship for 24 of 24 patients. In addition, the investigators also reported that for 83% of the subjects, the linear slope coefficients for the MMG amplitude were statistically similar to the slope coefficients for $\dot{V}o_2$ versus power output. Subsequent studies, however, have reported quadratic or cubic relationships between MMG amplitude versus output for cycle ergometry. More recently, Malek and colleagues[57] examined the relationship between MMG amplitude and excess postexercise oxygen consumption. The investigators reported that the time constant for MMG amplitude for the three superficial quadriceps femoris muscles were significantly different than the time constant for $\dot{V}o_2$.[57] Therefore, MMG and $\dot{V}o_2$ may not reflect a close relationship between the metabolic and mechanical properties of the muscle as hypothesized by Stout and colleagues.[55] These differences in the patterns of responses may be partly explained by fiber type composition or habitual exercise activity of the subjects.[58,59]

Recent studies, however, indicate no consistent patterns of responses for MMG frequency during incremental cycle[60] or knee-extensor ergometry.[61] However, muscle activation at $\dot{V}o_{2max}$ during cycle ergometry has been reported to reflect approximately 16% of MVC.[62] The lack of statistically significant changes in MMG frequency, therefore, may be due to reliance on motor unit recruitment rather than firing rate.[40,41]

SUMMARY

This article reviews recent studies using EMG and MMG to determine motor unit recruitment strategies of various muscles under different exercise paradigms. The results of these studies suggest that the use of EMG and MMG to determine muscle fatigue is robust. Future studies with clinical populations are needed, however, to determine the optimal use EMG and/or MMG for assessing muscle function in rehabilitative settings.

REFERENCES

1. Basmajian JV, De Luca CJ. Muscles alive, their functions revealed by electromyography. Baltimore (MD): Williams & Wilkins; 1985. p. xii, 561.
2. Beck TW, Housh TJ, Johnson GO, et al. Comparison of a piezoelectric contact sensor and an accelerometer for examining mechanomyographic amplitude and mean power frequency versus torque relationships during isokinetic and isometric muscle actions of the biceps brachii. J Electromyogr Kinesiol 2006; 16(4):324–35.
3. Coburn JW, Housh TJ, Malek MH, et al. Mechanomyographic and electromyographic responses to eccentric muscle contractions. Muscle Nerve 2006;33(5): 664–71.
4. Perry SR, Housh TJ, Johnson GO, et al. Mechanomyography, electromyography, heart rate, and ratings of perceived exertion during incremental cycle ergometry. J Sports Med Phys Fitness 2001;41(2):183–8.
5. Perry SR, Housh TJ, Weir JP, et al. Mean power frequency and amplitude of the mechanomyographic and electromyographic signals during incremental cycle ergometry. J Electromyogr Kinesiol 2001;11(4):299–305.
6. Perry-Rana SR, Housh TJ, Johnson GO, et al. MMG and EMG responses during fatiguing isokinetic muscle contractions at different velocities. Muscle Nerve 2002;26(3):367–73.
7. Matheson GO, Maffey-Ward L, Mooney M, et al. Vibromyography as a quantitative measure of muscle force production. Scand J Rehabil Med 1997;29(1):29–35.
8. Ebersole KT, Housh TJ, Johnson GO, et al. MMG and EMG responses of the superficial quadriceps femoris muscles. J Electromyogr Kinesiol 1999;9(3):219–27.
9. Shinohara M, Kouzaki M, Yoshihisa T, et al. Mechanomyogram from the different heads of the quadriceps muscle during incremental knee extension. Eur J Appl Physiol Occup Physiol 1998;78(4):289–95.
10. Eloranta V. Patterning of muscle activity in static knee extension. Electromyogr Clin Neurophysiol 1989;29(6):369–75.
11. Coburn JW, Housh TJ, Cramer JT, et al. Mechanomyographic and electromyographic responses of the vastus medialis muscle during isometric and concentric muscle actions. J Strength Cond Res 2005;19(2):412–20.
12. Woods JJ, Bigland-Ritchie B. Linear and non-linear surface EMG/force relationships in human muscles. An anatomical/functional argument for the existence of both. Am J Phys Med 1983;62(6):287–99.
13. Karlsson S, Gerdle B. Mean frequency and signal amplitude of the surface EMG of the quadriceps muscles increase with increasing torque—a study using the continuous wavelet transform. J Electromyogr Kinesiol 2001;11(2):131–40.

14. Kamen G, Caldwell GE. Physiology and interpretation of the electromyogram. J Clin Neurophysiol 1996;13(5):366–84.
15. McHugh MP, Tyler TF, Greenberg SC, et al. Differences in activation patterns between eccentric and concentric quadriceps contractions. J Sports Sci 2002; 20(2):83–91.
16. Nardone A, Schieppati M. Shift of activity from slow to fast muscle during voluntary lengthening contractions of the triceps surae muscles in humans. J Physiol 1988;395:363–81.
17. Nardone A, Romano C, Schieppati M. Selective recruitment of high-threshold human motor units during voluntary isotonic lengthening of active muscles. J Physiol 1989;409:451–71.
18. Komi PV, Kaneko M, Aura O. EMG activity of the leg extensor muscles with special reference to mechanical efficiency in concentric and eccentric exercise. Int J Sports Med 1987;8(Suppl 1):22–9.
19. Tesch PA, Dudley GA, Duvoisin MR, et al. Force and EMG signal patterns during repeated bouts of concentric or eccentric muscle actions. Acta Physiol Scand 1990;138(3):263–71.
20. McHugh MP, Connolly DA, Eston RG, et al. Electromyographic analysis of exercise resulting in symptoms of muscle damage. J Sports Sci 2000;18(3): 163–72.
21. deVries HA, Tichy MW, Housh TJ, et al. A method for estimating physical working capacity at the fatigue threshold (PWCFT). Ergonomics 1987;30(8): 1195–204.
22. Mielke M, Housh TJ, Malek MH, et al. Estimated times to exhaustion at the PWC V O2, PWC HRT, and VT. J Strength Cond Res 2008;22(6):2003–10.
23. Miller JM, Housh TJ, Coburn JW, et al. A proposed test for determining physical working capacity at the oxygen consumption threshold (PWCVO2). J Strength Cond Res 2004;18(3):618–24.
24. Camic CL, Housh TJ, Johnson GO, et al. An EMG frequency-based test for estimating the neuromuscular fatigue threshold during cycle ergometry. Eur J Appl Physiol 2010;108(2):337–45.
25. Lindstrom L, Kadefors R, Petersen I. An electromyographic index for localized muscle fatigue. J Appl Physiol 1977;43(4):750–4.
26. Williams DM, Sharma S, Bilodeau M. Neuromuscular fatigue of elbow flexor muscles of dominant and non-dominant arms in healthy humans. J Electromyogr Kinesiol 2002;12(4):287–94.
27. Callaghan MJ, McCarthy CJ, Oldham JA. Electromyographic fatigue characteristics of the quadriceps in patellofemoral pain syndrome. Man Ther 2001;6(1): 27–33.
28. Malek MH, Coburn JW, Weir JP, et al. The effects of innervation zone on electromyographic amplitude and mean power frequency during incremental cycle ergometry. J Neurosci Methods 2006;155(1):126–33.
29. Malek MH, Housh TJ, Coburn JW, et al. The effects of interelectrode distance on electromyographic amplitude and mean power frequency during incremental cycle ergometry. J Neurosci Methods 2006;151(2):139–47.
30. Malek MH, Coburn JW, Tedjasaputra V. Comparison of electromyographic responses for the superficial quadriceps muscles: cycle versus knee-extensor ergometry. Muscle Nerve 2009;39(6):810–8.
31. Richardson RS, Frank LR, Haseler LJ. Dynamic knee-extensor and cycle exercise: functional MRI of muscular activity. Int J Sports Med 1998;19(3): 182–7.

32. Hendrix CR, Housh TJ, Johnson GO, et al. The effect of epoch length on the electromyographic mean power frequency and amplitude versus time relationships. Electromyogr Clin Neurophysiol 2010;50(5):219–27.

33. Hendrix CR, Housh TJ, Camic CL, et al. Comparing electromyographic and mechanomyographic frequency-based fatigue thresholds to critical torque during isometric forearm flexion. J Neurosci Methods 2010;194(1):64–72.

34. Hendrix CR, Housh TJ, Mielke M, et al. Critical torque, estimated time to exhaustion, and anaerobic work capacity from linear and nonlinear mathematical models. Med Sci Sports Exerc 2009;41(12):2185–90.

35. Camic CL, Housh TJ, Hendrix CR, et al. The influence of the muscle fiber pennation angle and innervation zone on the identification of neuromuscular fatigue during cycle ergometry. J Electromyogr Kinesiol 2011;21(1):33–40.

36. Orizio C. Soundmyogram and EMG cross-spectrum during exhausting isometric contractions in humans. J Electromyogr Kinesiol 1992;2(3):141–9.

37. Orizio C. Muscle sound: bases for the introduction of a mechanomyographic signal in muscle studies. Crit Rev Biomed Eng 1993;21(3):201–43.

38. Gordon G, Holbourn H. The sounds from single motor units in a contracting muscle. J Physiol 1948;107:456–64.

39. Barry DT, Cole NM. Fluid mechanics of muscle vibrations. Biophys J 1988;53(6):899–905.

40. Beck TW, Housh TJ, Cramer JT, et al. Mechanomyographic amplitude and frequency responses during dynamic muscle actions: a comprehensive review. Biomed Eng Online 2005;4(1):67.

41. Beck TW, Housh TJ, Johnson GO, et al. Does the frequency content of the surface mechanomyographic signal reflect motor unit firing rates? A brief review. J Electromyogr Kinesiol 2007;17(1):1–13.

42. Coburn JW, Housh TJ, Cramer JT, et al. Mechanomyographic time and frequency domain responses of the vastus medialis muscle during submaximal to maximal isometric and isokinetic muscle actions. Electromyogr Clin Neurophysiol 2004;44(4):247–55.

43. Coburn JW, Housh TJ, Weir JP, et al. Mechanomyographic responses of the vastus medialis to isometric and eccentric muscle actions. Med Sci Sports Exerc 2004;36(11):1916–22.

44. Ebersole KT, Housh TJ, Johnson GO, et al. The effect of leg flexion angle on the mechanomyographic responses to isometric muscle actions. Eur J Appl Physiol Occup Physiol 1998;78(3):264–9.

45. Maton B, Petitjean M, Cnockaert JC. Phonomyogram and electromyogram relationships with isometric force reinvestigated in man. Eur J Appl Physiol Occup Physiol 1990;60(3):194–201.

46. Nonaka H, Mita K, Akataki K, et al. Mechanomyographic investigation of muscle contractile properties in preadolescent boys. Electromyogr Clin Neurophysiol 2000;40(5):287–93.

47. Stokes MJ, Dalton PA. Acoustic myographic activity increases linearly up to maximal voluntary isometric force in the human quadriceps muscle. J Neurol Sci 1991;101:163–7.

48. Marusiak J, Jaskolska A, Kisiel-Sajewicz K, et al. EMG and MMG activities of agonist and antagonist muscles in Parkinson's disease patients during absolute submaximal load holding. J Electromyogr Kinesiol 2009;19(5):903–14.

49. Akataki K, Mita K, Itoh K, et al. Acoustic and electrical activities during voluntary isometric contraction of biceps brachii muscles in patients with spastic cerebral palsy. Muscle Nerve 1996;19(10):1252–7.

50. Orizio C, Esposito F, Paganotti I, et al. Electrically-elicited surface mechanomyogram in myotonic dystrophy. Ital J Neurol Sci 1997;18(4):185–90.
51. Orizio C, Esposito F, Sansone V, et al. Muscle surface mechanical and electrical activities in myotonic dystrophy. Electromyogr Clin Neurophysiol 1997;37(4): 231–9.
52. Barry DT, Leonard JA Jr, Gitter AJ, et al. Acoustic myography as a control signal for an externally powered prosthesis. Arch Phys Med Rehabil 1986;67(4):267–9.
53. Housh TJ, Perry SR, Bull AJ, et al. Mechanomyographic and electromyographic responses during submaximal cycle ergometry. Eur J Appl Physiol 2000;83(4-5): 381–7.
54. Zuniga JM, Housh TJ, Camic CL, et al. The effects of skinfold thicknesses and innervation zone on the mechanomyographic signal during cycle ergometry. J Electromyogr Kinesiol 2011;21(5):789–94.
55. Stout JR, Housh TJ, Johnson GO, et al. Mechanomyography and oxygen consumption during incremental cycle ergometry. Eur J Appl Physiol Occup Physiol 1997;76(4):363–7.
56. Shinohara M, Kouzaki M, Yoshihisa T, et al. Mechanomyography of the human quadriceps muscle during incremental cycle ergometry. Eur J Appl Physiol 1997;76:314–9.
57. Malek MH, Coburn JW, Housh TJ, et al. Excess post-exercise oxygen consumption is not associated with mechanomyographic amplitude after incremental cycle ergometry in the quadriceps femoris muscles. Muscle Nerve 2011;44: 432–8.
58. Beck TW, Housh TJ, Fry AC, et al. The influence of muscle fiber type composition on the patterns of responses for electromyographic and mechanomyographic amplitude and mean power frequency during a fatiguing submaximal isometric muscle action. Electromyogr Clin Neurophysiol 2007;47(4-5):221–32.
59. Beck TW, Housh TJ, Fry AC, et al. The influence of myosin heavy chain isoform composition and training status on the patterns of responses for mechanomyographic amplitude versus isometric torque. J Strength Cond Res 2008;22(3): 818–25.
60. Malek MH, Coburn JW, York R, et al. Comparison of mechanomyographic sensors during incremental cycle ergometry for the quadriceps femoris. Muscle Nerve 2010;42(3):394–400.
61. Malek MH, Coburn JW, Tedjasaputra V. Comparison of mechanomyographic amplitude and mean power frequency for the rectus femoris muscle: cycle versus knee-extensor ergometry. J Neurosci Methods 2009;181(1):89–94.
62. Sjøgaard G. Force-velocity curve for bicycle work. In: Asmussen E, Jorgensen K, editors. Biomechanics VI-A. Baltimore (MD): University Park Press; 1978. p. 93–9.

Novel Concepts Integrated in Neuromuscular Assessments for Surgical Restoration of Arm and Hand Function in Tetraplegia

Jan Fridén, MD, PhD[a,b],*, Andreas Gohritz, MD[c]

KEYWORDS

- Tetraplegia • Spinal cord injury • Tendon transfer
- Novel concepts • Immediate activation • Combined procedure
- Nerve transfer

In the United States alone, approximately 225,000 to 300,000 persons live with a spinal cord injury (SCI), and about 12,000 new SCI injuries occur every year, mostly in young, healthy, and active individuals in their most productive years. More than 50% of all SCIs occur at the cervical level and lead to tetraplegia.[1]

Upper extremity function is, apart from the brain, the most important functional resource of tetraplegic patients and is judged to be the most desirable ability to regain after cervical SCI before bowel, bladder, sexual function, or walking ability.[2–6] Surgical rehabilitation of arm and hand abilities can indeed meet many of patient's requirements. Although regrettably greatly underused, tendon transfer surgery is a powerful

Funding for this project was provided by the Swedish Research Council Grant 11200, University of Gothenburg and Sahlgrenska University Hospital.

The authors have no financial disclosures.

[a] Department of Hand Surgery, Institute of Clinical Sciences, Sahlgrenska University Hospital, Sahlgrenska Academy at University of Gothenburg, Bruna Stråket 11, SE-413 45 Göteborg, Sweden

[b] Swiss Paraplegic Centre, Guido A. Zäch-Str. 1, CH-6207 Nottwil, Switzerland

[c] Department of Plastic, Hand and Reconstructive Surgery, Hannover Medical School, Carl-Neuberg-Str. 1, D-30625 Hannover, Germany

* Corresponding author. Department of Hand Surgery, Institute of Clinical Sciences, Sahlgrenska University Hospital, Sahlgrenska Academy at University of Gothenburg, Bruna Stråket 11, SE-413 45 Göteborg, Sweden.

E-mail address: jan.friden@orthop.gu.se

tool to improve upper extremity function, and an asset to enhance self-esteem and increase spontaneity.[7–10] Transfers can provide a certain amount of autonomy for persons with tetraplegia and allow them to regain meaningful roles and productive work. Restoration of hand function can eliminate the need for adaptive equipment for eating, personal care, catheterizing, and other activities of daily living.[11–13] Results from more than 500 cases in 14 studies were recently summarized, and revealed a mean increase of Medical Research Council score for elbow extension from 0 to 3.3 after reconstruction and a mean postoperative pinch strength of 2 kg, which markedly improved upper extremity usability.[10]

This article summarizes novel concepts of surgical restoration of arm and hand function based on neuromuscular assessment.

ANATOMY AND CLINICAL EXAMINATION
Muscle Testing

Surgical planning depends on preoperative evaluation of the upper extremity, and includes muscle strength tests according to the British Research Council system and International Classification of Surgery of the Hand in Tetraplegia (ICSHT) (**Tables 1** and **2**).[14]

The donor muscle must be healthy and of adequate strength (M4), preferably not injured or reinnervated, yet with limited available donor muscles; a weaker muscle (M3) may be considered for transfer. Optimally it should be synergistic, similar in architecture, and have an adequate soft-tissue bed along the route of transfer.[15,16]

Joint Range of Motion

Passive joint motion is a prerequisite for active and passive functional reconstruction. A tenodesis effect during wrist extension (hand closure), flexion (hand opening), and joint stability (primarily the thumb carpometacarpal [CMC] joint) is preferable but not required for reconstruction.

Sensibility Testing

Sensory examination focuses on cutaneous afferences of the hands with a 2-point discrimination, which should be 10 mm or better in the thumb for cutaneous control (Cu); otherwise ocular control (O) is required.

Table 1	
Muscle function according to British Research Council system	
Muscle Strength Grade	**Muscle Function**
M0	No active range of motion, no palpable muscle contraction
M1	No active range of motion, palpable muscle contraction only
M2	Reduced active range of motion—not against gravity, no muscle resistance
M3	Full active range of motion, no muscle resistance
M4	Full active range of motion, reduced muscle resistance
M5	Full active range of motion, normal muscle resistance

Table 2
International Classification of Surgery of the Hand in Tetraplegia

Group	Spinal Cord Segment	Possible Muscle Transfers	Possible Axon Sources for Nerve Transfers
0	≥C5	No transferable muscle below elbow	Musculocutaneous nerve branches to coracobrachialis and brachialis muscle
1	C5	Brachioradialis (BR)	Axillary nerve branches to deltoid and teres minor muscles
2	C6	+ Extensor carpi radialis longus (ECRL)	Radial nerve branches to supinator muscle
3	C6	+ Extensor carpi radialis brevis (ECRB)	
4	C6	+ Pronator teres (PT)	
5	C7	+ Flexor carpi radialis (FCR)	
6	C7	+ Extensor digitorum	
7	C7	+ Extensor pollicis longus	
8	C8	+ Flexor digitorum	Radial nerve branch to ECRB muscle
9	C8	No intrinsic hand muscles	
10 (X)		Exceptions	

Special aspects

Other aspects of neuromuscular examination include brachial plexus lesions and entrapment neuropathies, paralytic spine deformity, thoracoscapular stability, spasticity, contractures, stiffness, and instability of joints.[17–20] Pain and swelling are relative contraindications to surgery and need to be treated before reconstruction.

PLANNING OF RECONSTRUCTION

The main goals are reconstruction of elbow extension, grip function (flexion phase), and opening of the hand (extension phase). The most frequently used procedures to achieve patients' ability goals and an algorithm for surgical reconstruction based on International Classification (IC) are presented in **Tables 3** and **4**, respectively.

Reconstruction of Elbow Extension

Elbow extension is critical for overhead activities, weight shifting, and transfers, and greatly increases wheelchair propulsion and the workspace of the hand in space by 800%.[21–25] Elbow reconstruction should precede grip reconstruction because

- use of a hand that cannot reach out in space is very limited,
- elbow extension helps to stabilize the patient's trunk in the wheelchair,
- stability itself is a factor for more controlled use of the hand, and
- function of distal tendon transfers is improved, for example, brachioradialis (BR) muscle function (as a donor) requires a counteracting and stabilizing action from its antagonist, that is, elbow extension.

Two surgical procedures are advocated to restore active elbow extension:

1. Posterior deltoid-to-triceps transfer (**Fig. 1**)
2. Biceps-to-triceps transfer.

Table 3
Summary of possible surgical procedures (excluding nerve transfers) to achieve patients' ability goals

Ability Goal	Functional Goal	Procedure	Rehabilitation
Stabilizing elbow in space, reaching overhead objects, pushing wheelchair, stabilizing trunk	Elbow extension	Reconstruction of triceps function Posterior deltoid-triceps Biceps-triceps	 4-wk in cylinder cast with elbow fully extended 4-wk orthosis
Use of utensils, handwriting, pushing wheelchair	Grip	Reconstruction of grip Reconstruction of passive key grip BR-ECRB FPL-radius CMC I arthrodesis Reconstruction of active key grip BR-FPL CMC I arthrodesis Split FPL-EPL tenodesis	 4 wk with arm in cast with flexed thumb and wrist 4–10 wk active exercise 4 wk in orthosis with active key pinch but restriction of wrist extension
Reaching for objects, eg, cup or glass positioning of thumb and fingers for improved grasp control	Opening of the hand	Reconstruction of thumb and finger extensors Passive opening CMC I arthrodesis EPL to extensor retinaculum attachment Active opening PT-EDC and EPL/APL Reconstruction of intrinsics Zancolli-lasso tenodesis House tenodesis EDM-APB	 4 wk wrist and thumb in cast 4 wk wrist, fingers, and thumb in cast 4 wk of immobilization in intrinsic plus position. Thumb actively exercised 1st postoperative day

Abbreviations: APB, abductor pollicis brevis; APL, abductor pollicis longus; BR, brachioradialis; CMC, carpometacarpal; ECRB, extensor carpi radialis brevis; EDC, extensor digitorum communis; EDM, extensor digiti minimi; EPL, extensor pollicis longus; FPL, flexor pollicis longus; PT, pronator teres.

Posterior deltoid-to-triceps transfer reliably restores lost elbow extension in patients with C5/6 tetraplegia. Patient candidates for biceps-to-triceps transfer usually demonstrate intact and functional brachialis and supinator muscles, biceps spasticity, and elbow flexion contracture exceeding approximately 20°.[7,26] The result of reconstruction of elbow extension is generally very good, and provides the person with tetraplegia with improved arm control, useful in many daily activities (**Fig. 2**).

Reconstruction of Forearm Pronation

In patients affected by high-level tetraplegia (groups 0 and 1), impaired balance between functional forearm supinators and weakened or paralyzed pronators may produce supination contracture. Surgical options include:

a. Distal transposition of biceps tendon (rerouting), if necessary with interosseous membrane release[27]
b. Dorsal transposition of the BR during BR-to-flexor pollicis longus (FPL) transfer to achieve simultaneous thumb flexion and forearm pronation (**Fig. 3**)[28,29]
c. Derotation osteotomy of the radius.[27]

Reconstruction of Wrist Extension

Reconstruction of active wrist extension is of utmost importance because of the wrist-related tenodesis effect. If wrist extension is absent (IC groups 0 and 1), the BR (only IC group 1) can be transferred for wrist extension onto the extensor carpi radialis brevis (ECRB) to obtain a wrist extension without radial deviation (as if extensor carpi radialis longus [ECRL] is wrongly used).

Reconstruction of Grip Function

Tetraplegic patients usually have a spontaneous weak pinch between the thumb and index finger, depending on wrist extension/tenodesis grip. To produce a useful grip, preoperative planning must be based on patients' goals and wishes and thorough testing of muscle function, sensibility, and spasticity of the hand. In IC 2, the patient's active extension of the wrist depends only on the ECRL muscle; therefore, this muscle must not be used for a transfer in this group of patients. In IC 3 and higher, where active extension is supplied by both the ECRL and ECRB, the ECRL can be used for active transfers.[4]

Reconstruction of key pinch

Lateral pinch, termed key grip, is based on the fact that the hand opens by passive or active wrist flexion and closes by wrist extension, whereby the thumb pulp ideally should meet the radial side of the middle phalanx of index finger (**Fig. 4**). Prerequisites for passive key grip are wrist extension, minimum strength grade 3, forearm pronation, and acceptable relationship between thumb and index/long finger. Stabilizing procedures are split FPL–extensor pollicis longus (EPL), distal thumb tenodesis, and CMC I arthrodesis. Active key pinch is preferably achieved by BR-FPL tendon transfer (**Fig. 5**).[30,31]

Reconstruction of power grip: ECRL–flexor digitorum profundus (FDP) tendon transfer

Active whole-hand closure is powered by ECRL tendon transfer on the deep finger flexors 2 to 4, excluding the little finger, to prevent hyperflexion (**Fig. 6**).[32]

Reconstruction of Intrinsics

The purpose of interossei reconstruction is to secure MCP joint flexion. Key pinch can be achieved by positioning the index finger so that it is sufficiently flexed to meet the thumb, and also creating support by digits 3 to 5. Second, extension of the PIP joints is essential for grasp and release, and provides a more normal opening of the hand compared with reconstruction of extensor digitorum communis (EDC) function, giving an intrinsic minus type of opening. Passive interossei function of the fingers using passive tenodesis by tendon grafts in the lumbrical canals (house procedure) is shown in **Fig. 7**.[33] Restoration of palmar abduction of the thumb is illustrated in **Fig. 8**.

IC Group	Surgical Options	Alternatives
	Table 4 **Surgical algorithms according to International Classification (IC)**	
0	Abducted shoulder (AD transfer) Flexion contracture of the elbow (biceps tendon Z-tenotomy) Supinated but not contracted forearm (Zancolli: rerouting the biceps; check the presence of supinator muscle!) Fixed supination contracture (osteotomy of radius) Unstable or contracted wrist (wrist fusion)	
1	BR-to-ECRB for active wrist extension Split-thumb tenodesis Moberg's key pinch procedure	
2	BR-to-FPL for active key pinch Split-thumb tenodesis I. CMC fusion EPL tenodesis to the retinaculum	BR-to-FDP II–IV active grip Moberg's key pinch procedure Split-thumb tenodesis CMC I fusion EPL tenodesis to the retinaculum Zancolli-lasso procedure
3	BR-to-FPL ECRL-to-FDP II–IV Split-thumb tenodesis Zancolli-lasso or House intrinsic procedure CMC I fusion EPL tenodesis	BR-to-FDP II–IV Moberg's key pinch procedure Split-thumb tenodesis Zancolli-lasso or House intrinsic procedure CMC I fusion EPL tenodesis
4	BR-to-FPL ECRL-to-FDP II–IV Split-thumb tenodesis Zancolli-lasso or House intrinsic procedure CMC I fusion EPL tenodesis PT-to-FDS II–V (activated Zancolli lasso) or PT-to-FPL or PT transfer in extensor phase	
5	BR-to-FPL ECRL-to-FDP II–IV Split-thumb tenodesis Zancolli-lasso or House intrinsic procedure CMC I fusion EPL tenodesis PT-to-FDS II-V (activated Zancolli lasso) or PT transfer in extensor phase	PT-to-FPL ECRL-to-FDP II–IV Split-thumb tenodesis Zancolli-lasso or House intrinsic procedure BR-to-APB EPL tenodesis

(*continued on next page*)

Table 4 (continued)		
IC Group	**Surgical Options**	**Alternatives**
6	BR-to-FPL ECRL-to-FDP II–IV Split-thumb tenodesis Zancolli-lasso or House intrinsic procedure EDM-to-APB transfer EDC-to-EPL	PT-to-FPL ECRL-to-FDP II–IV Split-thumb tenodesis Zancolli-lasso or House intrinsic procedure BR-to-APB EDC-to-EPL ECU or FCU-to-FDS II–IV (activated Zancolli lasso)
7	BR-to-FPL ECRL-to-FDP II–IV Split-thumb tenodesis? Zancolli-lasso or House intrinsic procedure EDM-to-APB or EIP-to-APB or FCU-to-APB Activated Zancolli lasso (PT-to-FDS II–V)	PT-to-FPL BR-to-FDS II–IV ECRL-to-FDP II–IV Split-thumb tenodesis? Zancolli-lasso or House intrinsic procedure EDQ-to-APB or EIP-to-APB or FCU-to-APB or activated Zancolli lasso (BR-to-FDS II–V)
8	BR-to-FPL ECRB-activated APB Opponens plasty (EIP, EDM, FCU) Active Zancolli-lasso procedure (ECU) House intrinsic procedure	PT-to-FPL ECRB-activated APB Opponens plasty (EIP, EDM, FCU) Active Zancolli-lasso procedure (BR) House intrinsic procedure
9	Zancolli lasso House intrinsic procedure	
10	Pathologic postures (MP joints fixed in hyperextension, lack of any functioning intrinsic muscles, wrist fixed in either flexion or extension, etch) Release of contracted muscles, tendons, and joint capsules	

Abbreviations: APB, abductor pollicis brevis; APL, abductor pollicis longus; BR, brachioradialis; CMC, carpometacarpal; ECRB, extensor carpi radialis brevis; ECRL, extensor carpi radialis longus; ECU, extensor carpi ulnaris; EDC, extensor digitorum communis; EDM, extensor digiti minimi; EDQ, extensor digitorum quinti; EIP, extensor indicis proprius; EPL, extensor pollicis longus; FCU, flexor carpi ulnaris; FDP, flexor digitorum profundus; FDS, flexor digitorum superficialis; FPL, flexor pollicis longus; MP, metacarpophalangeal; PT, pronator teres.

Thumb palmar abduction can be restored by transferring extensor digiti minimi (EDM) to the insertion of abductor pollicis brevis (APB). For this reconstruction, M3 power of the EDM can be sufficient to increase the first web-space opening and to position the thumb along the radial index finger.[34]

Reconstruction of Hand Opening (Extensor Phase)

Reconstruction of hand opening is necessary to facilitate the ability to come around and grasp larger objects (eg, a bottle). Many tetraplegic patients do not have this ability because of "tenodesis grip," with adhesions of the finger flexors and insufficient stretching of the fingers even with good passive wrist flexion. Improvement of the opening of the hand is particularly necessary in patients with finger flexor spasticity

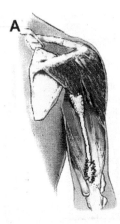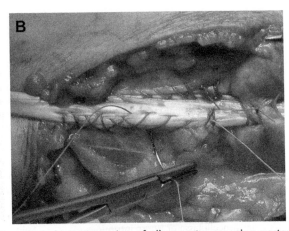

Fig. 1. Drawing demonstrating surgical reconstruction of elbow extensor using posterior deltoid to triceps via an interpositioning tibialis anterior tendon graft. (*A*) The posterior deltoid border is mobilized and the interval between middle and posterior deltoid identified. Care is taken to identify the posterior deltoid insertion that is subsequently detached along with the associated periosteum. A subcutaneous tunnel is created from the level of deltoid insertion to the distal triceps tendon via a dorsal incision to the level of olecranon. The distal deltoid tendon and the tendon graft are placed with an overlap of 5 cm and sutured to each other using 2/0 nonabsorbable running sutures along the sides of the graft and host tendons. (*B*) The distal graft insertion is created by threading the tendon graft through a hole made in the flat triceps tendon and sutured with overlap of 5 cm using 2/0 nonabsorbable running sutures up and down along both sides of the graft and host tendons.

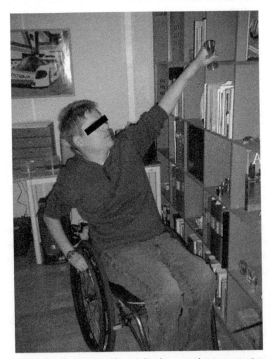

Fig. 2. Full elbow extension in overhead activity in a patient reconstructed with posterior deltoid to triceps 6 months earlier.

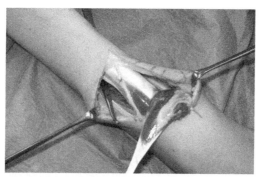

Fig. 3. Brachioradialis tendon is transferred dorsally and through the interosseous membrane (from dorsal to palmar muscle compartment) before being inserted into the flexor pollicis longus (FPL) tendon (not visible). Using this route, activation of the brachioradialis will power both thumb flexion and forearm pronation.

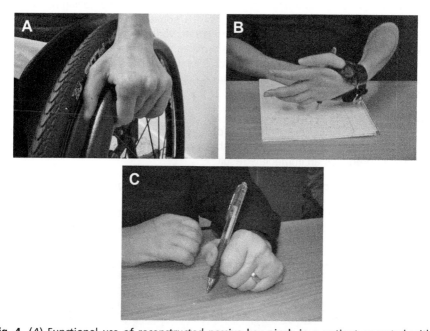

Fig. 4. (*A*) Functional use of reconstructed passive key pinch in a patient operated with strengthening of wrist extension by transfer of brachioradialis to extensor carpi radialis brevis (ECRB) and suturing of FPL into radius. By passively flexing the wrist the hand will open, and by actively extending the wrist (using brachioradialis) the thumb will flex and grasp the object (wheelchair driving ring) between thumb and index finger. By extending the wrist more, the magnitude of the key pinch is increased. (*B, C*) Hand function before and after reconstruction by transfer of brachioradialis (BR) to FPL and extensor carpi radialis longus (ECRL) to flexor digitorum profundus (FDP). A substantial improvement of hand control without need for a supporting brace is noted. These active transfers are combined with multiple tenodeses to optimize the position of the wrist, thumb, and fingers (described in detail under New Developments: Combined Procedures).

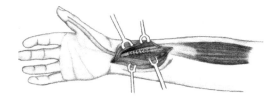

Fig. 5. Schematic representation of reconstruction of active key pinch by a BR to FPL tendon transfer.

whereby gravity or remaining finger extension strength cannot overpower the finger flexion spasticity.[35] This can be achieved by passive opening of the first commissure by EPL tenodesis to extensor retinaculum or forearm fascia (powered by active or passive wrist flexion), and active opening via tendon transfer by transferring pronator teres to EPL, abductor pollicis longus, and EDC (**Fig. 9**).

Additional Procedures in Spasticity

A common observation internationally in the past years is the increasing numbers of incomplete tetraplegics. These patients, with a somewhat new configuration and more complex functional loss, often demonstrate various degrees of spasticity and muscle-joint rearrangements.[36,37] Mild deformities primarily affect the PIP and distal interphalangeal (DIP) joints, whereas the MCP joints are usually spared; severe deformities may affect all finger joints. Certain surgical techniques have proved to be successful in additional spasticity[5]:

Littler release
In many cases, a partial resection of the oblique part of the extensor aponeurosis is enough; the insertion of the interossei on the proximal phalanx remains. The operation is rapid and produces an immediate result.[38]

Tendon lengthening of the extrinsic finger flexors (flexor digitorum superficialis [FDS]/FDP)
Tenotomies of the flexors are performed about 5 cm proximal to the carpal canal using a stair-step incision of 6 to 8 cm in length, which achieves a parallel sliding of both tendon stumps and subsequent prolongation of 2 to 3 cm.

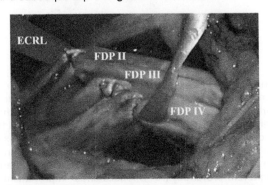

Fig. 6. Close-up of attachment sites for donor and recipient tendons. ECRL tendon is attached to FDP tendons II to IV to power finger flexion. To avoid small finger hyperflexion, FDP V is not included in this transfer.

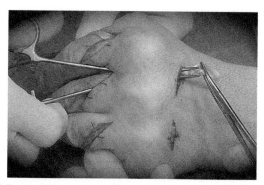

Fig. 7. A harvested flexor digitorum superficialis (FDS) tendon graft is brought through the lumbrical canal, that is, palmar to intermetacarpal ligaments and onto the extensor hood of the neighboring finger. This procedure secures flexion of the metacarpophalangeal and extension of the proximal interphalangeal joints. Two separate tendon loops are required to achieve this effect in digits II to V.

Additional procedures

In some cases other procedures may be required, such as release of muscle insertions, for example, of the adductor pollicis or pronator teres, or a teno-myotomy of the wrist flexors.

NEW DEVELOPMENTS
Combined Procedures: Active Flexor and Passive Extensor Phase with Intrinsic Reconstruction

Traditionally operations for flexors and extensors were separated, yet the authors have successfully combined procedures for active key pinch and finger flexion together with passive opening of hand as a one-stage operation. This reconstruction includes 7 individual operations performed in the following order: (1) split FPL-EPL distal thumb tenodesis, (2) reconstruction of passive interossei, (3) thumb CMC arthrodesis, (4) BR-FPL tendon transfer, (5) ECRL-FDP tendon transfer, (6) EPL tenodesis, and (7) extensor carpi

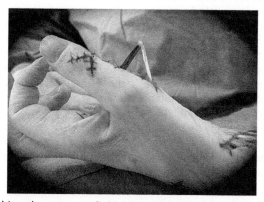

Fig. 8. After detaching the extensor digiti minimi (EDM) tendon from its insertion on the dorsum of small finger and tunneling it through the interosseous membrane, a straight line is secured through the interosseus membrane. The EDM tendon is then inserted into the abductor pollicis brevis muscle, and active palmar abduction of the thumb can be achieved.

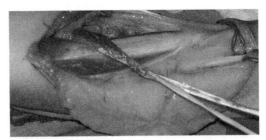

Fig. 9. Reconstruction of active finger extensors and thumb extensor using pronator teres as donor muscle. Tendon grafts are sutured to pronator teres before attaching it to the recipient tendons of thumb and finger extensors.

ulnaris (ECU) tenodesis. This reconstruction is termed the Alphabet or ABCDEFG procedure (Advanced Balanced Combined Digital Extensor Flexor Grip reconstruction) **(Table 5)**. To reduce the risk of adhesions after this extensive surgery and to facilitate relearning, the activation of transferred muscles with new functions requires early active postoperative training. One-stage reconstruction can reliably provide grip, grasp, and release function in persons with C6 tetraplegia. Patient compliance and satisfaction are high. Overall, this simultaneous reconstruction saves time and limits the need for immobilization; moreover, effort for patients and caregivers is less in comparison with the standard two-stage reconstructions. Incidence of complications is comparable with other published treatment modalities.[35]

Immediate Activation of Tendon Transfers

The most remarkable and effective strategy to improve function has been the consistent and immediate activation of transferred muscle after surgery. Early active training of new motors not only prevents the formation of adhesions but also facilitates the voluntary recruitment of motors powering new functions before swelling and immobilization-induced stiffness restrain muscle contractions. In addition, the patient will experience an early, spectacular, and inspiring effect of the reconstruction, which will help motivate training during the demanding and sometimes painful initial postoperative period. Early activation of the transferred muscles requires reliable tendon-to-tendon attachments. The authors have accumulated experience of hundreds of side-to-side attachments using running sutures back and forth along both sides and with a minimum of 5-cm overlap (see **Fig. 1**B).[39] This technique has proved to be extremely safe for allowing early active training and is now standard in our unit.[5,34,35] Tendon force measurements confirmed the assertion that the elbow joint need not be immobilized when the BR is used as a donor muscle in tendon transfer to the FPL, as the maximum passive tendon tension was only about 20 N in the authors' cadaveric model and the failure strength of this specific repair was more than 200 N.[40] The authors suggest that it is possible to consider performing multiple tendon transfers in a single stage, avoiding the adverse effect of immobilization. In brief, the day after surgery a removable splint replaces the cast and intermittent exercises commence **(Fig. 10)**. Training focuses on activating the donor muscles with slight external resistance.

Nerve Transfers

Additional reconstructive options could be achieved by nerve transfers, that is, extra-anatomic short-circuit between expendable donor nerve fascicles from above the SCI and the motor branch of a paralyzed muscle underneath. Nerve transfers have been established in recent years, especially in brachial plexus lesions, but rarely applied

Table 5
Advanced Balancing Combined Digital Extension Flexion Grip (ABCDEFG) Reconstruction

Order	Procedure	Type	Motor	Function	Effect
1	Split FPL-to-EPL	Tenodesis	Active[a]	Stabilize IP joint	Prevent hyperflexion of IP, Increase contact surface to index
2	Free tendon transplant (FDS IV) → extensor hood digits 2–3 and 4–5	Tenodesis	Passive[b]	Interossei[c]	Opening hand
3	CMC I	Arthrodesis	N/A	Fuse basis of the thumb and correct deformity	Secure thumb's approach against index during key pinch
4	BR-to-FPL	Tendon transfer	Active	Thumb flexion	Key pinch
5	ECRL-to-FDP II–IV	Tendon transfer	Active	Finger flexion	Power grasp
6	EPL-to-dorsal forearm fascia	Tenodesis	Passive[b]	Extend thumb	Opening hand
7	ECU-to-ulnar head	Tenodesis	Passive	Prevent radial deviation of wrist	Balance hand position at all types of grips

Abbreviations: APL, abductor pollicis longus; BR, brachioradialis; CMC, carpometacarpal; ECRL, extensor carpi radialis longus; ECU, extensor carpi ulnaris; EPL, extensor pollicis longus; FDS, flexor digitorum superficialis; FPL, flexor pollicis longus; (P)IP, (proximal) interphalangeal; MCP, metacarpophalangeal; N/A, not available.
[a] Powered by BR transferred to FPL.
[b] Powered by wrist flexion.
[c] Flexion of MCP and extension of PIP.

in tetraplegia. Ideally, nerve transfer means the coaptation of an expendable pure motor axon donor with the recipient branch over the shortest possible distance.[41] Theoretically, suitable donor nerves include

- axillary nerve (C5/6) branches to the posterior deltoid and teres minor to restore elbow extension,[42–45]
- radial nerve branches to the supinator (C6) or ECRB (C7)[46,47] for thumb or finger extension,
- musculocutaneous nerve branches to coracobrachialis or brachialis muscle,[42,43,48] and
- superficial radial nerve (C6) or lateral antebrachii cutaneous nerve (C5/6) for sensory restoration of the median nerve (first web space) in patients categorized as 0 (ocular control).[49]

Theoretically, nerve transfers in SCI may even be more effective in comparison with peripheral nerve injury because:

1. Recipient muscles with intact lower motoneuron preserve reflex arcs and do not become refractory to reinnervation/external stimulation after 18 to 24 months as after peripheral palsy

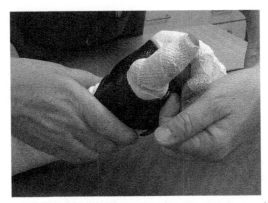

Fig. 10. Active training on the first postoperative day. Carpometacarpal arthrodesis of the thumb is protected with a splint, and the therapist stabilizes the wrist to prevent tenodesis-driven finger and thumb flexion. Photo shows active finger flexion powered by ECRL performed against light resistance applied by therapist.

2. Axon transfer to the intact donor nerve may allow highly selective neurotization by intraoperative fascicle stimulation of the intact recipient nerve
3. This may minimize the distance between donor and recipient and regeneration time.[43,44]

Advantages, when compared with peripheral nerve lesions, would be that in SCI both the donor and recipient nerves are intact and that the most appropriate fascicles could be precisely determined by intraoperative nerve stimulation.[1] If the lower motoneuron and spinal reflexes are intact, degeneration of the motor endplates will not occur and reinnervation remains theoretically for years by both external (FES) and internal (nerve transposition) stimulation. It is still unclear as to whether such a neural reconstruction is possible even years later or should be done as early as possible, that is, 3 to 6 months after SCI.[50] Furthermore, natural biomechanics of the extremity, force, and excursion of the original muscle are preserved and scar-induced motion restrictions are avoided without the need for extended periods of immobilization, a primary reason why appropriate candidates refuse muscle transfers. Axon transfers

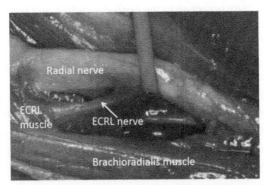

Fig. 11. Radial nerve and its motor branch to the ECRL muscle are exposed. Neurotization is obtained by transferring functioning musculocutaneous motor branch to brachialis muscle as donor to recipient ECRL motor nerve.

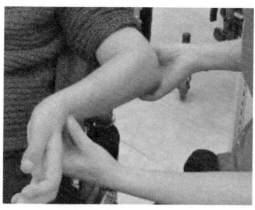

Fig. 12. Functional result 3 months after transfer of brachialis motor nerve into ECRL motor nerve. Patient can extend wrist unloaded (arm supported by assistant).

may even provide options for patients not amenable to conventional tendon transfers, including IC group 0.[1,43,44] Thus far, the authors have used the brachialis-to-ECRL selective transfer (BEST) procedure (**Fig. 11**) in 4 cases who all achieved muscular reinnervation, ranging from early palpable contraction to active wrist extension in a patient with complete paralysis below elbow level preoperatively (group 0) (**Fig. 12**).

Central plasticity may even enable independent activation of multiple target muscles by the same axons that originally controlled only a single function.[51] Nerve transfer may be a promising option to improve key muscle functions and sensory protection after SCI, especially in groups with very limited resources (such as IC groups 0–3). Further research should be directed at combining traditional algorithms with these new approaches.

ACKNOWLEDGMENTS

Multiple studies of tendon transfer biomechanics form the theoretical basis for several procedures presented in this paper. Several of these studies have been undertaken in Professor Richard L. Lieber's laboratory at the Department of Orthopaedic Surgery, UCSD, San Diego. The authors are indebted to Professor Lieber for his generous support and outstanding collaboration.

REFERENCES

1. Brown JM. Nerve transfers in tetraplegia I: background and technique. Surg Neurol Int 2011;2:121.
2. Moberg E. Surgical treatment for absent single-hand grip and elbow extension in quadriplegia. J Bone Joint Surg Am 1975;57(2):196–206.
3. Moberg E. The upper limb in tetraplegia. A new approach to surgical rehabilitation. Stuttgart: Thieme; 1978.
4. Hentz VR, Leclerq C. Surgical rehabilitation of the upper limb in tetraplegia. London: WB Saunders; 2002.
5. Fridén J, Reinholdt C. Current concepts in reconstruction of hand function in tetraplegia. Scand J Surg 2008;97(4):341–6.

6. Anderson KD, Fridén J, Lieber RL. Acceptable benefits and risks associated with surgically improving arm function in individuals living with cervical spinal cord injury. Spinal Cord 2009;47(4):334–8.
7. Fridén J. Reconstruction of elbow extension in tetraplegia. In: Fridén J, editor. Tendon transfers in reconstructive hand surgery. Oxford (UK): Taylor & Francis; 2005. p. 91–102.
8. Gohritz A, Fridén J, Herold C, et al. Tendon transposition to restore muscle function in the hand. Unfallchirurg 2007;110(9):759–76 [in German].
9. Ejeskär A. Reconstruction of grip function in tetraplegia. In: Fridén J, editor. Tendon transfers in reconstructive hand surgery. Oxford (UK): Taylor & Francis; 2005. p. 103–20.
10. Gohritz A, Fridén J, Spies M, et al. Nerve and muscle transfer surgery to restore paralyzed elbow function. Unfallchirurg 2008;111(2):85–101 [in German].
11. Hamou C, Shah NR, Di Ponio L, et al. Pinch and elbow extension restoration in people with tetraplegia: a systematic review of the literature. J Hand Surg Am 2009;34(4):692–9.
12. Wangdell J, Fridén J. Satisfaction and performance in patient selected goals after grip reconstruction in tetraplegia. J Hand Surg Eur Vol 2010;35(7):563–8.
13. Wangdell J, Fridén J. Performance of prioritized activities is not correlated with functional factors after grip reconstruction in tetraplegia. J Rehabil Med 2011; 43(7):626–30.
14. McDowell CL, Moberg EA, House JH. The second International Conference on Surgical Rehabilitation of the Upper Limb in Tetraplegia (quadriplegia). J Hand Surg 1986;11A(4):604–8.
15. Lieber RL, Fridén J. Functional and clinical significance of muscle architecture. Muscle Nerve 2000;23(11):1647–66.
16. Fridén J, Lieber RL. Clinical significance of skeletal muscle architecture. Clin Orthop Relat Res 2001;383:140–51.
17. Landi A, Mulcahey MJ, Caserta G, et al. Tetraplegia: update on assessment. Hand Clin 2002;18(3):377–89.
18. Landi A. Update on tetraplegia. J Hand Surg 2003;28B(3):196–204.
19. Mulcahey MJ, Hutchinson D, Kozin S. Assessment of upper limb in tetraplegia: considerations in evaluation and outcomes research. J Rehabil Res Dev 2007; 44(1):91–102.
20. Zlotolow DA. The role of the upper extremity surgeon in the management of tetraplegia. J Hand Surg Am 2011;36(5):929–35.
21. Fridén J, Ejeskar A, Dahlgren A, et al. Protection of the deltoid–to-triceps tendon transfer repair sites. J Hand Surg Am 2000;25(1):144–9.
22. Fridén J. New concepts in reconstruction of arm and hand function in tetraplegia—basic research and clinical application. Handchir Mikrochir Plast Chir 2005;37(4):223–9 [in German].
23. Endress RD, Hentz VR. Biceps-to-triceps transfer technique. J Hand Surg Am 2011;36(4):716–21.
24. Turcsanyí I, Fridén J. Shortened rehabilitation period using a modified surgical technique for reconstruction of lost elbow extension in tetraplegia. Scand J Plast Reconstr Surg Hand Surg 2010;44(3):156–62.
25. Lamberg AS, Fridén J. Changes in skills required for using a manual wheelchair after reconstructive hand surgery in tetraplegia. J Rehabil Med 2011;43(8): 714–9.
26. Kozin SH, D'Addesi L, Chafetz RS, et al. Biceps-to-triceps transfer for elbow extension in persons with tetraplegia. J Hand Surg Am 2010;35(6):968–75.

27. Coulet B, Boretto JG, Allieu Y, et al. Pronating osteotomy of the radius for forearm supination contracture in high-level tetraplegic patients: technique and results. J Bone Joint Surg Br 2010;92(6):828–34.
28. Ward SR, Peace WJ, Fridén J, et al. Dorsal transfer of the brachioradialis to the flexor pollicis longus enables simultaneous powering of key pinch and forearm pronation. J Hand Surg Am 2006;31(6):993–7.
29. Fridén J, Reinholdt C, Gohritz A, et al. Simultaneous powering of forearm pronation and key pinch in tetraplegia using a single muscle-tendon unit. J Hand Surg Eur Vol 2011. [Epub ahead of print].
30. Ejeskär A, Dahlgren A, Fridén J. Split distal flexor pollicis longus tenodesis: long-term results. Scand J Plast Reconstr Surg Hand Surg 2002;36(2):96–9.
31. Fridén J, Albrecht D, Lieber RL. Biomechanical analysis of the brachioradialis as a donor in tendon transfer. Clin Orthop Relat Res 2001;383:152–61.
32. Ejeskär A, Dahlgren A, Fridén J. Clinical and radiographic evaluation of surgical reconstruction of finger flexion in tetraplegia. J Hand Surg Am 2005;30(4): 842–9.
33. McCarthy CK, House JH, Van Heest A, et al. Intrinsic balancing in reconstruction of the tetraplegic hand. J Hand Surg Am 1997;22(4):596–604.
34. Fridén J, Gohritz A, Reinholdt C, et al. Restoration of active palmar abduction of the thumb in tetraplegia by tendon transfer of the extensor digiti minimi to abductor pollicis brevis. J Hand Surg Eur Vol 2011. [Epub ahead of print].
35. Fridén J, Reinholdt C, Turcsányii I, et al. A single-stage operation for reconstruction of hand flexion, extension and intrinsic function in tetraplegia—the alphabet procedure. Tech Hand Up Extr Surg 2011;15:230–5.
36. Fridén J, Lieber R. Spastic muscle cells are shorter and stiffer than normal cells. Muscle Nerve 2003;27(2):157–64.
37. Lieber RL, Fridén J. Spasticity causes a fundamental rearrangement of muscle-joint interaction. Muscle Nerve 2002;25(2):265–70.
38. Reinholdt C, Fridén J. Selective release of the digital extensor hood to reduce intrinsic tightness in tetraplegia. J Plast Surg Hand Surg 2011;45(2):83–9.
39. Brown SH, Hentzen ER, Kwan A, et al. Mechanical strength of the side-to-side versus Pulvertaft weave tendon repair. J Hand Surg Am 2010;35(4):540–5.
40. Fridén J, Shillito MC, Chehab EF, et al. Mechanical feasibility of immediate mobilization of the brachioradialis muscle after tendon transfer. J Hand Surg Am 2010; 35(9):1473–8.
41. Gohritz A, Turcsányi I, Fridén J. Handchirurgie bei Rückenmarkverletzungen (Tetraplegie). In: Towfigh H, Hierner R, Langer M, et al, editors. Handchirurgie. Heidelberg (Germany): Springer; 2011. p. 1673–94.
42. Gohritz A, Vogt PM, Fridén J. Restoring function in tetraplegia using innovative methods from peripheral nerve injury [abstract 13]. In: Abstracts of the 10th International Meeting on Surgical Rehabilitation of the Tetraplegic Upper Limb. Paris, September 20–22, 2010. p. 27.
43. Gohritz A, Vogt PM, Fridén J. Innovative methods from peripheral nerve surgery to improve upper extremity function in tetraplegia—literature review and anatomical feasibility. 11th Congress of the International Federation of Surgery of the Hand. Seoul, October 31–November 4, 2011.
44. Bertelli JA, Tacca CP, Winkelmann Duarte EC, et al. Transfer of axillary nerve branches to reconstruct elbow extension in tetraplegics: a laboratory investigation of surgical feasibility. Microsurgery 2011;31(5):376–81.
45. Bertelli JA, Ghizoni MF, Tacca CP. Transfer of the teres minor motor branch for triceps reinnervation in tetraplegia. J Neurosurg 2011;114(5):1457–60.

46. Bertelli JA, Tacca CP, Ghizoni MF, et al. Transfer of supinator motor branches to the posterior interosseous nerve to reconstruct thumb and finger extension in tetraplegia: case report. J Hand Surg Am 2010;35(10):1647–51.
47. Krasuski M, Kiwerski J. An analysis of the results of transferring the musculocutaneous nerve onto the median nerve in tetraplegics. Arch Orthop Trauma Surg 1991;111(1):32–3.
48. Bertelli JA, Mendes Lehm VL, Tacca CP, et al. Transfer of the distal terminal motor branch of the extensor carpi radialis brevis to the nerve of the flexor pollicis longus. An anatomical study and clinical application in a tetraplegic patient. Neurosurgery 2011. [Epub ahead of print].
49. Brown JM, Mackinnon SE. Nerve transfers in the forearm and hand. Hand Clin 2008;24(4):319–40.
50. Coulet B, Allieu Y, Chammas M. Injured metamere and functional surgery of the tetraplegic upper limb. Hand Clin 2002;18(3):399–412, 6.
51. Anastakis DJ, Malessy MJ, Chen R, et al. Cortical plasticity following nerve transfer in the upper extremity. Hand Clin 2008;24(4):425–44.

The Effects of Active and Passive Stretching on Muscle Length

Danny A. Riley, PhD*, J.M. Van Dyke, PhD

KEYWORDS

- Active stretching • Passive stretching • Muscle length

Skeletal muscle properties are dynamic and reflect the history of use over the past few days to weeks. The 4 major properties that determine the functional capacity are contractile strength, structural strength, endurance, and fiber length. This article focuses on length regulation and the effects of stretching. Stretching is widely practiced in clinical medicine and athletic activities. Poor outcomes have led clinicians and athletes to question the value of stretching but not to abandon the practice.[1,2] Are there physiologic benefits to the muscle tissue? The desired outcomes of length regulation are improvements in the range of motion and performance and the reductions of stiffness and pain.

The International Fitness Association Web site describes 7 stretching techniques, but these techniques can be broadly categorized as either passive, in which the lengthened muscle does not contract, or active, in which the muscle contracts at some point during the procedure. Confusion about the expected outcomes of stretching has arisen in part because active stretch has been misinterpreted as passive stretch in joint immobilization animal studies.[3,4] The immobilized muscles contract isometrically in the awake animal.[5–8] In this model, the addition or loss of series sarcomeres altering muscle fiber length definitely occurs in the presence of activity. The assertion that passive stretch alone can change muscle length has not been demonstrated. In this article, the authors discuss evidence that passive tension regulates muscle stiffness and pain tolerance, and muscle fiber length is changed only when components of contractile activity, not yet delineated, are present.

This work was supported in part by research funding from the Department of Physical Medicine and Rehabilitation Education and Research Fund (DAR) and Wisconsin Space Grant Consortium Graduate Fellowships, including the Dr Laurel Salton Clark Memorial Graduate Fellowship (JMVD).

Department of Cell Biology, Neurobiology & Anatomy, Medical College of Wisconsin, 8701 Watertown Plank Road, Milwaukee, WI 53226, USA

* Corresponding author.

E-mail address: dariley@mcw.edu

Phys Med Rehabil Clin N Am 23 (2012) 51–57

doi:10.1016/j.pmr.2011.11.006

The ability to adjust fiber length (sarcomere number) to meet the demands for force output at an optimal length is one of muscle's greatest strengths. Under abnormal demands, this adaptability turns into a weakness, because muscle debilitation can occur secondarily to disease, aging, and inactivity.[9] For example, healthy astronauts in superb physical condition were launched for 6-month missions aboard the International Space Station. Comparison of the preflight and postflight biopsies of soleus muscles revealed that, even with daily exercise, significant atrophy of slow fibers occurred.[10,11] The deconditioning put the astronauts at risk for inadequate mobility during emergency egress and heightened vulnerability to eccentric muscle contraction injury upon return to Earth.[12] Skylab investigations had demonstrated that during the first week of spaceflight, astronauts transitioned from the normal one-gravity standing posture to a microgravity, fetal-like floating posture with persistent plantarflexion foot drop.[13,14] The chronic plantarflexion posture decreases the working range of soleus. In a 35-day bed rest study in which plantarflexion bias was also present, the altered posture caused the reduction of muscle fiber length.[15] Upon reloading, the soleus fibers are hyperstretched, and the force output is reduced because of less overlap of thick and thin filaments and atrophy in fiber diameter. In this example, the muscle was normal before the event, and the maladaptation occurred secondarily to altered use. Interventions are needed to instruct the muscle to stay pre-event adapted.

WHAT IS KNOWN ABOUT MUSCLE LENGTH ADAPTATION?

Growth in muscle fiber length in neonates is required to keep pace with the expanding skeleton. The total number of muscle fibers appears to be present at birth in people and rats. As the neonates increase biomechanical activity, the working muscles grow in diameter. During the same period, elongation of the skeleton necessitates that the attached muscles keep pace in length by adding series sarcomeres.[16] Bone elongation ceases after puberty, but the ability of muscle to adapt fiber length persists.[17,18] Maladaptation of muscle length is common in the elderly suffering reduced mobility and bad posture.[19,20]

IS CONTRACTILE ACTIVITY NECESSARY TO ADJUST MUSCLE LENGTH?

The force output of a muscle cell depends on overlap of contractile filaments so that myosin cross bridges can bind to actin, hydrolyze adenosine triphosphate (ATP), and exert force. The number of sarcomeres in series is regulated to set optimal fiber length (L_o), the length at which the maximum number of cross bridges is possible, within the operating range of the muscle. What signals set L_o, and how is the number of series sarcomeres regulated? The results of numerous animal studies of muscle adapting to short and long lengths are consistent with contractile activity being required. Contractile activity continues at 10% to 60% of normal in rat soleus muscles hypershortened following tenotomy (simulating tendon rupture) or when statically shortened or lengthened by immobilization.[21,22] Contradicting the requirement for activity is the finding that the addition of sarcomeres proceeds in denervated muscles.[16] Nerve transection immediately removes motor neuron impulses and silences the muscle fibers. However, denervated fibers within a day or two begin fibrillation contractions at 2 to 20 Hz.[23,24] Thus, denervated muscle fibers are contracting, and the stretch is active. When the hindlimb muscles are completely silenced by spinal cord transection, but not denervated (no fibrillation), tenotomy-induced loss of series sarcomeres does not occur.[25] One interpretation, and certainly not the only possibility, is that the depolarization events of endplate-generated contractions and fibrillations raise intracellular free calcium from the sarcoplasmic reticulum. A logical conclusion is that calcium-dependent signaling pathways are required to regulate series sarcomere number.[26-28]

There may be a direct relationship between the level of contractile activity and the rate of sarcomere turnover. Compared with the slow soleus in the rat, the fast muscles (tibialis anterior, extensor digitorum longus) exhibit much less change in length during immobilization.[29] The contractile activity of fast muscles in both normal and immobilized conditions is very low, about 3% of soleus activity, and remains so after tenotomy or immobilization.[22] The lower activity correlates with the small changes in sarcomere number in fast muscles, whereas the high activity of slow muscles is associated with large changes. Fast and slow muscles were concluded to sense identical immobilization stimuli differently, but the amount of contractile activity may be the explanation.[29] Fewer contractions mean less elevation of cytoplasmic calcium and weaker signaling. Other investigators favor contractile tension as the major factor regulating sarcomere number.[8,30] While active tension cannot be dismissed, denervated fibers regulate sarcomere number, and the tensions generated during fibrillations are extremely small. Studies in which tension output was dramatically reduced chemically, but the elevation of cytoplasmic calcium remained high, showed that signaling activation persisted.[31] Tension reduction needs to be tested for the effects on series sarcomere regulation. Eliminating all activity halts sarcomere breakdown, and increasing activity increases breakdown.[25,32] The authors recently reported that passive daily stretch in rats does not prevent the loss of sarcomeres in tenotomized soleus muscles, but stretch plus contractile activity is effective.[33] The failure of passive stretch to prevent sarcomere loss in animal models is consistent with the large number of studies in people reporting that passive stretch produces little or no increase in muscle length (extensibility) based on joint angle excursion after weeks of treatment.[34-38] Thus, stretch plus an aspect of contractile activity is necessary for inducing series sarcomere turnover.

Some passive stretch studies in people report growth in muscle length.[39,40] Perhaps, the lengthening elevated cytoplasmic calcium by opening stretch-activated calcium channels.[41,42] Passive stretch in vivo may not activate these mechanisms when the magnitude of muscle lengthening is limited by the physical range of joint movement and the onset of stretch pain. However, if the L_o of the target muscle had been maladapted to a shorter length, then the in vivo range of movement may be sufficient for activation of calcium channels. Two joint muscles, like the hamstrings, can be lengthened by flexing the hip and extending the knee joint at the same time to achieve greater percentage stretches beyond L_o than are possible for normal one-joint muscles. Stretch pain may still limit the percentage of lengthening. Fortunately, daily passive stretch can increase stretch pain tolerance and allow greater lengthening.[34,37,43] Another factor to consider when evaluating whether stretch can increase muscle length is the position of L_o in the operating range. In biceps brachii, L_o is near the middle range, whereas in soleus and the wrist flexors/extensors, L_o is close to the end of the range.[44] Thus, predicting the effects of passive stretch in vivo requires consideration of the existing L_o point and range of motion permitted physiologically as well as stretch pain tolerance.

WHAT DOES PASSIVE STRETCH DO AND NOT DO?

While most studies on people report that passive stretch does not increase the range of motion to a functionally beneficial level, a substantial body of work shows that it reduces muscle stiffness and the pain associated with a large excursion stretches.[34,37,38,43] It is well-documented that passive stretch produces a transient reduction in stiffness (viscoelastic stress relaxation) that persists for 1 to 2 hours before returning to prestretch levels.[45,46] Other human investigations report that daily passive stretch of only 15 to 60 seconds reduces muscle stiffness in a 24-hour persistent manner.[47] When daily stretch is stopped, stiffness returns at the rate of 2% to 3% per day similar to the rate the effect was generated.[19,48] In 1 study involving 3 weeks of unsupervised of daily passive stretching, there was no reduction in stiffness (torque per joint angle degree), while in another study in which the daily passive stretching was more intense, stiffness was significantly decreased.[43,49] The authors performed a preliminary study of passive stretch on 5 healthy young males that also demonstrated reduced stiffness. The hamstring muscles were stretched 1 minute per day for 10 consecutive days using a Biodex dynamometer (Biodex Medical Systems, Shirley, NY, USA) to rotate the knee joint from −90° to −10° flexion, with the hip joint flexed 20° using the Magnusson model.[50] Daily measurements of dynamic stiffness revealed a progressive reduction in stiffness (**Fig. 1**). Passive stretch must be performed daily, because reversion begins in 24 hours. These findings imply that stiffness is a continuously adapting property of skeletal muscles, adjusting day to day to the experienced range of motion.

DOES REMODELING OF THE CONNECTIVE TISSUE DECREASE STIFFNESS?

The regulation of series sarcomere number is accomplished by the muscle fiber. Sarcomere number and composition influence series stiffness, but the major passive element is the connective tissue. Short- and long-term reductions in muscle tissue stiffness are reasonable expectations of connective tissue alterations. The ubiquitous fibroblast can respond to tension and remodel the connective tissue proteolytically

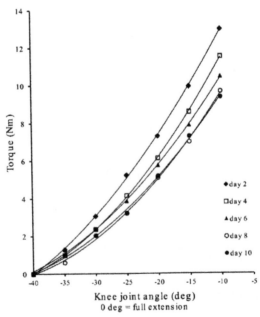

Fig. 1. Passive stretch of the hamstring muscles of normal young adults (1 min/d on 10 consecutive days) causes a progressive reduction in stiffness (ie, the torque required to passively rotate the knee joint to −10°). The stiffness curves (polynomial fit) are shown for days 2, 4, 6, 8, and 10.

and lower stiffness within a day.[51] In vitro, fibroblasts can change shape in minutes in response to tension by remodeling the cytoskeleton and lowering connective tissue stiffness.[52] Passive stretch of the human gastrocnemius generated extension of the connective tissue.[53] In muscle tissue, fibroblasts reside in the mysiums that enwrap muscle fibers, fascicles of muscle fibers and the whole muscle; tendons; the adventitia that encircle intramuscular blood vessels; and the neuriums that enwrap nerve fibers. Lengthening the muscle tissue stretches all of these connective tissue elements, with the fibroblast being the putative, common mechanoresponsive cell.[52]

SUMMARY

Clinical and animal research studies suggest that active stretch is required to increase muscle fiber length. Active stretch is effective, because cytoplasmic calcium is elevated during contractile activity. Passive stretch reduces stiffness and decreases stretch-induced pain. In normal subjects, the muscle stretching distance is limited in vivo by the joint range of motion. In abnormal hypershortened muscles, the degree of stretch permitted in vivo may be sufficient to raise intracellular calcium by turning on stretch-activated calcium channels. The effects of passive and active stretching vary within subjects depending on the position of L_o within the operating range of the target muscle. Stiffness is a continuously adapting property of skeletal muscles, adjusting day to day to the experienced range of motion.

REFERENCES

1. Katalinic OM, Harvey LA, Herbert RD. Effectiveness of stretch for the treatment and prevention of contractures in people with neurological conditions: a systematic review. Phys Ther 2011;91:11–24.
2. McHugh MP, Cosgrave CH. To stretch or not to stretch: the role of stretching in injury prevention and performance. Scand J Med Sci Sports 2010;20:169–81.
3. Goldspink DF. The influence of immobilization and stretch on protein turnover of rat skeletal muscle. J Physiol 1977;264:267–82.
4. Gomes AR, Cornachione A, Salvini TF, et al. Morphological effects of two protocols of passive stretch over the immobilized rat soleus muscle. J Anat 2007; 210:328–35.
5. Baewer DV, Hoffman M, Romatowski JG, et al. Passive stretch inhibits central corelike lesion formation in the soleus muscles of hindlimb-suspended unloaded rats. J Appl Physiol 2004;97:930–4.
6. Baewer DV, van Dyke JM, Bain JL, et al. Stretch reduces central core lesions and calcium build-up in tenotomized soleus. Muscle Nerve 2008;38:1563–71.
7. Giroux-Metges MA, Pennec JP, Petit J, et al. Effects of immobilizing a single muscle on the morphology and the activation of its muscle fibers. Exp Neurol 2005;194:495–505.
8. Williams PE, Goldspink G. Changes in sarcomere length and physiological properties in immobilized muscle. J Anat 1978;127:459–68.
9. Evans WJ, Paolisso G, Abbatecola AM, et al. Frailty and muscle metabolism dysregulation in the elderly. Biogerontology 2010;11:527–36.
10. Fitts RH, Trappe SW, Costill DL, et al. Prolonged space flight-induced alterations in the structure and function of human skeletal muscle fibres. J Physiol 2010;588: 3567–92.
11. Trappe S, Costill D, Gallagher P, et al. Exercise in space: human skeletal muscle after 6 months aboard the International Space Station. J Appl Physiol 2009;106: 1159–68.

12. Riley DA, Bain JL, Thompson JL, et al. Decreased thin filament density and length in human atrophic soleus muscle fibers after spaceflight. J Appl Physiol 2000;88: 567–72.

13. Clement G, Lestienne F. Adaptive modifications of postural attitude in conditions of weightlessness. Exp Brain Res 1988;72:381–9.

14. Tengwall R, Jackson J, Kimura T, et al. Human posture in zero gravity. Curr Anthropol 1982;23:657–66.

15. de Boer MD, Seynnes OR, di Prampero PE, et al. Effect of 5 weeks horizontal bed rest on human muscle thickness and architecture of weight bearing and nonweight-bearing muscles. Eur J Appl Physiol 2008;104:401–7.

16. Williams PE, Goldspink G. The effect of denervation and dystrophy on the adaptation of sarcomere number to the functional length of the muscle in young and adult mice. J Anat 1976;122:455–65.

17. Boakes JL, Foran J, Ward SR, et al. Muscle adaptation by serial sarcomere addition 1 year after femoral lengthening. Clin Orthop Relat Res 2007;456:250–3.

18. Lynn R, Morgan DL. Decline running produces more sarcomeres in rat vastus intermedius muscle fibers than does incline running. J Appl Physiol 1994;77: 1439–44.

19. Feland JB, Myrer JW, Schulthies SS, et al. The effect of duration of stretching of the hamstring muscle group for increasing range of motion in people aged 65 years or older. Phys Ther 2001;81:1110–7.

20. Light KE, Nuzik S, Personius W, et al. Low-load prolonged stretch vs. high-load brief stretch in treating knee contractures. Phys Ther 1984;64:330–3.

21. Elder GC, Toner LV. Muscle shortening induced by tenotomy does not reduce activity levels in rat soleus. J Physiol 1998;512:251–65.

22. Hnik P, Vejsada R, Goldspink DF, et al. Quantitative evaluation of electromyogram activity in rat extensor and flexor muscles immobilized at different lengths. Exp Neurol 1985;88:515–28.

23. Heaton JT, Kobler JB. Use of muscle fibrillation for tracking nerve regeneration. Muscle Nerve 2005;31:235–41.

24. Salafsky B, Bell J, Prewitt MA. Development of fibrillation potentials in denervated fast and slow skeletal muscle. Am J Physiol 1968;215:637–43.

25. Karpati G, Carpenter S, Eisen AA. Experimental core-like lesions and nemaline rods. A correlative morphological and physiological study. Arch Neurol 1972; 27:237–51.

26. Chin ER. Role of Ca^{2+}/calmodulin-dependent kinases in skeletal muscle plasticity. J Appl Physiol 2005;99:414–23.

27. Coffey VG, Hawley JA. The molecular bases of training adaptation. Sports Med 2007;37:737–63.

28. Koulmann N, Bigard AX. Interaction between signalling pathways involved in skeletal muscle responses to endurance exercise. Pflugers Arch 2006;452: 125–39.

29. Spector SA, Simard CP, Fournier M, et al. Architectural alterations of rat hind-limb skeletal muscles immobilized at different lengths. Exp Neurol 1982;76:94–110.

30. Herring SW, Grimm AF, Grimm BR. Regulation of sarcomere number in skeletal muscle: a comparison of hypotheses. Muscle Nerve 1984;7:161–73.

31. Dentel JN, Blanchard SG, Ankrapp DP, et al. Inhibition of cross-bridge formation has no effect on contraction-associated phosphorylation of p38 MAPK in mouse skeletal muscle. Am J Physiol Cell Physiol 2005;288:C824–30.

32. McMinn RM, Vrbova G. Motoneurone activity as a cause of degeneration in the soleus muscle of the rabbit. Q J Exp Physiol Cogn Med Sci 1967;52:411–5.

33. Van Dyke JM, Bain JLW, Riley DA. Preserving sarcomere number after tenotomy requires stretch and contraction. Muscle Nerve 2011. DOI: 10.1002/mus.22286.
34. Ben M, Harvey LA. Regular stretch does not increase muscle extensibility: a randomized controlled trial. Scand J Med Sci Sports 2010;20:136–44.
35. Halbertsma JP, van Bolhuis SI, Goeken LN. Sport stretching: effect on passive muscle stiffness of short hamstrings. Arch Phys Med Rehabil 1996;77:688–92.
36. Higgs F, Winter SL. The effect of a four-week proprioceptive neuromuscular facilitation stretching program on isokinetic torque production. J Strength Cond Res 2009;23:1442–7.
37. Law RY, Harvey LA, Nicholas MK, et al. Stretch exercises increase tolerance to stretch in patients with chronic musculoskeletal pain: a randomized controlled trial. Phys Ther 2009;89:1016–26.
38. Weppler CH, Magnusson SP. Increasing muscle extensibility: a matter of increasing length or modifying sensation? Phys Ther 2010;90:438–49.
39. Gajdosik RL. Effects of static stretching on the maximal length and resistance to passive stretch of short hamstring muscles. J Orthop Sports Phys Ther 1991;14:250–5.
40. Reid DA, McNair PJ. Passive force, angle, and stiffness changes after stretching of hamstring muscles. Med Sci Sports Exerc 2004;36:1944–8.
41. Armstrong RB, Duan C, Delp MD, et al. Elevations in rat soleus muscle [Ca2+] with passive stretch. J Appl Physiol 1993;74:2990–7.
42. Snowdowne KW. The effect of stretch on sarcoplasmic free calcium of frog skeletal muscle at rest. Biochim Biophys Acta 1986;862:441–4.
43. Magnusson SP, Simonsen EB, Aagaard P, et al. A mechanism for altered flexibility in human skeletal muscle. J Physiol 1996;497:291–8.
44. Lieber RL, Friden J. Musculoskeletal balance of the human wrist elucidated using intraoperative laser diffraction. J Electromyogr Kinesiol 1998;8:93–100.
45. Magnusson SP, Simonsen EB, Aagaard P, et al. Biomechanical responses to repeated stretches in human hamstring muscle in vivo. Am J Sports Med 1996;24:622–8.
46. Ryan ED, Beck TW, Herda TJ, et al. The time course of musculotendinous stiffness responses following different durations of passive stretching. J Orthop Sports Phys Ther 2008;38:632–9.
47. Bandy WD, Irion JM, Briggler M. The effect of static stretch and dynamic range of motion training on the flexibility of the hamstring muscles. J Orthop Sports Phys Ther 1998;27:295–300.
48. Willy RW, Kyle BA, Moore SA, et al. Effect of cessation and resumption of static hamstring muscle stretching on joint range of motion. J Orthop Sports Phys Ther 2001;31:138–44.
49. Guissard N, Duchateau J. Effect of static stretch training on neural and mechanical properties of the human plantar–flexor muscles. Muscle Nerve 2004;29:248–55.
50. Magnusson SP. Passive properties of human skeletal muscle during stretch maneuvers. A review. Scand J Med Sci Sports 1998;8:65–77.
51. van Griensven M, Zeichen J, Skutek M, et al. Cyclic mechanical strain induces NO production in human patellar tendon fibroblasts—a possible role for remodelling and pathological transformation. Exp Toxicol Pathol 2003;54:335–8.
52. Langevin HM, Bouffard NA, Fox JR, et al. Fibroblast cytoskeletal remodeling contributes to connective tissue tension. J Cell Physiol 2011;226:1166–75.
53. Morse CI, Degens H, Seynnes OR, et al. The acute effect of stretching on the passive stiffness of the human gastrocnemius muscle tendon unit. J Physiol 2008;586:97–106.

Hypohomocysteinemia: A Potentially Treatable Cause of Peripheral Neuropathology?

Clark E. Cullen, MD[a,b], Gregory T. Carter, MD, MS[c,*],
Michael D. Weiss, MD[d], Peter A. Grant, MD[e],
David Scott Saperstein, MD[f]

KEYWORDS

- Neuromuscular disease • Peripheral neuropathy
- Homocysteine deficiency • Hypohomocysteinemia • Nutrition
- Folate

Homocysteine is a homologue of the amino acid cysteine, differing by an additional methylene ($-CH_2-$) group. It is synthesized from methionine by the removal of its terminal $C\varepsilon$ methyl group.[1] Homocysteine can be converted into cysteine or recycled into methionine, via pathways that are facilitated by B vitamins. Detection of abnormal levels of homocysteine has been linked to cardiovascular disease and inflammatory bowel disease.[2–10] Homocysteine-lowering interventions in people with or without preexisting cardiovascular disease does not reduce the risk of nonfatal or fatal myocardial infarction or stroke.[11] Elevated plasma homocysteine levels are associated with an increased risk of atherosclerosis and thrombosis, as well as a variety of other pathologies such as birth defects, Alzheimer disease and other dementias, osteoporosis, diabetes, and renal disease.[12]

Homocysteine metabolism is catalyzed by several enzymes that require B vitamins as cofactors, and homocysteine levels are particularly responsive to folate status. The predictive power of plasma homocysteine level as a risk factor for atherothrombotic

[a] Sunstone Medical Research, LLC 1904 East Barnett Road, Medford, OR 97504, USA
[b] PO Box 756, Ashland, OR 97520, USA
[c] Muscular Dystrophy Association, Regional Neuromuscular Center, 410 Providence Lane, Building 2, Olympia, WA 98506, USA
[d] Division and Electrodiagnostic Laboratory, Department of Neurology, University Washington Medical Center, 1959 North East Pacific Street, Box 356115, Seattle, WA 98195, USA
[e] 473 Murphy Road, Medford, OR 97504, USA
[f] Phoenix Neurological Associates Ltd, 5090 North 40th Street, Suite 250, Phoenix, AZ 85018, USA
* Corresponding author.
E-mail address: gtcarter@uw.edu

Phys Med Rehabil Clin N Am 23 (2012) 59–65
doi:10.1016/j.pmr.2011.11.001
1047-9651/12/$ – see front matter © 2012 Elsevier Inc. All rights reserved.

disorders raised the appealing hypothesis that reduction of homocysteine levels by vitamin supplementation might result in a commensurate reduction in the risk of atherothrombotic events.[12,13] Unfortunately, most clinical trials failed to show a significant benefit of vitamin supplementation on cardiovascular events, despite significant lowering of plasma homocysteine levels.[13] Thus it is not clear whether homocysteine actually plays a causal role in many pathologies with which it is associated, or whether it is instead a marker for some other underlying mechanism. A large body of data links hyperhomocysteinemia and folate status with oxidant stress.[14–18]

Homocysteine is synthesized from dietary methionine and cannot be obtained directly from the diet. Plasma homocysteine concentration is actually inversely related to intake and plasma levels of folate, vitamin B6, and vitamin B12.[14] Homocysteine metabolism is important for two crucial biochemical pathways: remethylation, which is the focus of this article, and transsulfuration.[14] Transsulfuration, the vitamin B6–dependent sulfuration of homocysteine to cysteine, requires pyridoxal-5′-phosphate, the vitamin B6 coenzyme. Remethylation requires folic acid and vitamin B12 coenzymes, and involves the methylation and recycling of homocysteine to methionine, then to the eventual formation of S-adenosylmethionine (SAMe). SAMe is a major donor of methyl groups for reactions involving methyltransferases throughout the body, and the principal donor in the brain.[16,17] The methylation of homocysteine to methionine is accomplished by methionine synthase, a B12-dependent enzyme that uses 5-methylfolate, an essential cofactor, as the methyl donor. 5-Methylfolate is formed from folic acid through a series of steps with methylenetetrahydrofolate reductase (MTHFR), the enzyme at the rate-limiting step.[19–21] Two common mutations of the MTHFR gene sequence (A128C and C677T) occur in 10% to 20% of the United States population, and are the most common of the known inborn errors of metabolism.[20] Elevated homocysteine is considered a marker for the magnitude of dysfunction at this step (**Fig. 1**).

Deficiencies of vitamin B12 or folic acid, or abnormalities caused by mutations in these and other enzymes in this metabolic sequence, result in derangements of this process and are associated with peripheral neuropathy (PN) as well as with various other central nervous system (CNS) disorders including depression and dementia.[4,5] Treatment of vitamin B12 or folic acid deficiency with replacement may result in improvement or resolution of the neuropathic process. Often homocysteine levels are elevated in these deranged states and, again, elevation of homocysteine has been considered important evidence for the presence of metabolic derangement.

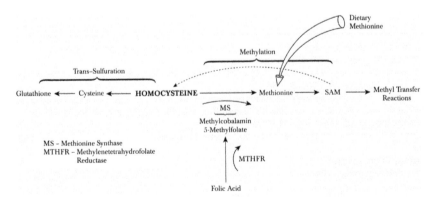

Fig. 1. Metabolic pathways of homocysteine. Note the irreversible transsulfuration pathway. SAM, S-adenosylmethionine.

Because homocysteine is continuously replenished via dietary methionine, the overall level in the blood must be determined by processes other than the ongoing recycling of these two amino acids alone. These other processes determine the ultimate catabolic fate of dietary methionine, in which the transsulfuration pathway could play a significant role. In humans, however, data suggest that it is difficult to assess any dose-response curve in terms of vitamin replacement.[21–23] For example, a daily dose of 25 mg of vitamin B6 taken orally for 10 days reduces plasma folate but does not affect basal and postprandial homocysteine levels. This fact suggests the existence of either normal cellular folate availability or possibly increased transsulfuration to compensate for impaired homocysteine remethylation.

Further complicating the picture is a theorized metabolic methylfolate trap, hypothesizing that 5-methyltetrahydrofolate (5MTHF) becomes metabolically trapped.[24] This trap arises because 5MTHF can neither be metabolized via the methionine synthase pathway nor reconverted to its precursor, methylenetetrahydrofolate (see **Fig. 1**). Other manifestations of the methylfolate trap include cellular folate loss resulting from reduced overall methylation. One report noted that global DNA methylation was 22% lower in a patient with vitamin B12 deficiency who was homozygous for the (MTHFR) C677T mutation.[24]

CLINICAL RAMIFICATIONS
Case Study

Reduced levels of homocysteine, or hypohomocysteinemia (HH), resulting from variations in the aforementioned pathways, may represent a pathologic state not previously elucidated. This state would result in consequences similar to those of other derangements of the single carbon cycle, through diminished levels of SAMe and reduced methylation capacity. This scenario is clinically relevant, as it raises the possibility that a neuropathy secondary to or associated with HH is pathologically possible and is potentially treatable by dietary methionine supplementation.

To illustrate this, the clinical course of a 75-year-old woman with an idiopathic peripheral neuropathy (IPN) and HH who responded to oral methionine treatment is presented. The patient presented several years previously with complaints of burning, tingling, and numbness in her feet. In addition she also noted cramping in her lower extremities, and a feeling that her "legs were like dead." There were no complaints of dysautonomia. She was otherwise in good overall health, with no history of diabetes or other neuroendocrine or metabolic disorders. On initial examination she appeared well-nourished but demonstrated atrophic shiny skin. On neurologic examination, her cranial nerves were normal. On motor examination, her muscle bulk and tone were relatively preserved, although she had absent deep tendon reflexes. She also showed significant muscle weakness, more than expected for the degree of atrophy. She exhibited symmetric mild distal predominant weakness in the upper and lower extremities. Her laboratory workup revealed a homocysteine level of 3.6 μmol/L (normal range 6–10 μmol/L), a vitamin B12 level of 605 pg/mL (normal range 150–750 pg/mL), and an MTHFR polymorphism with heterozygosity of the A1298C mutation. Folate status at this time was not known. She was begun on methylfolate 7.5 mg daily, SAMe 400 mg twice daily, and methionine 1500 mg twice daily. Over the next 4 months (assessed at initial assessment, then at 2 and 4 months) her electrodiagnostic testing (EDx) showed either stability or improvement in all parameters, including increasing amplitudes and decreasing latencies. The most striking improvements included her fibular (peroneal) sensory nerve action potential (SNAP) amplitudes, which increased on the left side from 3.7 to 4.7 and then finally 9 μV on serial EDx studies; on the right side, the values increased from 4 to 8 and then to 8.3 µV. Her fibular (peroneal) compound motor action potential (CMAP) amplitude, measured on the right side only, increased from 1.8 to 3.8 and then to 5 mV. Peroneal distal sensory latencies decreased from 5.0 to 4.1 and then to 3.6 ms on the left, and from 4.4 to 4.2 and then to 3.4 ms on the right. Over that same time, her homocysteine level rose to 7.9 µmol/L. She also reported subjective improvement and she had minimal residual neuropathic symptoms.

Retrospective Review

Provoked by these observations, a subsequent retrospective data search of the electronic health record database of a larger, tertiary medical group in southern Oregon was implemented, assessing data for the past 10 years. The data were collected from all patients born before 1965 who had at least one office encounter with a group provider and at least one homocysteine level in the stated range. These results are summarized in **Table 1**. The study included a total of 37,442 patients. Of this group, 1547 patients carried the diagnosis of IPN (International Classification of Diseases–9 code = 356.9). Of the patients who were found to have an abnormally low homocysteine level below 6 µmol/L, 5.9% had IPN compared with 0.6% of patients without IPN ($P<.0001$ by χ^2 test with Yates correction). Overall, 86 of 210 (41%) patients with an abnormally low homocysteine level had IPN. These observations indicate that although reduced levels of homocysteine are uncommon in the general population, there is a striking relationship between hypohomocysteinemia and the incidence of IPN.

DISCUSSION

Whether all patients with IPN and HH will show clinical improvement with methionine supplementation remains to be studied. There are confounding comorbidities and possible alternative explanations, but the risk/benefit ratio associated with methionine treatment weighs heavily in favor of further investigation. To date there is simply not enough available clinical data from which to draw any hard and fast conclusions about the relationship between risk of acquired IPN, HH, and MTHFR polymorphisms. Nevertheless, the available data suggest some provoking possibilities that warrant further investigation. Typically MTHFR polymorphisms are not considered clinically relevant unless homocysteine levels are abnormal. The preliminary data discussed here challenge that assumption. While not suggesting that MTHFR abnormalities cause HH, the data do point to a need to quantitatively assess the correlation between abnormal levels of homocysteine and polymorphism in MTHFR-pathway genes and

Table 1
Homocysteine levels in patients carrying the diagnosis of idiopathic peripheral neuropathy (IPN) versus controls without neuropathy

Homocysteine Level (µmol/L) (normal range 6–10 µmol/L)	No. of Patients Without IPN	No. of Patients With IPN (%)
4–5.1	180	66 (36)
3–4	22	14 (64)
<3	8[a]	[a]6 (75)

[a] History regarding the presence of neuropathy in 2 of these 8 patients was unobtainable. These 6 patients with available history all had the diagnosis of neuropathy. The total number of patients was 37,442, of whom 1547 (4%) carried the diagnosis of IPN (International Classification of Diseases–9 code = 356.9).

associated cofactors in the overall population. Which other nutritional, environmental, and/or genetic factors contribute to either elevated or lowered levels of homocysteine also remain to be better elucidated.

It is possible that there are abnormalities in this process related to a relative vitamin B12 deficiency that are not adequately assessed by measuring homocysteine levels, or even methylmalonic acid, as an independent surrogate marker. Yet the consequences of the same processes that lead to abnormal levels of homocysteine also appear to lead to diminished methylation capacity, and this in turn may be what leads to the development of neuropathology.

The PN associated with HH may be viewed in the context of a broader neurodegenerative picture, which also includes dementia and depression, similar to the spectrum of vitamin B12 deficiency. The neuropathologic sequelae of vitamin B12 deficiency have been attributed to altered DNA synthesis, yet vitamin B12 itself plays no direct role in DNA biosynthesis. The previously mentioned methylfolate trap hypothesis could provide the explanation for this. The final common pathophysiologic deficit in all of these neuropathic scenarios could be reduced global DNA methylation, which has been demonstrated in animal models.[17,25] However, the pathologic consequences of diminished methylation are widespread, as DNA mismatch repair, cell cycle regulation in postmitotic neurons, and neurogenesis are all influenced by DNA methylation.[26] Moreover, the consequences of abnormal methylation have not been adequately separated from the consequences of the toxic effects of abnormal levels of homocysteine, either elevated or lowered. It is possible that the power of studies showing pathology associated with elevated homocysteine has been weakened by placing people with abnormal methylation related to functionally low homocysteine in the "normal" group, which would reduce the apparent magnitude of the disease burden difference between the subjects with hyperhomocysteinemia and those with HH because both states produce similar associated pathology. If reduced methylation is the real problem then, at least in some disease states, homocysteine may be an insufficient marker for pathology.

There are studies that show benefit in the treatment of neuropathy associated with diabetes from the use of methylfolate and methylcobalamin.[27–29] There is also evidence of the benefit of the use of methylfolate in depression.[30,31] These studies did not stratify treatment effects with identification of any known derangement (eg, MTHFR polymorphisms). Thus the beneficial effects might mainly occur in the subset of patients with diabetic neuropathy or depressed patients who also have derangements in single carbon metabolism. Recently, Iskander and colleagues[17] demonstrated the relationship of folic acid to DNA methylation and nerve regeneration following injury, suggesting an epigenetic mechanism for both neuropathology and subsequent regeneration.

There are many unanswered questions. If oral therapy with a cocktail of methylfolate, SAMe, and methionine were to be studied, what would be the appropriate dosing range? Would all ingredients be necessary? What might be the exact mechanism of any observed benefit? Benefits might be derived from single or multiple effects of the interventions. For example, the biosynthesis of creatine is dependent on methylation via methionine and SAMe, and creatine is known to have positive effects on strength independent of other cofactors.[32] Testing for these metabolic products is also challenging. At present there are commercially available blood tests for the known MTHFR polymorphisms, although testing for methionine, SAMe, or methylfolate levels may only be measured in a research setting. The possibility that HH is a potentially treatable cause of IPN is compelling enough to warrant a more rigorous evaluation of the possibility that HH as a pathologic state should be added to the differential diagnosis of PN. Such a demonstration would reinforce the importance of future research regarding the impact of derangements in DNA methylation on other neuropathologic disease states. A more expansive appreciation of the prevalence of methylation defects in the etiology of PN should enhance the appreciation of peripheral and central neuropathologic consequences of inborn errors of metabolism that are less severe and more indolent in their progression than the classic, severe versions that manifest in childhood. This development could potentially lead to treatment paradigms that result in actual partial or complete restoration of neurophysiologic function and thus to represent a huge change in the current clinical approach to IPN, which is now largely rehabilitative and palliative. While not conclusive, there is enough emerging evidence to warrant further studies aimed at investigating the linkage between HH, MTHFR polymorphisms, and increased risk for PN.

REFERENCES

1. Postiglione A, Milan G, Ruocco A, et al. Plasma folate, vitamin B-12, and total homocysteine and homozygosity for the C677T mutation of the 5,10-methylene tetrahydrofolate reductase gene in patients with Alzheimer's dementia. A case-control study. Gerontology 2001;47(6):324–9.
2. Oussalah A, Guéant JL, Peyrin-Biroulet L. Meta-analysis: hyperhomocysteinaemia in inflammatory bowel diseases. Aliment Pharmacol Ther 2011;34(10):1173–84.
3. Metz J. Cobalamin deficiency and the pathogenesis of nervous system disease. Annu Rev Nutr 1992;12:59–79.
4. Mischoulon D, Raab MF. The role of folate in depression and dementia. J Clin Psychiatry 2007;68(Suppl 10):28–33.
5. Anello G, Guéant-Rodríguez RM, Bosco P, et al. Homocysteine and methylenetetrahydrofolate reductase polymorphism in Alzheimer's disease. Neuroreport 2004;15(5):859–61.
6. Bottiglieri T, Hyland K, Reynolds EH. The clinical potential of admetionine (S-adenosylmethionine) in neurologic disorders. Drugs 1994;48(2):137–52.
7. Smith DA, Smith SM, de Jager CA, et al. Homocysteine-lowering by B vitamins slows the rate of accelerated brain atrophy in mild cognitive impairment: a randomized controlled trial. PLoS One 2010;5(9):e12244.
8. Bottiglieri T. Homocysteine and folate metabolism in depression. Prog Neuropsychopharmacol Biol Psychiatry 2005;29:1103–12.
9. Morris SA, Jacques PF. Folate and neurologic function: epidemiologic perspective. In: Bailey LB, editor. Folate in health and disease. Boca Raton (FL): Taylor and Francis Group; 2010. p. 330–3.
10. Zhou YH, Tang JY, Wu MJ, et al. Effect of folic acid supplementation on cardiovascular outcomes: a systematic review and meta-analysis. PLoS One 2011; 6(9):e25142.
11. Martí-Carvajal AJ, Solà I, Lathyris D, et al. Homocysteine lowering interventions for preventing cardiovascular events. Cochrane Database Syst Rev 2009;4. CD006612.
12. van Guldener C, Stehouwer CD. Homocysteine-lowering treatment: an overview. Expert Opin Pharmacother 2001;2(9):1449–60.
13. Albert CM, Cook NR, Gaziano JM, et al. Effect of folic acid and B vitamins on risk of cardiovascular events and total mortality among women at high risk for cardiovascular disease: a randomized trial. JAMA 2008;299(17):2027–36.
14. Selhub J. Public health significance of elevated homocysteine. Food Nutr Bull 2008;29(Suppl 2):S116–25.

15. Bottiglieri T, Reynolds E. Folate and neurologic disease: basic mechanisms. In: Bailey L, editor. Folate in health and disease. Boca Raton (FL): Taylor and Francis Group, LLC; CRC Press; 2010. p. 355–80.
16. Batey RT. Recognition of S-adenosylmethionine by riboswitches. Wiley Interdiscip Rev RNA 2011;2(2):299–311.
17. Iskandar BJ, Rizk E, Meier B, et al. Folate regulation of axonal regeneration in the rodent central nervous system through DNA methylation. J Clin Invest 2010; 120(5):1603–16.
18. Lawrance AK, Racine J, Deng L, et al. Complete deficiency of methylenetetrahydrofolate reductase in mice is associated with impaired retinal function and variable mortality, hematological profiles, and reproductive outcomes. J Inherit Metab Dis 2011;34(1):147–57.
19. Leclerc D, Rozen R. Molecular genetics of MTHFR: polymorphisms are not all benign. Med Sci (Paris) 2007;23(3):297–302.
20. Rummel T, Suormala T, Häberle J, et al. Intermediate hyperhomocysteinaemia and compound heterozygosity for the common variant c.677C>T and a MTHFR gene mutation. J Inherit Metab Dis 2007;30(3):401.
21. Bosy-Westphal A, Holzapfel A, Czech N, et al. Plasma folate but not vitamin B(12) or homocysteine concentrations are reduced after short-term vitamin B(6) supplementation. Ann Nutr Metab 2001;45(6):255–8.
22. Hoffman M. Hypothesis: hyperhomocysteinemia is an indicator of oxidant stress. Med Hypotheses 2011;77(6):1088–93.
23. Bader N, Bosy-Westphal A, Koch A, et al. Influence of vitamin C and E supplementation on oxidative stress induced by hyperbaric oxygen in healthy men. Ann Nutr Metab 2006;50(3):173–6.
24. Smulders YM, Smith DE, Kok RM, et al. Cellular folate vitamer distribution during and after correction of vitamin B12 deficiency: a case for the methylfolate trap. Br J Haematol 2006;132(5):623–9.
25. Aoyama K, Suh SW, Hamby AM, et al. Neuronal glutathione deficiency and age-dependent neurodegeneration in the EAAC1 deficient mouse. Nat Neurosci 2005;9:119–26.
26. Bird A. Putting the DNA back into DNA methylation. Nat Genet 2011;43(11): 1050–1.
27. Watkins D, Ru M, Hwang HY, et al. Hyperhomocysteinemia due to methionine synthase deficiency, cblG structure of the MTR gene, genotype diversity, and recognition of a common mutation, p1173L. Am J Hum Genet 2002;71:143–53.
28. Ukinc K, Ersoz HO, Karahan C, et al. Methyltetrahydrofolate reductase C677T gene mutation and hyperhomocysteinemia as a novel risk factor for diabetic nephropathy. Endocrine 2009;36(2):255–61.
29. Walker MJ Jr, Morris LM, Cheng D. Improvement of cutaneous sensitivity in diabetic peripheral neuropathy with combination L-methylfolate, methylcobalamin, and pyridoxal 5′-phosphate. Rev Neurol Dis 2010;7(4):132–9.
30. Ginsberg LD, Oubre AY, Daoud YA. L-methylfolate plus SSRI or SNRI from treatment initiation compared to SSRI or SNRI monotherapy in a major depressive episode. Innov Clin Neurosci 2011;8(1):19–28.
31. Bottiglieri T, Laundy M, Crellin R, et al. Homocysteine, folate, methylation, and monoamine metabolism in depression. J Neurol Neurosurg Psychiatry 2000;69: 228–32.
32. Head SI, Greenaway B, Chan S. Incubating isolated mouse EDL muscles with creatine improves force production and twitch kinetics in fatigue due to reduction in ionic strength. PLoS One 2011;6(8):e22742.

Regional and Whole-Body Dual-Energy X-Ray Absorptiometry to Guide Treatment and Monitor Disease Progression in Neuromuscular Disease

Andrew J. Skalsky, MD[a],*, Jay J. Han, MD[b],
Richard T. Abresch, MS[b], Craig M. McDonald, MD[b]

KEYWORDS

• DEXA • Body composition • Lean mass • Fat mass

Body composition is often altered in neuromuscular diseases. Better characterization may help not only to better understand disease processes but also to aid in clinical management. Current imaging modalities can estimate both regional and whole-body composition.

DUAL-ENERGY X-RAY ABSORPTIOMETRY

Dual-energy x-ray absorptiometry or dual-emission x-ray absorptiometry (DEXA) is a means of measuring body composition. Two x-ray beams with different energy levels, one high and one low energy beam, are aimed at the patient. The radiation that passes through the tissue is measured for each beam. Body composition can be determined from the absorption of each beam by different body tissues. When soft tissue absorption is subtracted out, the bone mineral DEXA is determined. DEXA is, by far, the most widely used technique for bone mineral density measurements. Although DEXA is used primarily to evaluate bone mineral density in clinical practice, it can also be used to measure or estimate total body mass, lean soft tissue mass, bone mineral content, and fat mass.

[a] Department of Pediatrics, University of California San Diego, Rady Children's Hospital and Health Center, 3020 Children's Way, MC 5096, San Diego, CA 92123, USA
[b] Department of Physical Medicine and Rehabilitation, University of California Davis, 4860 Y Street, Suite 3850, Sacramento, CA 95817, USA
* Corresponding author.
E-mail address: askalsky@rchsd.org

Phys Med Rehabil Clin N Am 23 (2012) 67–73
doi:10.1016/j.pmr.2011.11.007
1047-9651/12/$ – see front matter © 2012 Elsevier Inc. All rights reserved.

REGIONAL DEXA

Regional DEXA applies the same concepts as whole-body DEXA but is limited to defined body regions. This technique is widely used for the assessment of bone mineral density and is most often performed on the lower spine and hips. However, regional DEXA can also be used to assess regional body composition of limbs or any other defined body region (**Fig. 1**). This assessment can be helpful to determine if the changes in body composition are primarily appendicular, axial, or a complex combination. Another potential advantage of regional DEXA would be in the setting of a focal treatment such as the implantation of stem cells. Following the region of interest serially over time may identify an increase in muscle mass or lean tissue that would have been lost in whole-body evaluations.

ADVANTAGES OF DEXA

DEXA is relatively easy to perform, and the amount of radiation exposure is low. The technique is considered to be cheap, accessible, and able to provide accurate estimations of body composition.[1] The radiation received by the patient is usually less than that of a transatlantic airline flight or similar to approximately one-twentieth that of a standard chest radiograph but varies from patient to patient. A regional and whole-body DEXA scan can be performed in less than 5 minutes, whereas it takes at least 30 to 60 minutes to acquire whole-body magnetic resonance imaging (MRI) data.[2]

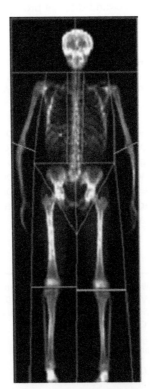

Fig. 1. Anatomic delineations used for regional body composition assessment.

McDonald and colleagues[3] found multifrequency bioelectric impedance analysis to be accurate in normal subjects, but it underestimated lean tissue mass and overestimated fat tissue mass in patients with Duchenne muscular dystrophy (DMD) compared with DEXA. Multifrequency bioelectric impedance analysis can only estimate whole-body composition. In comparison, DEXA has the capacity to estimate both whole-body and regional composition. Skinfold thickness measurements have also been used to estimate body composition. Mok and colleagues[4] found that skinfold thickness measurements overestimate the fat-free mass in DMD, which results in an underestimation of the body fat percentage. This same study found bioelectric impedance analysis to be similar to DEXA. This differs from the findings of McDonald and colleagues. Bioelectric impedance has been shown to accurately predict fat-free mass and lean tissue mass in normal controls. The boys with DMD studied by Mok and colleagues were younger than the population evaluated by McDonald and colleagues, which would suggest less disease progression and less deviation from control body composition. This may account for the contradictory findings.

DISADVANTAGES OF DEXA

Although it very accurately measures mineral content and lean soft tissue mass, DEXA may skew the calculation of fat mass because of its method of indirectly calculating fat mass by subtracting lean soft tissue mass and mineral content, which are the elements DEXA actually measures. In addition, lean soft tissue mass as measured by DEXA is an overestimate of muscle mass. The reason for the overestimation is that lean tissue includes multiple nonmuscle compartments (ie, skin, connective tissue, and the fat-free portion of adipose tissue).[5] Skin accounts for approximately 10% of lean soft tissue mass.[6] The overestimation of muscle mass is magnified in dystrophic muscle because muscle is replaced by fibrous connective tissue. Both skeletal muscle and fibrous connective tissue are lean soft tissue mass.

Additionally, a traditional 2-dimensional DEXA scan is not able to account for anterior and posterior compartments despite its regional compartmentalization capability given that it is a 2-dimensional imaging modality. To more accurately assess 3-dimensional body composition, a 3-dimensional imaging modality, such as computed tomography (CT) or MRI, is needed. MRI provides the additional benefits of distinguishing between intramuscular and extramuscular lipid content using hydrogen-1 magnetic resonance spectroscopy[7] as well as information regarding the quality of muscle tissues in vivo using sodium-23 MRI.[8]

Bone mineral density assessed by DEXA is actually the measure of bone mineral content in a given 2-dimensional area (normally the outline of the osseous structure), thus calculating the apparent bone mineral density. This differs from the actual 3-dimensional volume of the bone being measured, so the values cannot be directly compared with other methods of assessing 3-dimensional bone mineral density such as quantitative CT (QCT). QCT is capable of measuring the bone's volume and therefore is not susceptible to the confounding effect of apparent bone size in the way that DEXA is susceptible. Although a standard CT scanner can be used to assess bone mineral density, the radiation exposure is much higher and the cost is substantially greater than with DEXA. These reasons currently limit QCT from being used in general practice for the measurement of bone density and likely limit 3-dimensional technology in the assessment of whole-body or regional body composition. Despite the apparent limitations of a 2-dimensional imaging modality, DEXA technology has been applied to bone mineral density quite successfully. As with any imaging modality, severe joint contractures and scoliosis can distort body composition estimates.

DEXA IN NEUROMUSCULAR DISEASES

In neuromuscular diseases, DEXA has already been shown to have an excellent correlation with other established and validated methods of measuring lean body mass.[9] DEXA has also been used in clinical trials in neuromuscular disorders. Kissel and colleagues[10] showed that albuterol increases lean tissue mass in facioscapulohumeral dystrophy (FSHD) by DEXA measurements. However, the same trial did not show an improvement in global strength or function. The use of regional DEXA may provide additional insight into this contradictory result by determining if there was primarily appendicular, axial, or a combined increase in lean tissue mass.

Several studies have used DEXA to demonstrate significantly increased body fat mass and percentage as well as significantly decreased lean tissue mass in comparison with anthropometrically similar controls.[3,9,11–14] The authors[12,13] have shown that the decrease in regional lean tissue mass and the increase in regional fat mass correlate with the stereotyped pattern of weakness. In DMD, the most altered region in comparison with controls was the thigh. There was no significant difference detected in the lower leg. This finding is consistent with what is noticed clinically.[13] Likewise, in FSHD, the regions most altered in comparison with controls were the lower leg and upper arm, which corresponds to the typical pattern of weakness observed in FSHD. Similarly, the forearm composition was not different because these muscle groups tend to be relatively spared in FSHD.[12] In comparison with controls in both the authors' studies, the whole-body fat mass was significantly increased and the whole-body lean tissue mass was significantly decreased in both DMD and FSHD despite similar body mass index (BMI) and anthropometric values. Additional work by Pruna and colleagues[11] demonstrated aberrant regional and whole-body composition in myotonic dystrophy type 1 using DEXA. As in DMD and FSHD, there was an increase in fat mass and a decrease in fat-free mass when compared with controls. This pattern of change in body composition matched clinical severity. There was also increased muscular disability rating, decreased motor function, and decreased vital capacity with increased fat mass. The investigators also found that the use of BMI greatly underestimated the whole-body fat mass and was not an accurate index of overweight or obesity in myotonic dystrophy. Because of these findings, multiple investigators have concluded that BMI is not an appropriate index in neuromuscular disorders because it greatly underestimates the amount of fat mass in comparison with the general population.[11–13]

There have also been several studies comparing lean tissue mass with strength and functional measures.[12–14] By using regional lean tissue mass and strength measures, it has been determined that the strength per lean tissue mass decreases with disease progression in muscular dystrophies, whereas it remains constant in able-bodied controls. This ratio may provide a macroscopic evaluation of in vivo muscle contractility function in addition to muscle mass assessment. This finding correlates with what is observed and known clinically.

In boys with DMD using home mechanical ventilation, the measured resting energy expenditure (mREE) was significantly lower than the control population and also lower than what would have been predicted using the Harris and Benedict equation. However, the mREE and the predicted resting energy expenditure (REE) were better matched when taking lean tissue mass into consideration.[15] This study suggests that even in the advanced stages of a muscular dystrophy, the caloric requirements can be accurately predicted if body composition is known and taken into consideration. This further supports the use of DEXA to obtain an accurate assessment of body composition to guide caloric needs of individuals with neuromuscular diseases.

CLINICAL APPLICATIONS OF DEXA

The consensus statement for standard of care in spinal muscular atrophy states, "children with spinal muscular atrophy (SMA) may have acceptable fat mass but plot as underweight based on weight/height criteria due to a decrease in lean body mass. Hence, normal body mass indexes may not represent ideal weights for children with spinal muscular atrophy. Decreased activity and lean body mass will lead to reduced resting energy expenditure and increased risk of obesity... The goal is to maintain each child on his or her own growth velocity. Growth velocity curves (weight, height/length, weight/height) followed over a period of time are, for the most part, the most accurate indicator of nutritional status."[16] Having a more precise approach to caloric requirements based on actual body composition may reduce the epidemic of obesity among individuals with neuromuscular diseases.

DEXA Guiding Treatment

Age, height, weight, and BMI are often used to estimate caloric needs in the general population. Reliance on the same measures in neuromuscular diseases often results in an overestimation of calories. This becomes especially important when clinicians rely on the physical appearance of an individual with a neuromuscular disease to guide caloric needs. Many clinicians feel uncomfortable with adult patients with neuromuscular diseases and low BMIs (<18.5). However, given the perturbations in body fat and lean tissue, a low BMI may still represent a body composition with relatively increased body fat percentage in individuals with neuromuscular disease. For example, based on the DEXA data from the authors' previous publications, to achieve a similar body fat percentage as a control man with a weight of 70 kg and BMI of 23, an adult man with FSHD of the same height would likely weigh only 57 kg, which would result in a BMI of 18.4. A similar trend was observed in DMD. For a comparable body fat percentage to a 10-year-old able-bodied boy at the 50th percentile for weight-for-age, a boy with DMD would likely be below the 10th percentile weight-for-age. The use of DEXA in neuromuscular diseases can more appropriately estimate the caloric needs by estimating the mass of metabolically active tissue or lean tissue mass.

Direct measurement of REE is one of the most accurate methods of estimating daily caloric requirements. However, this measurement is costly, labor intensive, time consuming, and not feasible as a practical ambulatory setting clinical tool. Several studies have measured the REE in boys with DMD.[15,17–19] In DMD, it has been shown that REE decreases with time after 10 years of age. This may relate to the progressive loss of metabolically active lean tissue mass.[17]

Zanardi and colleagues[18] investigated the relationship of REE to whole-body weight and fat-free mass in younger boys (ages, 6–12 years) with DMD. Their results show similar REE per kilogram total body weight for boys with DMD to controls but with a high variance. The investigators concluded that the development of obesity in children with DMD is not primarily because of a low REE but because of other causes such as a reduction in physical activity and/or overfeeding. The study also found a high correlation between fat-free mass and REE (r = 0.899; P = .001) in boys with DMD despite varied body composition. Although there was an even stronger correlation between total body weight and REE (r = 0.948; P<.001), there was a much smaller coefficient of variation for REE/fat-free mass versus REE/total body weight (0.10 vs 0.21). Thus, estimating caloric needs in DMD based on fat-free mass should yield fairly accurate results.

Body composition affects not only nutritional needs but also medication pharmacokinetics. With the increase in percentage of body fat, there is a corresponding decrease in the percentage of body free water. In individuals with neuromuscular diseases, blood levels of water-soluble medications will be higher than expected because there is less body water to distribute into. Likewise, fat-soluble medications stay in the body much longer because there is more fat for storage of the medication. This distribution may result in increasingly complicated balance between therapeutic effects and side effects of medications in treating neuromuscular diseases. This complicated balance is especially true in treating DMD, whereby fat-soluble cortico-steroids are the current standard of care and are also associated with an additional increase in body fat.[20] In the future, more effective treatments for neuromuscular diseases will become available. Assessing body composition with DEXA will allow more appropriate dosing guidance and limit toxic side effects that result from altered pharmacokinetics due to perturbed body composition.

DEXA Monitoring Disease Progression

Whole-body DEXA has been used in previous neuromuscular clinical trials.[4,10] It has also been shown to be sensitive to change. As mentioned previously, Kissel and colleagues[10] found a significant change in lean tissue mass even though no changes in strength or function were detected. Similarly, over the 5-month trial period evaluating the efficacy of glutamate in DMD, Mok and colleagues[4] found DEXA sensitive to change in fat tissue mass despite only a mean weight gain of 1.1 kg.

Having a sensitive outcome measure such as change in lean tissue mass is especially important for assessing change in the later stages of neuromuscular diseases during which measures based on function or strength are no longer attainable. The use of regional body composition measures, especially lean tissue mass, along with strength assessments can help determine if disease progression is primarily because of sarcopenia or muscle atrophy or decreased function of the lean tissue contractility mechanism. Although both are likely partially responsible, determining if sarcopenia or decreased contractility is predominantly responsible for disease progression may help guide future targeted treatments for various neuromuscular diseases.

SUMMARY

Whole-body DEXA when combined with regional data is a safe, noninvasive, cost-effective, time-efficient measure of both disease progression as well as monitors intervention efficacy in neuromuscular disease. Further work in the area of regional DEXA and strength measures may offer additional insight into the pathophysiology of the stereotyped patterns of weakness clinically observed in various neuromuscular diseases.

REFERENCES

1. Gilsanz V. Bone density in children: a review of the available techniques and indications. Eur J Radiol 1998;26(2):177–82.
2. Ross R. Advances in the application of imaging methods in applied and clinical physiology. Acta Diabetol 2003;40(Suppl 1):S45–50.
3. McDonald CM, Carter GT, Abresch RT, et al. Body composition and water compartment measurements in boys with Duchenne muscular dystrophy. Am J Phys Med Rehabil 2005;84:483–91.
4. Mok E, Letellier G, Cuisset JM, et al. Assessing change in body composition in children with Duchenne muscular dystrophy: anthropometry and bioelectrical

impedance analysis versus dual-energy X-ray absorptiometry. Clin Nutr 2010; 29(5):633–8.

5. Wang W, Wang Z, Faith MS, et al. Regional skeletal muscle measurement: evaluation of new dual-energy X-ray absorptiometry model. J Appl Physiol 1999;87: 1163–71.

6. Snyder WS, Cook MJ, Nasset ES, et al. Report of the task group on reference man. Oxford (UK): Pergamon Press; 1975.

7. Boesch C, Slotboom J, Hoppeler H, et al. In vivo determination of intramyocellular lipids in human muscle by means of localized 1H-MR-spectroscopy. Magn Reson Med 1997;37:484–93.

8. Constantinides CD, Gillen JS, Boada FE, et al. Human skeletal muscle: sodium MR imaging and quantification-potential applications in exercise and disease. Radiology 2000;216(2):559–68.

9. Forbes GB, Griggs RC, Moxley RT 3rd, et al. K-40 and dual-energy X-ray absorptiometry estimates of lean weight compared. Normals and patients with neuromuscular disease. Ann N Y Acad Sci 2000;904:111–4.

10. Kissel JT, McDermott MP, Mendell JR, FSH-DY Group, et al. Randomized, double-blind, placebo-controlled trial of albuterol in facioscapulohumeral dystrophy. Neurology 2001;57(8):1434–40.

11. Pruna L, Chatelin J, Pascal-Vigneron V, et al. Regional body composition and functional impairment in patients with myotonic dystrophy. Muscle Nerve 2011; 44(4):503–8.

12. Skalsky AJ, Abresch RT, Han JJ, et al. The relationship between regional body composition and quantitative strength in facioscapulohumeral muscular dystrophy (FSHD). Neuromuscul Disord 2008;18(11):873–80.

13. Skalsky AJ, Han JJ, Abresch RT, et al. Assessment of regional body composition with dual-energy X-ray absorptiometry in Duchenne muscular dystrophy: correlation of regional lean mass and quantitative strength. Muscle Nerve 2009;39(5): 647–51.

14. Palmieri MD, Bertorini MD, Griffin JW, et al. Assessment of whole body composition with dual energy X-ray absorptiometry in Duchenne muscular dystrophy: correlation of lean body mass with muscle function. Muscle Nerve 1996;19: 777–9.

15. Gonzalez-Bermejo J, Lofaso F, Falaize L, et al. Resting energy expenditure in Duchenne patients using home mechanical ventilation. Eur Respir J 2005; 25(4):682–7.

16. Wang CH, Finkel RS, Bertini ES, Participants of the International Conference on SMA Standard of Care, et al. Consensus statement for standard of care in spinal muscular atrophy. J Child Neurol 2007;22(8):1027–49.

17. Shimizu-Fujiwara M, Komaki H, Nakagawa E, et al. Decreased resting energy expenditure in patients with Duchenne muscular dystrophy. Brain Dev 2011. [Epub ahead of print].

18. Zanardi MC, Tagliabue A, Orcesi S, et al. Body composition and energy expenditure in Duchenne muscular dystrophy. Eur J Clin Nutr 2003;57(2):273–8.

19. Hankard R, Gottrand F, Turck D, et al. Resting energy expenditure and energy substrate utilization in children with Duchenne muscular dystrophy. Pediatr Res 1996;40(1):29–33.

20. Bushby K, Finkel R, Birnkrant DJ, et al. Diagnosis and management of Duchenne muscular dystrophy, part 1: diagnosis, and pharmacological and psychosocial management [review]. Lancet Neurol 2010;9(1):77–93.

Establishing Clinical End Points of Respiratory Function in Large Animals for Clinical Translation

Melissa A. Goddard, BSc[a], Erin L. Mitchell, DVM[b],
Barbara K. Smith, PhD, PT[c], Martin K. Childers, DO, PhD[a,d],*

KEYWORDS

- X-linked myotubular myopathy
- Respiratory impedance plethysmography • XLMTM dog
- Respiratory dysfunction

This article serves to describe the need for animal models and, more specifically, a canine model, to accurately define and establish clinical end points for the treatment of neuromuscular disease (NMD) in humans. Characterization of respiratory involvement in NMDs is needed, and the canine model can be used to asses, define, characterize and establish efficacy of new therapeutic modalities.

RESPIRATORY ASSESSMENT IN NMD PATIENTS

Although the genetic etiology, pathophysiology, and disease course varies vastly between the inherited NMDs, a common clinical feature is impaired ventilatory function. Respiratory muscle dysfunction increases the rate of pulmonary complications and death, and is a major factor in respiratory failure.[1,2] Respiratory failure is the primary cause of mortality for many inherited NMDs.[3]

Although a common attribute of neuromuscular compromise is the predominance of respiratory insufficiency,[4] the pathology, clinical signs, onset, and response to

[a] Wake Forest Institute for Regenerative Medicine, Wake Forest University, Winston-Salem, NC, USA
[b] Department of Physical Therapy, University of Florida, Gainesville, FL, USA
[c] Animal Resources Program, Wake Forest University, Winston-Salem, NC, USA
[d] Section of PM&R, Department of Neurology, School of Medicine, Wake Forest University Health Sciences, Room 258, Dean Biomedical Research Building, 391 Technology Way, Winston-Salem, NC 27101, USA
* Corresponding author. Section of PM&R, Department of Neurology, School of Medicine, Wake Forest University Health Sciences, Room 258, Dean Biomedical Research Building, 391 Technology Way, Winston-Salem, NC 27101.
E-mail address: mchilder@wfubmc.edu

Phys Med Rehabil Clin N Am 23 (2012) 75–94
doi:10.1016/j.pmr.2011.11.017
1047-9651/12/$ – see front matter

medical management vary vastly between NMD diagnoses. For example, patients with Pompe disease may be distinguished from other NMDs by a relatively earlier involvement of ventilatory weakness, with a preservation of locomotor function.[5] As a result, the time course and pattern of ventilatory muscle weakness differs between the NMDs. Vital capacity declines by greater than 8% per year in Duchenne muscular dystrophy (DMD) after the age of 12,[6] yet inspiratory strength remains preserved to a greater degree than expiratory strength.[7,8] In DMD and amyotrophic lateral sclerosis (ALS), maximal inspiratory and expiratory pressures correlate equally with unassisted cough peak flows.[8,9] By contrast, the rate of decline in global ventilatory function varies vastly between patients with Pompe disease, but is characterized by predominant diaphragm muscle weakness.[5,10,11] Intercostal and diaphragm muscle involvement are differentially affected among spinal muscular atrophy variants[12] and may not occur at all in the mildest, adult-onset phenotype.[13]

Pulmonary pressures generally decline prior to a loss of forced expiratory volumes in most NMDs,[14] making strength a more sensitive index of respiratory function. Because both the inspiratory and expiratory muscles can be affected by NMD, it is important to conduct regular assessments of ventilatory muscle function. Different aspects of ventilatory muscle function can be discerned during assessments of resting tidal breathing, respiratory challenges with external loads, hypercapnia or hypoxia, muscle strength and endurance testing, and forced expiratory maneuvers, as well as during evoked contractions.

INSPIRATORY MUSCLE WEAKNESS

Early declines in respiratory muscle strength may go undetected by patients with NMD, because their overall activity levels often decline concurrently, and tidal breathing requires only a small proportion of the pressure capacity of the system. As a result, significant decreases in strength may occur before an appreciable change in vital capacity.[15] In patients with generalized NMD, a 25% or greater decrease in vital capacity between the upright and supine postures has been shown to predict significant diaphragm muscle weakness.[16] The weakened inspiratory pump has been associated with a stiffened chest wall and increased lung elastic loads, microatelectasis, reduced long volumes with restrictive pulmonary function impairment, CO_2 retention, and rapid, shallow breathing pattern.[17] In addition, patients with NMD and respiratory muscle weakness may have a greater susceptibility to fatigue.

Weakness of the respiratory pump can be measured as a decrease in its pressure-generating capacity. In many NMDs the strength of the respiratory pump is poorly correlated with that of the limb muscles,[10,18] and should be evaluated separately. Volitional pressure generation can be expressed as the maximal transdiaphragmatic pressure, described later.

Maximal Inspiratory Pressure

Maximal inspiratory pressure (MIP) measures the global pressure capacity of the inspiratory muscle pump at the mouth or tracheostomy opening. It is a noninvasive test with established reference values for age and gender, in both children and adults.[19,20] MIP can be influenced by lung volume and is typically measured from residual volume. Accurate measurements may also be challenging for patients who are mechanically ventilated or have difficulty consistently following commands. In these cases, valid maximal efforts can be obtained with short bouts of inspiratory occlusions.[21,22]

Nasal Sniff Pressure

Alternatively, nasal sniff pressures mimic a natural motor function, and maximal sniff maneuvers correlate well with MIP measurements at both the mouth and esophagus.[23] In patients with NMD and severe ventilatory weakness, sniff pressure correlates well with restrictions in vital capacity[24] related to pulmonary restrictive disease and/or progression of diaphragm dysfunction. Whereas MIP is a static maneuver, sniff is quasi-isometric, and different inspiratory muscle recruitment patterns have been noted during each maneuver.[25] Thus, the combined use of MIP and maximal sniff pressures may prove valuable for accurate diagnosis of weakness and longitudinal follow-up of patients with NMD.[26,27]

Transdiaphragmatic Pressure

The presence of specific diaphragm muscle weakness can be determined by the transdiaphragmatic pressure (Pdi) gradient. Balloon catheters or microtransducers placed in the esophagus (Pes) and stomach (Pga) can be used to estimate abdominal and pleural pressures. In healthy individuals, Pes becomes more negative during inspiration whereas Pga becomes more positive. Pdi can be evaluated during maximal voluntary inspiratory maneuvers or during contractions evoked by electrical or magnetic stimulation. In addition, Pdi during tidal breathing and inspiratory challenges may identify the fatigability of the diaphragm muscle.[28] The use of esophageal manometry can provide a greater insight into specific diaphragm muscle weakness but the procedure is invasive, and catheter placement may be poorly tolerated by patients.

Diaphragmatic paralysis results in an upward movement of the diaphragm, resulting in a negative Pga during inspiration. As a result, the Pdi approaches zero. This process is accompanied by asynchronous, paradoxic breathing. The timing and extent of the chest and abdominal wall movements can be quantified during tidal breathing, as well as maximal efforts, by respiratory inductance plethysmography.

Evoked Phrenic Motor Unit Function

Nonvolitional assessments of diaphragm contractile function reduce the variability of voluntary, maximal-effort maneuvers and remove the role of patient cooperation from the examination. Diaphragm contractions can be elicited by supramaximal electrical or magnetic stimulation of the phrenic nerves and be measured by Pdi or electromyogram (EMG) responses. In patients with DMD and severe diaphragm dysfunction, diaphragm electrophysiological responses remained present even when Pdi responses to phrenic stimulation could not be detected. The diaphragm motor responses revealed a normal to elevated ventilatory drive despite an undetectable Pdi.[29] In conjunction with needle EMG activity at rest and during graded contractions, the electrophysiological features elicited during phrenic stimulation can differentiate patients with an isolated neural pathology from those with a purely muscular impairment or a mixed pathology.[30]

INSPIRATORY MUSCLE FATIGUE

Inspiratory muscle weakness yields a progressive reduction in expansion of lung and chest wall during inhalation, resulting in a gradually reduced compliance and relative increase in the mechanical load during breathing. An imbalance between breathing loads and the pressure-generating capacity of the respiratory pump can lead to fatigue and ventilatory failure.[31] The pressure-time index (PTI) can estimate the threshold for diaphragm fatigue. The PTI consists of two components: the relative pressure required of the diaphragm to generate a tidal breath and the portion of the respiratory cycle spent in inspiration. In healthy individuals, the fatigue threshold is a PTI in excess of 0.15.[32] When relative breathing loads increase, patients with neuromuscular weakness may shorten inspiratory time and lower Pdi to minimize the work of breathing. However, this strategy of rapid, shallow breathing has been associated with an increased elastic load of the lung and hypercapnia.[33] It has been shown that the PTI threshold for fatigue may be closer to 0.10 to 0.12 for patients with quadriplegia,[34] and a low fatigue threshold is also thought to apply to patients with chronic NMD.[31]

EXPIRATORY MUSCLE DYSFUNCTION

Expiratory muscle weakness results in a reduced ability to lower volume below functional residual capacity, resulting in declines of expiratory reserve volume and residual volume. Patients become less capable of producing the intrathoracic pressures necessary to generate effective cough flows and clear lung secretions. An inability to clear airway secretions Is a serious problem in neuromuscular dysfunction, and is associated with an increased risk of mortality.[35] Maximal expiratory pressure (MEP) is a noninvasive estimate of expiratory muscle strength, typically measured from total lung capacity (TLC). MEP is the expiratory equivalent of MIP, and the advantages and limitations of the MEP maneuver are similar to those of MIP. Although MEP decreases with the progression of NMD,[33] it has not been found to be an independent predictor of hypercapnia.[36] MEP is a significant predictor of peak cough flow in patients with DMD and ALS.[8] Cough gastric pressure has been found to correlate well with MEP and may better differentiate weakness from technical difficulties when MEP is reduced.[37]

Congenital NMD with Severe Respiratory Dysfunction: A Description of XLMTM in Humans

XLMTM, classified as a congenital myopathy, is an inherited disease transmitted on the X chromosome. It is characterized by marked muscle weakness, hypotonia, and feeding and breathing difficulties in male infants. Many XLMTM patients die during their first year of life, due to respiratory insufficiency.[38] Affected infants may also present at birth with hypotonia, external ophthalmoplegia, and macrosomia. Female carriers do not display symptoms of the disease unless affected with other X-linked disorders.[39,40] The incidence of XLMTM in humans is estimated to be 1 in 50,000 male births.[41] Patients who survive past birth often have prolonged ventilator dependence and delayed motor milestones, but usually have intact intelligence.[42] Long-term survivors of the disease (>1 year), appear to be at risk for medical complications involving other organ systems in addition to complications derived from being partially or completely ventilator dependent.[42]

Diagnosis of XLMTM typically follows a muscle biopsy in which characteristic muscle histopathology has been identified as small, rounded muscle fibers with centrally located nuclei surrounded by a halo devoid of contractile elements and sarcoplasmic disorganization, reminiscent of the fetal stage of skeletal muscle, hence the name myotubular myopathy.[39,43] The muscle fibers contain abnormal mitochondria,[44] and type I fiber hypotrophy is present in patients afflicted with XLMTM.[39] This histopathology does not appear to change significantly during the course of the disease, despite clinical deterioration.

Animal Models of XLMTM

To more fully define the progression and understanding of the mechanism and pathogenesis of human disease, a well-defined animal model is necessary.[45] Animal models also allow for the development of therapeutic strategies that more accurately reflect disease severity and immunologic problems. A relevant animal model, and therefore species used, would be one in which the biological response to therapy would be expected to mimic the human response. Safety and efficacy data are needed prior to entry of any therapeutic agents into clinical trials.[46] Some animal models of NMD appear as true counterparts to human disorders; others resemble but do not duplicate disease in humans. Still others require further study to determine the degree of compatibility.[47]

Zebrafish and murine models of XLMTM have been recently established.[48,49] The discovery, further classification, and additional testing of a recently discovered canine model of XLMTM has broadened the field for this disease. These models have played an important role in understanding the pathogenesis of how loss of myotubularin leads to respiratory weakness and death.[45] Together these various species with myotubularin deficiency can be used to demonstrate different aspects of muscle maturation, maintenance, growth, and development. Findings in animals can lead to direct clinical translation, application, and use and refinement of diagnostic and therapeutic modalities for XLMTM patients. **Tables 1–3** compare and contrast the existing models of XLMTM.

Appropriate use of each species can be guided by several preclinical considerations. For example, the small size of mice guarantees that reagents can be produced in sufficient quantity and facilitates delivery of reagent in high doses.[50] However, there are other aspects that may be more accurately performed in a larger model because of physiology,[51] therapeutic feasibility and monitoring, and toxicity. If delivering therapeutic agents, large volumes may be required for translation to human medicine, which becomes impractical in mice.[50] The larger canine model allows for studies of safety and efficacy to be performed, and dose-escalation studies are more easily executed. Specifically, this becomes important when considering intramuscular injections of gene-therapy vectors. For example, direct injection of plasmid DNA into muscles for gene therapy is more practical, feasible, and plausible when using the canine model as opposed to the murine model of XLMTM, and this holds especially true for respiratory muscle injections to test for therapeutic efficiency. The ability to provide additional medical and nutritional support to affected dogs as opposed to mice may allow the model to survive longer periods of time, thus allowing long-term evaluation to establish the typical chronologic sequence of clinical and histologic signs for XLMTM.[52] **Box 1** describes in further detail the relative advantages and disadvantages of the canine model of XLMTM.

Description of Neuromuscular Disorders in Dogs

In contrast to the congenital myopathies, most of the muscular dystrophies recognized in dogs are caused by a genetic mutation in the dystrophin gene, which is located on the X chromosome. Thus, these disorders are inherited as X-linked recessive traits, clinically apparent in male dogs and transmitted by clinically asymptomatic female dogs.[61] Canine X-linked muscular dystrophy has been identified in Golden Retrievers, Irish Terriers, Samoyeds, Miniature Schnauzers, German Short-Haired Pointers, Rottweilers, Pembroke Welsh Corgi, and Belgian Shepherds.[62] The Golden Retriever model of Canine X-Linked Muscular Dystrophy (GRMD) is well established and has been characterized over many years.[59,63–65] Additional colonies of dogs with well-characterized clinical and histopathological characteristics of muscular dystrophy have been developed in Japan (CXMDJ), in which beagles were crossed with affected Golden Retrievers.[66] The addition of the beagle to the line allowed for a canine model that was more appropriately sized for muscular dystrophy and more

Table 1
Comparison of XLMTM animal models: genotypic and phenotypic features

	Zebrafish	Mouse	Mouse	Canine
	Morpholino Knockdown	Myotubularin-Deficient KO (*Mtm1* KO)	HSA Mutant	
Descriptor	Genetically modified	Genetically modified	Genetically modified	Naturally occurring, spontaneous
Gene loci	Not available	MTM1	Deletion of MTM1 exon 4	MTM1
Mutation	Antisense morpholino used to interrupt MTM1 transcription	Frameshift mutation		Missense variation
Expression	Both males and females	Sex linked: seen in the hemizygous male	Sex linked: seen in the hemizygous male	Sex linked: seen in the hemizygous male
Phenotype	Rapidly fatal	Rapidly fatal	Severe and rapidly fatal	Progressive
Screening	Phenotypic appearance	Tail snip		Cheek swab
Genetic manipulability	Functional gene knockdown			

easily handled.[53] This size manipulation is an example of what can be done in the XLMTM Labrador.

Description of XLMTM in Dogs

X-Linked myotubular myopathy was identified in Labrador retrievers as missense mutation in the MTM1 gene on the short arm of the X chromosome.[45] Generalized muscle atrophy, weakness, diminished spinal reflexes, and abnormal ability to eat and drink was reported in affected littermates in Canada.[61] Male dogs afflicted with XLMTM display temporal muscle mass loss, dropped-jaw appearance (likely due to weakness of masticatory muscles),[45] hindlimb muscle atrophy, contracture of hind distal and middle phalanges, a shortened, choppy, and stilted gait, and inability to stand for any length of time progressing to inability to rise or stand without assistance. Puppies appear clinically normal at birth, and subtle signs of disease start to appear at approximately 8 to 10 weeks of age. In the authors' experience, XLMTM dogs appear to have normal mentation up to the time of euthanasia. In addition, unaffected female and male dogs and female carrier dogs do not display any of the aforementioned clinical signs.

Affected dogs are generally euthanized between 3 and 6 months of age, due to the lack of intensive supportive care often present in affected humans. The dogs do not receive intubation for respiratory support or gastrotomy-tube feedings for nutritional support. This course differs from that of human XLMTM, in which the myopathy is relatively nonprogressive despite being severe at birth.[45] In dogs, paradoxic breathing is apparent at the first measurement of respiratory function, at approximately 10 weeks

Table 2
Comparison of XLMTM animal models: clinical and histologic features

	Zebrafish	Mouse	Mouse	Canine
Clinical features	Diminished spontaneous contractions of embryo Inability to hatch from chorion Dorsal curvature through back of tail (instead of normal flat or C-shaped dorsum) Bent and/or foreshortened tails Small heads Abnormally shaped yolk balls Reduced body extension	Growth impairment Kyphosis Hindlimb muscle paralysis	Growth impairment Kyphosis Hindlimb muscle paralysis	Generalized muscle atrophy Weakness Diminished spinal reflexes Normal ability to eat and drink Temporal muscle mass loss Dropped-jaw appearance Hindlimb muscle atrophy Contracture of hind distal and middle phalanges Shortened, choppy, stilted gait Inability to stand for any length of time progressing to inability to rise or stand without assistance
Histopathologic features	Small muscle fibers (50%) Large unusual and mislocalized nuclei Sarcoplasmic disorganization Myofiber hypotrophy	Generalized myopathy with fiber size variation Type I muscle fiber hypotrophy Progressive accumulation of paracentral or central nuclei in muscle fibers Necklace fibers	Nuclei originating mainly from myofibers and from fibroblasts, muscle satellite cells, endothelial and Schwann cells	Excessive variability in myofiber size Variable numbers of myofibers containing prominent internal nuclei Necklace fibers Subsarcolemmal rings and central changes
Respiratory function	Not tested			Paradoxic breathing

Table 3
Comparison of XLMTM animal models: use as a model

	Zebrafish	Mouse	Canine
Average litter size	Large	6–9	7
Affected animal average life span		7–9 wk/6–14 wk	14–19 wk
Time to detection of disease	Within 48–72 h postfertilization	4 wk	9–10 wk
Reproducibility	High	High	Dependent on Mendelian genetics
Muscle differentiation	At primary myogenesis	Complete at birth	4 wk postpartum
Appropriate use	Small molecule therapeutic testing Rapid testing of therapeutic strategies	Early therapeutic development Proof of concept Understanding function of myotubularin Gene therapy trials	Better reflection of disease severity Better reflection of immunologic problems associated with therapeutic development strategies Proof of concept Pre-FDA clinical trials

Abbreviation: FDA, Food and Drug Administration.

of age (Mitchell and Childers, unpublished observations, 2011). It is not certain currently whether paradoxic breathing is present before this age, as it has yet to be studied. From the first display of muscle weakness, most clinically apparent between 12 and 16 weeks of age, the puppies are hand-fed their daily caloric intake. Care is taken to ensure that they are able to rise on their own to urinate and defecate. Progressive skeletal muscle weakness leading to the inability to rise without assistance is the reason why dogs are euthanized between 16 and 19 weeks of age.

RESPIRATORY ASSESSMENT IN THE DOG

Given that respiratory dysfunction contributes to the shortened life span and compromised quality of life of XLMTM patients, and that long-term mechanical ventilation can cause complications[42] and may lead to damage of the diaphragm,[67] the ability to evaluate respiratory function and study pathologic changes related to the weakened diaphragm is of great value in an appropriately analogous animal model of XLMTM. There are two ways that this can be measured: by assessing respiratory function as a whole or by taking a direct look at the strength and function of the diaphragm muscle.

Several of the currently used means of examining respiratory function in animal models were developed to detect side effects of new drugs under development.[46] Some methods can be used only in rodents, and those available for use in larger animal models like the dog may have various disadvantages. These methods may be of limited use in anesthetized animals, restricting the length of time and number of intervals available to the investigator for study; other issues can include difficulties in calibrating and using the equipment, which may require a highly skilled operator. However, there are approaches that allow for the respiratory assessment of larger unanesthetized animals.

Plethysmography Chambers

One method is the assessment of restrained animals using a plethysmograph chamber, whereby the animal is either completely enclosed except for the head in a "head-out" chamber or, conversely, only the head is enclosed in a "head-in" chamber. While this allows for data collection in conscious animals and for whole-body measurement, the use of restraints introduces stress, which can affect the accuracy of results. In addition, there is some issue with sensitivity when used with large animals such as the dog, given the relatively small size of the measured change in comparison with the size of the chamber.[46]

Pneumotachometer

A second approach is a facemask or helmet with an attached air-flow meter known as a pneumotachometer, used with sling restraint of the dog. The pneumotachometer detects changes in air volume by measuring pressure changes across the device during inspiration and expiration, and these measures of air flow over time can be used to calculate values such as tidal volume, respiratory rate, and minute ventilation. Restraint stress is a factor when using the pneumotachometer, as with the plethysmograph chamber, but one advantage of pneumatography is that it provides a direct measurement of respiration and air flow. Therefore, it is often used when calibrating or assessing the effectiveness of, or in conjunction with, more indirect types of apparatus such as impedance bands, described next.

Invasive Respiratory Impedance

One of these indirect methods is the use of implanted impedance leads. These leads consist of a long coil of wire through which a low, constant electrical current is transmitted. The leads can be surgically inserted in a large animal and wrapped across the thorax or abdomen. As the animal breathes the coils are stretched, and a change in electrical resistance or impedance occurs. These resistance changes in the implanted coils correspond directly with the length of change during respiration. This change in electrical resistance is subsequently converted to volume changes, provided that a known amount of gas exchange can be used to calibrate the equipment. Thus, impedance technology can be used to measure even small changes in abdominal or thoracic volume during respiration.[68,69]

In invasive respiratory impedance the impedance device is placed in the pleural cavity, with the leads implanted into the intercostal space, This technique has been shown to be a relatively sensitive and accurate way of measuring respiratory function in dogs. In addition, it can be used both in anesthetized and in ambulatory, awake dogs, and allows for continual data collection over a fairly long period of time.[68] However, implantation of the leads is a surgical procedure, thus requiring additional surgical and anesthetic equipment.

Noninvasive Respiratory Impedance Plethysmography

The authors identified respiratory impedance plethysmography (RIP) as an effective means of assessing respiratory dysfunction and related diaphragmatic weakness in dogs with NMD. RIP offers many of the advantages of alternative techniques, especially implanted devices, but avoids many of their disadvantages. Here dogs are fitted with jackets, which hold the RIP bands in place throughout the experiment. RIP and electrocardiographic leads are connected to a telemetry device, which also records movement. Thus, data from the chest wall, heart, and whole-body movement can all be collected simultaneously and analyzed in real time.

Box 1
Advantages and disadvantages of the canine model of XLMTM

Advantages

- Genetic testing: cheek swab rather than tail snip; less pain and distress to animal
- Long life span
  - Long-term observations for therapeutic effectiveness, disease progression, and side effects
- Size
  - Human equipment to be used in research environment (no specialized equipment)
  - Respiratory impedance bands easily placed
  - Image quality better and easier to obtain
  - Quantifiable respiratory rate and pattern by direct visualization (allows secondary confirmation with respiratory impedance bands)
  - Able to take multiple muscle biopsies for characterization/progression of disease and response to therapeutics (from same muscle belly)[45]
- Attitude/good temperament[53,54]
  - Ease of handling and restraint
- Well-established protocols for sedation and anesthesia, maintenance of such
  - Easy to anesthetize
- Large database of normal values known for breed[55,56]
  - Respiratory rate, heart rate, tidal volume, clinical chemistry, complete blood cell count
- Transition to clinical studies for Food and Drug Administration applications
- May reduce number of animals needed for study to generate a more definitive data set[53]
- Artificial insemination for breeding purposes[57,58]
  - Ability to modify size of animal model in further generations
- Similarity to human respiratory function values (especially pediatrics)
  - Anatomic
    - Lung lobes, trachea, bronchi, and anatomic positioning of diaphragm[56]
  - Physiologic
    - Respiratory rate and pattern, sensitivity to pharmacologic agents[55]
- Naturally occurring mutation[45]
  - Avoids technical issues of genetically modified animals
    - Unexpected downstream effects
    - Loss or change of modification in later generations
- May uncover problems not appreciated in inbred strains of laboratory mice[59]
- Species-specific transgenes available[50]

Disadvantages

- Size
- Limited availability
- Life span
- Cost of upkeep/supplies (anesthesia, drugs)[60]

- Small litter sizes/longer gestation/longer time to wean
- Genetic variation within breed
- Expense of maintaining breeding colony
- Quadruped (does not lack instability of upper body, as do humans afflicted with disorder)
- May require larger quantities of test reagents to see significant effects[50]

The authors also collected measures of inspiratory and expiratory air flow using a pneumotachometer, to assess the relative fidelity of the RIP bands and to quantify the volumetric band data. Air flow can be measured directly with a pneumotachometer and a transducer. A pneumotachometer converts the flow of gases through it into a proportional signal of pressure difference. The authors found this noninvasive method of plethysmography to be quite accurate and sensitive; changes in band volume reflected simultaneously recorded changes in air flow across the pneumotachometer (**Fig. 1**).

As XLMTM is a myopathy that results in profound and fatal weakness of the respiratory muscles in patients, the respiratory dysfunction in XLMTM can be attributed to the increasing diaphragmatic weakness over the course of the disease. The authors hypothesize that differences exist between thoracic and abdominal mechanics for affected and unaffected individuals. The authors observed that XLMTM dogs display a "paradoxic" breathing pattern whereby thoracic motions are out of phase with those of the abdomen, particularly during respiratory challenge. By contrast, the thoracic and abdominal muscles move together during respiration in normal dogs. The

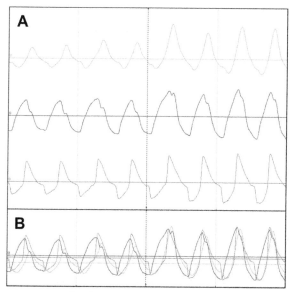

Fig. 1. Simultaneous outputs for the RIP bands and the flow pneumatograph, as measured in a normal dog. Note changes in the wave form from the left to the right, due to the administration of a respiratory stimulant doxapram. (*A*) The upper trace represents thoracic measures, the middle trace is obtained from the abdominal band, and the bottom trace represents pneumotach data. (*B*) Overlay of the 3 outputs.

sensitivity of RIP bands allows for comparative analysis of thoracic and abdominal contributions to changes in lung volume. Respiratory software (lox version 2.5.1.10, EMKA Technologies Inc, Falls Church, VA) records not only individual values for thoracic and abdominal contributions to total lung volume but also sums the total values. Therefore, measures can be expressed both as absolute measures of thoracic or abdominal values and as percentages of the whole. Accordingly, the authors have used RIP to provide a measure of progressive diaphragmatic weakness in the XLMTM dog. Other advantages of respiratory impedance plethysmography are that it is noninvasive and is unaffected by atmospheric conditions such as temperature and humidity. It should be noted that there are provisions in the software to record these details.

Transdiaphragmatic Pressure

A direct assessment of the pressure gradient above and below the diaphragm (transdiaphragmatic pressure) can be used to assess the strength of this critical respiratory muscle. As previously discussed, pressure changes are an established way of assessing strength and endurance of the diaphragm of human patients in the clinic, as well as its fatigability, and are therefore an autologous method in the dog.[28,70,71] For this technique balloon pressure catheters are placed above and below the diaphragm, the first placed at the mid-thoracic esophagus and the second in the stomach (**Fig. 2**). The esophageal balloon catheter is inflated with 0.5 mL of air and the gastric balloon with 1 mL of air.[72] Pressure change at each balloon, caused by movement of the diaphragm, is converted by a pressure transducer into a measured electrical signal, which generates a recorded waveform (**Fig. 3**).

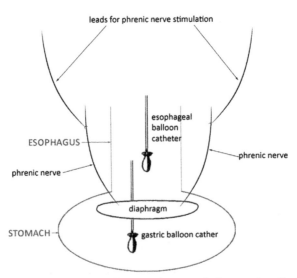

Fig. 2. Placement of each of the balloon catheters relative to the diaphragm for the measurement of transdiaphragmatic pressure in the dog. Phrenic nerve stimulation causes the diaphragm to contract, and results in pressure changes above and below this muscle. Pressure changes are proportional to the force elicited by the contracting diaphragm. This method provides an assessment of strength in the diaphragm muscle of the dog.

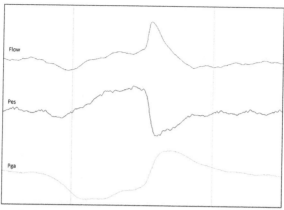

Fig. 3. Screenshot of observed esophageal (Pes) and gastric (Pga) pressures, as compared with flow data collected by the pneumatograph at 40-Hz (for 3 seconds) stimulation of the phrenic nerve in an XLMTM dog.

Transdiaphragmatic pressure (Pdi) is then calculated as the differences between gastric (Pga) and esophageal (Pes) pressures:

$$Pdi = Pga - Pes$$

The authors induced contraction of the diaphragm using phrenic nerve stimulation. Under general gas anesthesia, 2 50-mm 26-gauge pin electrodes were placed percutaneously into the sternothyroideus muscle bellies for bilateral stimulation of the phrenic nerve. Accurate placement of the electrodes was ensured by measuring twitch responses using a Grass stimulator. Voluntary respiration was temporarily suspended and apnea induced with a single bolus dose of intravenous anesthetic propofol, and twitch confirmed visually as a rapid change in either Pga or Pes. Once placement was confirmed, simultaneous bilateral phrenic nerve stimulation was performed, first at 1 Hz and then from 10 to 80 Hz in 10-Hz increments.

Though useful, the authors found this method to have limited application in the canine XLMTM model. First, because of the need for dissection to isolate and stimulate the phrenic nerves, this method often can only be used in terminal experiments. Such placement of the leads requires trained personnel with the necessary surgical skill and experience. The authors succeeded in percutaneous placement of the leads with variable reliability, and this method added considerable time and complexity to the procedure. Ensuring that the leads remained in place during the course of the experiment is challenging, both in the surgical and percutaneous placements, often requiring 2 or more people to manually hold both electrodes in place. Shifting of the balloons, especially the gastric balloon, during stimulation can affect the data. Movement of the catheters during stimulation can be mitigated by creating various catheter designs or by making changes in placement order of the electrodes versus the catheters, and by including restraint techniques such as taping to the surgical table, the mouth, or the muzzle of the dog. However, those catheters sturdy enough to remain in position are typically not sensitive enough to appreciably register pressure changes, while the more sensitive balloons rarely remain in position. As such, obtaining a consistent result using this method can prove challenging.

In the authors' initial experiments of respiratory function, dogs were challenged with the respiratory stimulant doxapram. Doxapram is thought to act on the respiratory centers of the central nervous system; in particular it acts on the carotid chemoreceptors and subsequently causes stimulation of the respiratory center,[73] but may also have some peripheral activity.[74] It is known to increase respiratory rate and tidal volumes, and this response is dependent on the size of the administered dose. Doxapram's short duration of action and rapid metabolism made it a suitable choice for these studies.[75]

The authors administered doxapram by intravenous bolus to test dogs both at single and in escalating doses. Using the RIP bands in conjunction with flow plethysmography (calibrated using a 1-L supersyringe), data were collected in anesthetized dogs. Measures included tidal volume, respiratory rate, inspiratory and expiratory flow, and thoracic and abdominal volume changes. Data were collected in a total of 6 dogs at 3 time points, including a terminal end point. RIP values, obtained at a baseline before the administration of doxapram and then after each dose, were analyzed using the software ecgAUTO v2.8.1.25 (EMKA Technologies Inc), while Iox software was used to analyze pneumatographic values. Point values obtained for a fixed interval of time were also compared between affected dogs and their unaffected control littermates to identify potential trends and changes over time.

The authors found significant differences ($P = .05$) between wild-type and XLMTM dogs in tidal volume, respiratory rate, and the calculated minute ventilation for pneumatograph-derived and RIP-derived values, trends that were maintained at each of the 3 time points at which data were collected. The sensitivity and accuracy of the RIP technique were also demonstrated, illustrated by the close agreement between pneumatograph and RIP measures (**Fig. 4**); this is also supported by visual analysis of the raw traces (see **Fig. 1**).

In this model of XLMTM, respiratory dysfunction is most clearly illustrated by 3 measures:

1. The inspiratory and expiratory flow rates (**Fig. 5**A, B)
2. The inspiratory and expiratory durations, especially the inspiratory duration (see **Fig. 5**C, D)
3. The percent abdominal contribution to the volume change due to respiration (see **Fig. 5**E).

Air-flow rates are significantly reduced in affected animals (see **Fig. 5**) despite significantly higher inspiratory durations. Most noticeably, inspiratory duration decreases in the XLMTM dog following doxapram stimulation, demonstrating the marked differences observed in the wild-type littermate control. This finding is consistent with respiratory muscle weakness, which renders the XLMTM dogs unable to respond normally to respiratory challenge. Moreover, increased respiratory flow, reduced inspiratory duration, and a return to a normal response to respiratory challenge can be measured and used as clinical indicators of improved respiratory function after treatment.

Using the RIP bands the thoracic and abdominal measures can be examined separately, both as absolute values and in terms of what percentage change in the total volume can be attributed to a change at either the thoracic or the abdominal band. This analysis allows one to determine whether observed changes are due to diaphragmatic weakness, as indicated by the abdominal band. In affected dogs, the fractional abdominal contribution decreases under the effects of respiratory stimulation; this is markedly different from what occurs in wild-type dogs, where respiratory challenge causes an increased abdominal contribution. The abdominal contribution to total volume falls to values significantly lower than those observed in normal wild-type littermates. Thus, the authors attribute the observed respiratory dysfunction to loss of strength in the diaphragm. The percentage of abdominal contribution to the tidal

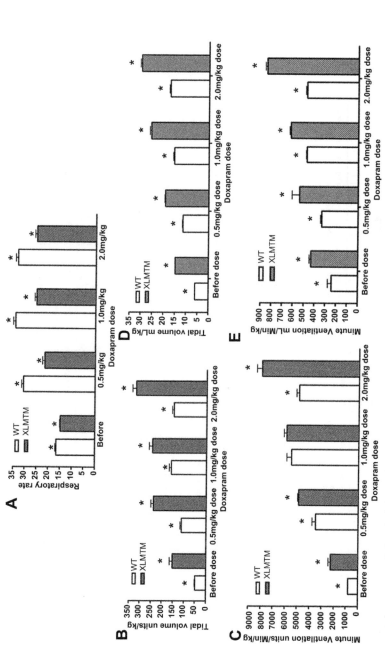

Fig. 4. Measures taken over serially administered doxapram doses, in affected XLMTM and unaffected wild-type (WT) control dogs. (*A–C*) Impedance-derived values of respiratory rate (*A*), tidal volume (*B*), and minute ventilation (*C*) (n = 3 for each group, for a total of 6 animals). Respiratory and minute ventilation are here expressed as the arbitrary "mL" units assigned by the Iox program, and represent relative values. (*D, E*) Pneumotach-derived values of tidal volume (*D*) and minute ventilation (*E*) (n = 1 for each group, for a total of 2 animals). Values here are actual, as calibrated by 1-L supersyringe at the time of collection.

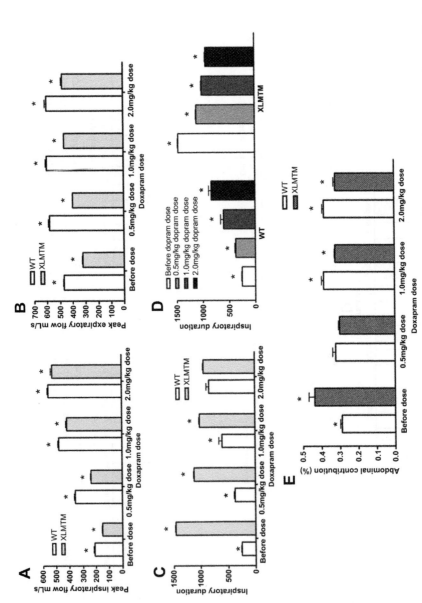

Fig. 5. (A, B) Pneumatometer-derived values of peak inspiratory and expiratory flow, as well as inspiratory duration compared across the dosage (C) and between each group (D) (n = 1 for each group, for a total of 2 animals). (E) Impedance-derived values of the abdominal contribution to respiration, expressed as a percentage.

volume can be used as a preclinical end point in the course of investigating new drugs or treatments.

SUMMARY

Animal models of NMDs (such as XLMTM) have been established and subsequently defined. Some models (such as the mouse) play critical roles in identifying associated pathology, investigating the biological mechanisms of the disease, and determining the safety and efficacy of potential treatments. However, their ability to accurately recreate the state of the disease in the patient can be limited, due to size or to the means by which the disease state must be approximated; this holds particularly true in the case of the assessment of respiratory dysfunction associated with NMDs. Methods used to assess respiratory function must be accurate and sensitive enough to measure subtle changes over the progression of the disease. The ability to follow changes allows for the evaluation of treatment outcomes for NMD. The XLMTM dog, as a naturally occurring, large animal model, is a suitable analogue of the XLMTM patient. The size of the dog provides the opportunity to use techniques that are prohibited in smaller models such as the mouse. Indeed, many of the methods used to measure inspiratory and expiratory muscle weakness in the clinic can be applied to the dog model to improve translational applications of tested treatments. When coupled with RIP, quantitative descriptions of respiratory efficacy establish preclinical end points for the testing of new therapeutics.

REFERENCES

1. Mehta S. Neuromuscular disease causing acute respiratory failure. Respir Care 2006;51(9):1016–21 [discussion: 1021–3].
2. Shahrizaila N, Kinnear WJ, Wills AJ. Respiratory involvement in inherited primary muscle conditions. J Neurol Neurosurg Psychiatry 2006;77(10):1108–15.
3. Racca F, Del Sorbo L, Mongini T, et al. Respiratory management of acute respiratory failure in neuromuscular diseases. Minerva Anestesiol 2010;76(1):51–62.
4. Howard RS, Wiles CM, Hirsch NP, et al. Respiratory involvement in primary muscle disorders: assessment and management. Q J Med 1993;86(3):175–89.
5. Mellies U, Lofaso F. Pompe disease: a neuromuscular disease with respiratory muscle involvement. Respir Med 2009;103(4):477–84.
6. Hahn A, Bach JR, Delaubier A, et al. Clinical implications of maximal respiratory pressure determinations for individuals with Duchenne muscular dystrophy. Arch Phys Med Rehabil 1997;78(1):1–6.
7. Bach JR, O'Brien J, Krotenberg R, et al. Management of end stage respiratory failure in Duchenne muscular dystrophy. Muscle Nerve 1987;10(2):177–82.
8. Park JH, Kang SW, Lee SC, et al. How respiratory muscle strength correlates with cough capacity in patients with respiratory muscle weakness. Yonsei Med J 2010; 51(3):392–7.
9. Kang SW, Kang YS, Sohn HS, et al. Respiratory muscle strength and cough capacity in patients with Duchenne muscular dystrophy. Yonsei Med J 2006; 47(2):184–90.
10. Pellegrini N, Laforet P, Orlikowski D, et al. Respiratory insufficiency and limb muscle weakness in adults with Pompe's disease. Eur Respir J 2005;26(6): 1024–31.
11. Wokke JH, Escolar DM, Pestronk A, et al. Clinical features of late-onset Pompe disease: a prospective cohort study. Muscle Nerve 2008;38(4):1236–45.

12. Kaindl AM, Guenther UP, Rudnik-Schoneborn S, et al. Spinal muscular atrophy with respiratory distress type 1 (SMARD1). J Child Neurol 2008;23(2):199–204.
13. Piepers S, van den Berg LH, Brugman F, et al. A natural history study of late onset spinal muscular atrophy types 3b and 4. J Neurol 2008;255(9):1400–4.
14. Griggs RC, Donohoe KM, Utell MJ, et al. Evaluation of pulmonary function in neuromuscular disease. Arch Neurol 1981;38(1):9–12.
15. Braun NM, Arora NS, Rochester DF. Respiratory muscle and pulmonary function in polymyositis and other proximal myopathies. Thorax 1983;38(8):616–23.
16. Fromageot C, Lofaso F, Annane D, et al. Supine fall in lung volumes in the assessment of diaphragmatic weakness in neuromuscular disorders. Arch Phys Med Rehabil 2001;82(1):123–8.
17. Allen J. Pulmonary complications of neuromuscular disease: a respiratory mechanics perspective. Paediatr Respir Rev 2010;11(1):18–23.
18. Vincken W, Elleker MG, Cosio MG. Determinants of respiratory muscle weakness in stable chronic neuromuscular disorders. Am J Med 1987;82(1):53–8.
19. Black LF, Hyatt RE. Maximal respiratory pressures: normal values and relationship to age and sex. Am Rev Respir Dis 1969;99(5):696–702.
20. Wilson SH, Cooke NT, Edwards RH, et al. Predicted normal values for maximal respiratory pressures in Caucasian adults and children. Thorax 1984;39(7): 535–8.
21. Harikumar G, Moxham J, Greenough A, et al. Measurement of maximal inspiratory pressure in ventilated children. Pediatr Pulmonol 2008;43(11):1085–91.
22. Truwit JD, Marini JJ. Validation of a technique to assess maximal inspiratory pressure in poorly cooperative patients. Chest 1992;102(4):1216–9.
23. ATS/ERS. ATS/ERS Statement on respiratory muscle testing. Am J Respir Crit Care Med 2002;166(4):518–624.
24. Hart N, Polkey MI, Sharshar T, et al. Limitations of sniff nasal pressure in patients with severe neuromuscular weakness. J Neurol Neurosurg Psychiatry 2003; 74(12):1685–7.
25. Nava S, Ambrosino N, Crotti P, et al. Recruitment of some respiratory muscles during three maximal inspiratory manoeuvres. Thorax 1993;48(7):702–7.
26. Terzi N, Orlikowski D, Fermanian C, et al. Measuring inspiratory muscle strength in neuromuscular disease: one test or two? Eur Respir J 2008;31(1):93–8.
27. Steier J, Kaul S, Seymour J, et al. The value of multiple tests of respiratory muscle strength. Thorax 2007;62(11):975–80.
28. de Torres JP, Talamo C, Aguirre-Jaime A, et al. Electromyographic validation of the mouth pressure-time index: a noninvasive assessment of inspiratory muscle load. Respir Med 2003;97(9):1006–13.
29. Beck J, Weinberg J, Hamnegard CH, et al. Diaphragmatic function in advanced Duchenne muscular dystrophy. Neuromuscul Disord 2006;16(3):161–7.
30. Bolton CF. Phrenic nerve conduction studies: technical aspects and normative data. Muscle Nerve 2008;38(6):1658–9.
31. Perrin C, Unterborn JN, Ambrosio CD, et al. Pulmonary complications of chronic neuromuscular diseases and their management. Muscle Nerve 2004;29(1):5–27.
32. Bellemare F, Grassino A. Effect of pressure and timing of contraction on human diaphragm fatigue. J Appl Physiol 1982;53(5):1190–5.
33. Misuri G, Lanini B, Gigliotti F, et al. Mechanism of CO(2) retention in patients with neuromuscular disease. Chest 2000;117(2):447–53.
34. Nava S, Rubini F, Zanotti E, et al. The tension-time index of the diaphragm revisited in quadriplegic patients with diaphragm pacing. Am J Respir Crit Care Med 1996;153(4 Pt 1):1322–7.

35. Chaudri MB, Liu C, Hubbard R, et al. Relationship between supramaximal flow during cough and mortality in motor neurone disease. Eur Respir J 2002;19(3): 434–8.

36. Polkey MI, Lyall RA, Green M, et al. Expiratory muscle function in amyotrophic lateral sclerosis. Am J Respir Crit Care Med 1998;158(3):734–41.

37. Man WD, Kyroussis D, Fleming TA, et al. Cough gastric pressure and maximum expiratory mouth pressure in humans. Am J Respir Crit Care Med 2003;168(6): 714–7.

38. Noguchi S, Fujita M, Murayama K, et al. Gene expression analyses in X-linked myotubular myopathy. Neurology 2005;65(5):732–7.

39. Jungbluth H, Wallgren-Pettersson C, Laporte J. Centronuclear (myotubular) myopathy. Orphanet J Rare Dis 2008;3:26.

40. Laporte J, Biancalana V, Tanner SM, et al. MTM1 mutations in X-linked myotubular myopathy. Hum Mutat 2000;15(5):393–409.

41. Mruk DD, Cheng CY. The myotubularin family of lipid phosphatases in disease and in spermatogenesis. Biochem J 2011;433(2):253–62.

42. Herman GE, Finegold M, Zhao W, et al. Medical complications in long-term survivors with X-linked myotubular myopathy. J Pediatr 1999;134(2):206–14.

43. Spiro AJ, Shy GM, Gonatas NK. Myotubular myopathy. Persistence of fetal muscle in an adolescent boy. Arch Neurol 1966;14(1):1–14.

44. Fardeau M. Congenital myopathies. In: Mastaglia FL, Detchant LWO, editors. Skeletal muscle pathology. Edinburgh (UK); New York: Churchill Livingstone; 1992. p. 1177.

45. Beggs AH, Böhm J, Snead E, et al. MTM1 mutation associated with X-linked myotubular myopathy in Labrador Retrievers. Proc Natl Acad Sci U S A 2010; 107(33):14697–702.

46. Murphy DJ. Comprehensive non-clinical respiratory evaluation of promising new drugs. Toxicol Appl Pharmacol 2005;207(Suppl 2):414–24.

47. Cummings JF. Nervous system. In: Andrews EJ, Ward BC, Altman NH, editors. Spontaneous animal models of human disease. vol. 2. New York: Academic Press; 1997. p. 109.

48. Dowling JJ, Vreede AP, Low SE, et al. Loss of myotubularin function results in T-tubule disorganization in zebrafish and human myotubular myopathy. PLoS Genet 2009;5(2):e1000372.

49. Buj-Bello A, Laugel V, Messaddeq N, et al. The lipid phosphatase myotubularin is essential for skeletal muscle maintenance but not for myogenesis in mice. Proc Natl Acad Sci U S A 2002;99(23):15060–5.

50. Arruda VR, Stedman HH, Nichols TC, et al. Regional intravascular delivery of AAV-2-F.IX to skeletal muscle achieves long-term correction of hemophilia B in a large animal model. Blood 2005;105(9):3458–64.

51. Zhang G, Budker V, Wolff JA. High levels of foreign gene expression in hepatocytes after tail vein injections of naked plasmid DNA. Hum Gene Ther 1999; 10(10):1735–7.

52. Jungbluth H, Wallgren-Pettersson C, Laporte JF, et al. 164th ENMC International workshop: 6th workshop on centronuclear (myotubular) myopathies, 16-18th January 2009, Naarden, The Netherlands. Neuromuscul Disord 2009;19(10): 721–9.

53. Shimatsu Y, Katagiri K, Furuta T, et al. Canine X-linked muscular dystrophy in Japan (CXMDJ). Exp Anim 2003;52(2):93–7.

54. Hrapkiewicz K, Medina L. Clinical laboratory animal medicine. 3rd edition. Ames: Blackwell Publishing; 2007.

55. Cunningham J. Textbook of veterinary physiology. 2nd edition. Philadelphia: W.B. Saunders Company; 1997.

56. Evans HE. Miller's anatomy of the dog. 3rd edition. Philadelphia: W.B. Saunders Company; 1993.

57. Johnston S, Kustiritz M, Olson P. Canine and feline theriogenology. St. Louis: W.B. Saunders Company; 2001.

58. Feldman EC, Nelson RW. Canine and feline endocrinology and reproduction. 3rd edition. St. Louis: W.B. Saunders; 2004.

59. Cooper BJ, Winand NJ, Stedman H, et al. The homologue of the Duchenne locus is defective in X-linked muscular dystrophy of dogs. Nature 1988;334(6178): 154–6.

60. Paoloni M, Khanna C. Translation of new cancer treatments from pet dogs to humans. Nat Rev Cancer 2008;8(2):147–56.

61. Cosford KL, Taylor SM, Thompson L, et al. A possible new inherited myopathy in a young Labrador retriever. Can Vet J 2008;49(4):393–7.

62. Shelton GD. Neuromuscular disorders affecting young dogs and cats. Vet Neurol Neurosurg J 1999;1(1):1.

63. Valentine BA, Cooper BJ, de Lahunta A, et al. Canine X-linked muscular dystrophy. An animal model of Duchenne muscular dystrophy: clinical studies. J Neurol Sci 1988;88(1–3):69–81.

64. Kornegay JN, Tuler SM, Miller DM, et al. Muscular dystrophy in a litter of golden retriever dogs. Muscle Nerve 1988;11(10):1056–64.

65. Kornegay JN, Bogan JR, Bogan DJ, et al. Golden retriever muscular dystrophy (GRMD): Developing and maintaining a colony and physiological functional measurements. Methods Mol Biol 2011;709:105–23.

66. Shimatsu Y, Yoshimura M, Yuasa K, et al. Major clinical and histopathological characteristics of canine X-linked muscular dystrophy in Japan, CXMDJ. Acta Myol 2005;24(2):145–54.

67. Jaber S, Petrof BJ, Jung B, et al. Rapidly progressive diaphragmatic weakness and injury during mechanical ventilation in humans. Am J Respir Crit Care Med 2011;183(3):364–71.

68. Kearney K, Metea M, Gleason T, et al. Evaluation of respiratory function in freely moving Beagle dogs using implanted impedance technology. J Pharmacol Toxicol Methods 2010;62(2):119–26.

69. Murphy DJ, Renninger JP, Schramek D. Respiratory inductive plethysmography as a method for measuring ventilatory parameters in conscious, non-restrained dogs. J Pharmacol Toxicol Methods 2010;62(1):47–53.

70. Marini JJ, Rodriguez RM, Lamb V. Bedside estimation of the inspiratory work of breathing during mechanical ventilation. Chest 1986;89(1):56–63.

71. Laghi F, Cattapan SE, Jubran A, et al. Is weaning failure caused by low-frequency fatigue of the diaphragm? Am J Respir Crit Care Med 2003;167(2):120–7.

72. Hubmayr RD, Sprung J, Nelson S. Determinants of transdiaphragmatic pressure in dogs. J Appl Physiol 1990;69(6):2050–6.

73. Papich MG. Saunders. In: Winkel A, acquisitions editor, Slaten, M, development editor. Handbook of veterinary drugs. St Louis (MO): W.B. Saunders; 2007. p. 22.

74. Muir W, Hubbell J. Handbook of veterinary anesthesia. 3rd edition. St Louis: Mosby; 2000.

75. Yost CS. A new look at the respiratory stimulant doxapram. CNS Drug Rev 2006; 12(3–4):236–49.

New Opportunities and Novel Paradigms to Support Neuromuscular Research

Richard Lieber, PhD[a,b,c,]*, Samuel Ward, PT, PhD[a,c,d],
Lawrence Frank, PhD[b,d], Simon Schenk, PhD[a]

KEYWORDS

- Rehabilitation research • Muscle research • Muscle histology
- Muscle biomechanics • Muscle imaging • Muscle metabolism

Key Points

1. Understand the organizational structure and function of the National Skeletal Muscle Research Center (NSMRC)

2. Identify potential opportunities for collaboration with the NSMRC for clinicians interested in muscle research

---

Rehabilitation clinician-scientists often encounter a variety of primary and secondary diseases that are associated with skeletal muscle. Although muscular dystrophy, sarcopenia, and tendinitis are familiar skeletal muscle problems, diseases with cerebrovascular, coronary artery, and arthritic causes also affect skeletal muscle. Perhaps most importantly, most rehabilitation treatment strategies, regardless of the clinical entity, are directed toward or through skeletal muscle. Currently, scientific investigations in rehabilitation lack state-of-the-art, quantitative tools for measuring acute and chronic skeletal muscle changes. It is unreasonable to expect rehabilitation clinician-scientists to master the myriad of techniques necessary to study skeletal muscle or to put them in proper perspective when choosing methods. To address this methodological and knowledge void, The Medical Rehabilitation Research Infrastructure Network

---

This work was supported in part by NSMRC R24 HD650837.

[a] Department of Orthopaedic Surgery, University of California San Diego, 9500 Gilman Drive (Mail Code 0863), La Jolla, San Diego, CA 92093, USA
[b] Research Service, VA San Diego Healthcare System, San Diego, CA, USA
[c] Department of Bioengineering, University of California San Diego, San Diego, CA, USA
[d] Department of Radiology, University of California San Diego, San Diego, CA, USA
* Corresponding author. Department of Orthopaedic Surgery, University of California San Diego, 9500 Gilman Drive (Mail Code 0863), La Jolla, San Diego, CA 92093.
E-mail address: rlieber@ucsd.edu

Phys Med Rehabil Clin N Am 23 (2012) 95–105
doi:10.1016/j.pmr.2011.11.015
1047-9651/12/$ – see front matter Published by Elsevier Inc.

(MRRIN), funded by The National Institute of Child Health and Human Development (NICHD), through the National Center for Medical Rehabilitation Research (NCMRR), the National Institute for Neurologic Disorders and Stroke (NINDS), and the National Institute of Biomedical Imaging and Bioengineering (NIBIB), was created to facilitate access for physicians to experts, technology, and resources from scientific fields related to medical rehabilitation.

The MRRIN comprises 7 research centers, including the NSMRC of the University of California, San Diego (UCSD). The NSMRC consists of 5 core units that span 3 departmental boundaries and 2 schools within the university. The 5 cores are Muscle Histology, Muscle Biomechanics, Muscle Imaging, Muscle Metabolism, and Program Administration. The program is structured to foster cooperation and synergy across cores (**Fig. 1**). This organization facilitates interaction among the program faculty and minimizes the overhead needed to accomplish rehabilitation research. Each of these cores is a strong research force at the UCSD and within the international research community. Thus, the strength of this infrastructure program is that it leverages existing strongholds of muscle research at UCSD and makes these resources readily available to the rehabilitation community within the United States. Another strength of the program is that it is based at UCSD, which is a major research University in the United States, and worldwide.

The NSMRC has been successful in equipping rehabilitation medicine professionals with the necessary tools to study muscle in the context of clinical problems and in attracting scientists to study skeletal muscle in a rehabilitation context. Since its inception in July 2005, the NSMRC has offered 6 symposia, and joined with such prestigious organizations as the Rehabilitation Institute of Chicago and the American

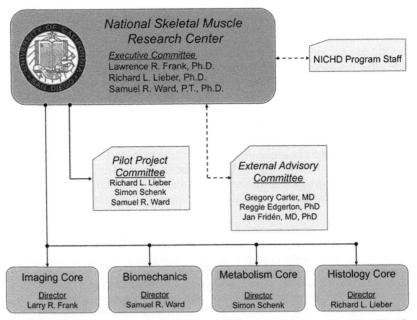

Fig. 1. Organizational chart for the NSMRC. This center crosses 3 departments and 2 schools within the University of California, San Diego (UCSD). The program is accountable to UCSD as well as to the National Institutes of Health (NIH)/NICHD program staff, and the external advisory committee. Accountability and 2-way communication are indicated by the dashed connecting lines. This structure has functioned effectively since July 2005. The Administration Core interacts with each scientific core as well as all other committees and is thus not explicitly shown.

Physical Therapy Association to sponsor 2 additional symposia. The NSMRC has also played a supporting role for several other NICHD-funded centers across the United States to provide muscle expertise or to train core directors. In addition, and most importantly, in the past 6 years, the program has funded $625,000 in pilot projects for 25 faculty members at 13 universities across the United States, resulting in many publications and National Institutes of Health (NIH) grant submissions. Although it was expected that career advancement and improved productivity would result from these pilot projects, some of the more subjective effects (prestige of independent funding, making scientific connections, learning and applying state-of-the-art methodologies) are almost equally important.

CORE DESCRIPTIONS
Histology Core

Skeletal muscle histology has a long and distinguished presence at the UCSD. Under the direction of Dr Richard Lieber and housed in the UCSD Department of Orthopaedic Surgery, skeletal muscle studies have been produced in large number since 1981. From the early studies describing skeletal muscle from normal and diseased tissues,[1] to more recent studies that show more subtle changes that occur in skeletal muscle after injury from exercise or disease (as reported in Refs.[2,3]), the Histology Core has been at the forefront of the development of new methodologies and new approaches to studying skeletal muscle tissue (**Fig. 2**). Many tools are available to the Histology Core. Traditional histologic methods such as paraffin embedding, frozen sectioning, and traditional histologic stains are available. However, the Histology Core is also able to perform immunohistochemical staining and correlate antibody stains with quantitative approaches and composition even on a single-cell basis. As an example

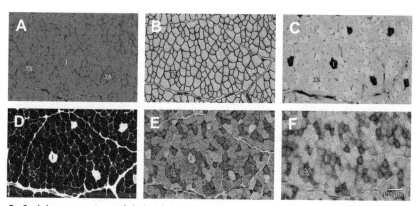

Fig. 2. Serial cross sections of skeletal muscle under various staining conditions. (*A*) Hematoxylin and eosin, showing general muscle fiber morphology. (*B*) Dystrophin immunohistochemistry showing the sarcolemmal association of this protein. (*C*) Myofibrillar ATPase under acid preincubation conditions. Under these conditions, slow fibers stain darkly, as do the extracellular capillaries, whereas fast fibers stain lightly. (*D*) Myofibrillar ATPase under alkaline preincubation conditions. Under these conditions, slow fibers stain lightly, whereas fast fibers stain darkly. Note that in both panels (*C*) and (*D*), fast fiber staining intensity occurs at 2 levels. (*E*) Immunohistochemical reaction for fast myosin heavy chain antibody. In rat skeletal muscle, this antibody (SC71) stains type 2A fibers darkly and type 2X fibers more lightly, and is negative for types 2B and 1 fibers. (*F*) Succinate dehydrogenase (SDH), used to show muscle fiber oxidative capacity. (*Modified from* Lieber RL. Skeletal muscle structure, function, and plasticity. 3rd edition. Philadelphia: Lippincott Williams & Wilkins; 2010; with permission.)

of this technically demanding approach, the MRRPM NSMRC quantified the amount of various myosin heavy chains present in single cells of frog skeletal muscle fibers using correlative immunohistochemistry, quantitative Western blots, and reverse transcription/polymerase chain reaction (RT/PCR).[4] There is thus virtually no protein structure or complex within skeletal muscle that cannot currently be studied by the Histology Core at the structural level, at least with the aid of the light microscope. In addition, the Histology Core has performed detailed quantitative analysis of skeletal muscle ultrastructure in exercised tissue[5] and transgenic animal models.[6] It has also combined forces with the Imaging Core and Biomechanics Core to develop methods for real-time imaging of single muscle cells during biomechanical loading.[7,8] The Histology Core was used by 17 of the 25 projects supported by our infrastructure program from July 2005 to September 2011, making it the most heavily used core.

Biomechanics Core

The muscle Biomechanics Core uses numerous approaches for biomechanical testing of muscles and muscle-related structures in a variety of settings. The Biomechanics Core is flexible and powerful in its ability to perform routine and advanced biomechanical studies. For example, standard facilities for performing laser diffraction of isolated skeletal muscles permit muscle architectural determination.[9,10] Measurement of muscle architecture describes the most important single structural feature of a muscle that predicts function.[11] To determine muscle architectural properties, fixed tissues are harvested, processed, and small bundles are isolated from the muscles. Muscle fiber bundles (consisting of 5–50 muscle fibers) are isolated and then sarcomere length (SL) of the isolated fiber bundles is determined by laser diffraction (**Fig. 3**). This line of research has been extremely fruitful and was one of the main reasons that the Biomechanics Core received the 2003 Nicolas Andry Award from the Association for Bone and Joint Surgeons.[12]

Imaging Core

The Imaging Core consists of some of the most diverse and powerful sets of tools available within the program, capable of imaging both anatomy and physiology from the whole body to the cellular level. State-of-the-art 3T GE human and 7T Bruker animal magnetic resonance imaging (MRI) research scanners are located at the UCSD Center for Functional MRI (CFMRI). The CFMRI has research agreements with both GE and Bruker that allow researchers to develop novel MRI acquisition methods (pulse sequences) using proprietary scanner software and hardware, making this a unique environment for collaborative development of novel, cutting-edge muscle MRI methodologies. Resources are also available within the UCSD Department of Radiology for other imaging modalities, such as positron emission tomography (PET), including the cyclotron for generation of high-energy particles.

UCSD is renowned for its collaborative efforts that routinely cross departmental boundaries. For example, state-of-the-art imaging facilities are housed in the UCSD Department of Radiology (MRI, computed tomography, PET, ultrasound), Department of Bioengineering (atomic force microscope, scanning electron microscopy, three-dimensional [3D] histologic reconstruction), and Department of Orthopedic Surgery (light, electron, and confocal microscopy), which facilitates the application of multimodal imaging, sophisticated image analysis, and high-end visualization to a wide range of clinical and basic science problems. All MRI facilities are available for use in human rehabilitation and animal experimentation. Although structural imaging is typically performed using a 1.5-T imaging system, the NSMRC's access to state-of-the-art 3-T systems allows the achievement of higher quality in anatomic imaging and

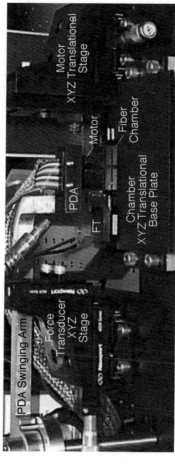

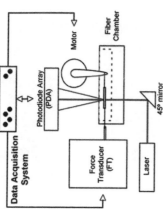

Fig. 3. Apparatus used for a single fiber, a small fiber bundle, or even whole-muscle mechanical studies. A specimen is flanked on either side by a force transducer (FT) and motor in a chamber of physiologic solution. The specimen is transilluminated by an optical laser that creates a diffraction pattern (*red lines*) that is incident on a photodiode array (PDA). Devices are synchronized and data acquired at rates ranging from 1000 Hz (force) to 100 kHz (PDA) to guard against signal aliasing.

provides unique opportunities to probe physiologic processes. Pulse sequences such as 3D fast spoiled gradient echo (using the following parameters: repetition time, 7.7 milliseconds; echo time, 2.2 milliseconds; flip angle, 60°; number of excitations, 2; field of view, 12×12 cm; matrix, 512×512; slice thickness, 1 mm) yield voxel resolutions of 0.23×0.23×1 mm and contrasts highly enough to rapidly and accurately digitally separate (ie, segment) tissues of interest, from which can be derived geometric properties such as volume and surface area. This type of imaging may allow researchers to acquire and analyze musculoskeletal structures in ways that were previously not possible. Using these imaging, segmentation, and reconstruction algorithms, whole muscles from humans can be analyzed and archived for future studies (**Fig. 4**).

Muscle Metabolism Core

Lifestyle diseases (eg, insulin resistance and type 2 diabetes), musculoskeletal injury (eg, rotator cuff tear), and musculoskeletal diseases (eg, muscular dystrophy) are associated with alterations in skeletal muscle metabolism.[13,14] In many cases, the metabolic machinery is so deranged that intramuscular fat tissue accumulates. Improving muscle function and capacity is a central tenet of successful rehabilitation and, because skeletal muscle metabolism is intimately linked to muscle function, metabolism is intimately linked with rehabilitation. Accordingly, to design effective rehabilitation strategies, it is important to understand the response of muscle metabolic networks to disease and altered recruitment patterns.

To address these types of issues, the Muscle Metabolism Core was created. The goal of the Metabolism Core is to permit investigators to undertake state-of-the-art research related to skeletal muscle metabolism with an integrative, translational, bench-to-bedside approach. The core specializes in many facets of the metabolic phenotyping of skeletal muscle, both in vivo, ex vivo, and in vitro. Examples of such human-based and animal-based approaches include the assessment of whole-body substrate metabolism, the metabolism of specific substrates (such as glucose, fatty acids, and amino acids), and the use of a variety of validated biochemical techniques.

To allow investigators to more clearly identify their research needs, the Metabolism Core is divided into 3 primary areas of investigation: clinical and integrative research, basic science animal research (**Fig. 5**), and biochemical research.

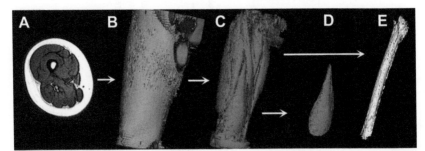

Fig. 4. Example of segmentation used to render and calculate muscle volume for a vastus medialis. (*A*) Serial contiguous slices are acquired. (*B*) Serial images are reconstructed into the entire thigh. (*C*) Muscles are distinguished from the other tissues to represent total muscle volume. (*D*) Vastus medialis muscle is isolated from the entire muscle volume and volume calculated. (*E*) Bone length may also be obtained from the MRI reconstruction to yield scaling parameters between muscle properties and skeletal dimensions.

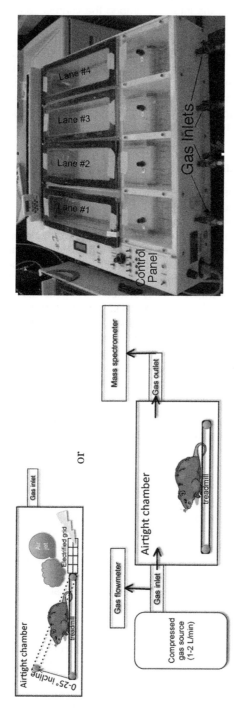

Fig. 5. Exercise training and/or physiologic testing (ie, maximal running speed, endurance run time) is performed on one of two 4-lane rodent treadmills (allowing up to 8 rodents to be trained/tested simultaneously). Treadmills also have motor lift device to increase treadmill incline (0°–25°). Measurement of oxygen (O_2) consumption and carbon dioxide (CO_2) production during exercise is made using a custom-designed airtight metabolic chamber made by modifying a motorized treadmill. Inspired and expired O_2 and CO_2 concentrations can be continuously measured using a mass spectrometer (Perkin-Elmer 1100, Pomona, CA, USA) and recorded (Acknowledge 3.7.1., Biopac Systems, Inc., Santa Barbara, CA, USA). Relative humidity and chamber temperature are also recorded from the gas outflow at the rear of the treadmill.

Administration Core

The Administration Core acts as the interface among the various cores and as the communication link with the university and the rehabilitation investigators throughout the country who require our infrastructure. The Administration Core is responsible for maintaining excellent communication among the core directors, for scheduling meetings among the core directors, and for assuring regulatory compliance for all animal and human subject protocols required to perform the experiments proposed by rehabilitation investigators. The information technology (IT) division of the Administration Core is responsible for the regular updating of the center's Web page. Currently, the Web page receives about 1000 hits per week.

NSMRC OPPORTUNITIES FOR REHABILITATION RESEARCHERS

The target clinical professionals for the NSMRC are physical therapists, physiatrists, neurologists, and occupational therapists. In addition, bioengineers, rehabilitation engineers, neuroscientists, and exercise physiologists are targeted. All of these researchers are interested in the restoration or improvement of movement after loss of function. The loss of function might be caused by such factors as postoperative muscle atrophy, stroke, spinal cord injury, head injury, chronic type II diabetes, peripheral nerve injury, or general trauma. All of these conditions result in loss of function that is caused, at least in part, by a decreased ability of muscles to generate force, or in the adaptation of muscle to a new pattern of use. Thus, the rehabilitation professional must have a basic background in systemic physiology and basic principles of motor control. Detailed knowledge of biomechanics or muscle is not required. One of the benefits of the NSMRC is the access to research professionals who can assist rehabilitation professionals with definition of important experimental variables as well as experimental design itself. The goal of the NSMRC is to be directly accessible to the average academic clinician and rehabilitation professional.

THE NSMRC SHARES ITS EXPERTISE IN MUSCLE WITH THE REHABILITATION COMMUNITY

Evidence of the commitment to teaching in rehabilitation is the third edition of Dr Lieber's[15] textbook entitled *Skeletal Muscle Structure, Function and Plasticity: Implications for Rehabilitation and Sports Medicine*. This book is presented in a user-friendly manner, in which the goal is to transmit the information in a clear and consistent manner, not to impress the reader with breadth or depth of knowledge. The NSMRC believes this is a critical educational attitude at a time when so many physicians have become disenfranchised from state-of-the-art research simply because of a lack of modern vocabulary. The textbook also serves as the foundation of the retreats/courses and Web-based educational seminars (ie, Webinars) offered by the NSMRC. Retreats/courses are held in La Jolla (CA) approximately twice per year. Past courses titles include *Functional Restoration of the Stroke Survivor, Skeletal Muscle Imaging, Basic Science and Application of Tendon Transfer Surgery, Mechanism Underlying Disordered Movement*, and *Workshop on Multi-Scale Muscle Mechanics*. Webinars are offered once per year; upcoming Webinars include *Fundamentals of MRI Physics, Fundamentals of Diffusion Tensor Imaging, Skeletal Muscle Histology Basics, Fundamentals of Human Exercise Physiology*, and *Fundamentals of Human Biomechanics*. Retreats/courses and Webinars are advertised in appropriate journals and on the NSMRC Web page.

The core directors consider the pilot project program to be the single most significant and most enjoyable part of the program because the funds awarded to (primarily)
young investigators provide a jump start to their careers for which they are very appre-
ciative. Pilot projects also permit the core directors to be involved in the academic
careers of these individuals in a mentor role.

During the previous funding cycle, 27 grants were awarded that averaged $23,221
for a total of $626,967 (about 35% of the total direct costs of the grant) and were
distributed across the cores fairly evenly. Most pilot projects were discussed with at
least 2 core directors. Seventy-five percent of the projects resulted in publication
and 45% resulted in submission of an NIH grant.

Criteria used to prioritize pilot project applications are presented in **Fig. 6**. Note that
the main purpose of this pilot project funding program is to generate sufficient data to
enable NIH funding of the resulting research. Thus, applicants are queried regarding the
ultimate funding goal. In addition, they are asked to provide a list of similar topics that
have been funded by the NIH based on a review of the CRISP (Computer Retrieval of
Information on Scientific Projects) database (http://crisp.cit.nih.gov) to give them

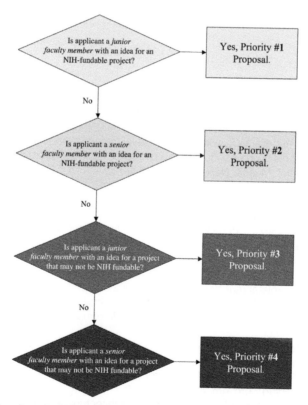

Fig. 6. Algorithm for prioritizing the pilot projects from rank #1 to rank #4. This secondary
ranking procedure establishes the priority for funding because projects from junior investigators tend to be emphasized and projects from investigators familiar with the core tend to
be emphasized. The net effect is to increase pilot project opportunities from junior faculty
with significant expertise in some aspect of muscle research (imaging, physiology, biomechanics, or metabolism). In all cases, the NSMRC is vigilant to define the level of grant
and manuscript productivity resulting from each pilot project.

experience on the database and to ensure that they are forward-thinking in their proposals. All of our policies were created to maintain the spirit of the R24 request for applications (RFA), which states:

> *There should be a formal process to solicit and review pilot proposals, and evaluate their potential to develop into successful NIH applications. Researchers associated with the infrastructure grant may be considered for pilot funding, but first priority should be researchers from other locations. The distribution of pilot funding will require negotiating with secondary institutions to transfer grant funds in the most efficient manner...*

Lastly, sabbatical opportunities available through the NSMRC are advertised strategically in professional journals and posted at the appropriate scientific meetings. As with pilot projects, applicants must have an MD and/or PhD degree and be in a rehabilitation-related field.

The NSMRC core directors invite interested researchers and clinicians to contact them regarding potential opportunities for collaboration. Please contact them with any questions through the NSMRC Web site at http://muscle.ucsd.edu/NSMRC/home.shtml.

REFERENCES

1. Lieber RL. Skeletal muscle adaptability II: muscle properties following spinal-cord injury. Dev Med Child Neurol 1986;28:533–42, 662–70.
2. Fridén J, Lieber RL, Thornell LE. Subtle indications of muscle damage following eccentric contractions. Acta Physiol Scand 1991;142:523–4.
3. Lieber RL, Runesson E, Einarsson F, et al. Inferior mechanical properties of spastic muscle bundles due to hypertrophic but compromised extracellular matrix material. Muscle Nerve 2003;28:464–71.
4. Lutz GJ, Cuizon DB, Ryan AF, et al. Four novel myosin heavy chain transcripts in *Rana pipiens* single muscle fibres define a molecular basis for muscle fibre types in the frog. J Physiol (Lond) 1998;508:667–80.
5. Mishra DK, Fridén J, Schmitz MC, et al. Antiinflammatory medication after muscle injury. A treatment resulting in short-term improvement but subsequent loss of muscle function. J Bone Joint Surg Am 1995;77:1510–9.
6. Shah S, Fridén J, Su FC, et al. Evidence for increased mobility of myofibrils in desmin null skeletal muscles. J Exp Biol 2002;205:321–5.
7. Shah SB, Davis J, Weisleder N, et al. Structural and functional roles of desmin in mouse skeletal muscle during passive deformation. Biophys J 2004;86: 2993–3008.
8. Shah S, Lieber RL. Real-time imaging and mechanical measurement of muscle cytoskeletal proteins. J Histochem Cytochem 2003;51:19–29.
9. Lieber RL, Fazeli BM, Botte MJ. Architecture of selected wrist flexor and extensor muscles. J Hand Surg Am 1990;15:244–50.
10. Lieber RL, Jacobson MD, Fazeli BM, et al. Architecture of selected muscles of the arm and forearm: anatomy and implications for tendon transfer. J Hand Surg Am 1992;17:787–98.
11. Lieber RL, Fridén J. Functional and clinical significance of skeletal muscle architecture. Muscle Nerve 2000;23:1647–66.
12. Lieber RL, Friden J. Implications of muscle design on surgical reconstruction of upper extremities. Clin Orthop Relat Res 2004;(419):267–79.

13. Savage DB, Petersen KF, Shulman GI. Disordered lipid metabolism and the pathogenesis of insulin resistance. Physiol Rev 2007;87:507–20.
14. Rubino LJ, Stills HF Jr, Sprott DC, et al. Fatty infiltration of the torn rotator cuff worsens over time in a rabbit model. Arthroscopy 2007;23:717–22.
15. Lieber R. Skeletal muscle structure, function, and plasticity: implications for rehabilitation and sports medicine. 2nd edition. Philadelphia: Lippincott Williams & Wilkins; 2002.

Skeletal Muscle Edema in Muscular Dystrophy: Clinical and Diagnostic Implications

Sandra L. Poliachik, PhD[a,b,*], Seth D. Friedman, PhD[c],
Gregory T. Carter, MD, MS[d], Shawn E. Parnell, MD[a,b],
Dennis W. Shaw, MD[a,b]

KEYWORDS

- Muscular dystrophy • MRI • Myoedema
- Neuromuscular disease

Numerous major forms of muscular dystrophy have been identified.[1] The type of muscular dystrophy influences the progression of muscle degradation and the pattern of muscle involvement (**Table 1**). An increasing number of defects in specific genes have been identified as the underlying cause of different forms of muscular dystrophy. Many of these genes encode for components of transmembrane and membrane-associated proteins that form a structural linkage between the F-actin cytoskeleton and the extracellular matrix in muscle. One example of this is the dystrophin–glycoprotein complex (DGC), an assembly of proteins that are organized into three subcomponents: the cytoskeletal proteins, sarcoglycans, and sarcospan.[2,3] Several of the subtypes of limb girdle muscular dystrophy (LGMD) arise from primary mutations in genes encoding components of this complex. At least four sarcoglycan subunits (α, β, γ, and δ subunits) are present in muscle, and mutations here also result in a form of muscular dystrophy. Alpha laminin-2 (LAMA2) is a basement membrane

This work was supported by a grant from the Friends of FSH Research.
[a] Department of Radiology, Seattle Children's Hospital, 4800 Sand Point Way NE, L-shaped Room, R-5417, Seattle, WA 98105, USA
[b] Seattle Children's Center for Clinical and Translational Research, Seattle Children's Hospital, 4800 Sand Point Way NE, L-shaped Room, R-5417, Seattle, WA 98105, USA
[c] Department of Radiology, Center for Clinical and Translational Research, Seattle Children's Hospital, Seattle, WA, USA
[d] Muscular Dystrophy Association, Regional Neuromuscular Center, 410 Providence Lane, Building 2, Olympia, WA 98506, USA
* Corresponding author. Department of Radiology, Seattle Children's Hospital, 4800 Sand Point Way NE, L-shaped Room, R-5417, Seattle, WA 98105.
E-mail address: sandra.poliachik@seattlechildrens.org

Phys Med Rehabil Clin N Am 23 (2012) 107–122
doi:10.1016/j.pmr.2011.11.016
1047-9651/12/$ – see front matter © 2012 Elsevier Inc. All rights reserved.

Table 1
Types of muscular dystrophy and general pattern of progression

Type	Typical Age of Onset	Muscles Affected
Myotonic	20–30 y	Facial, neck, forearm, cardiac
Duchenne	Childhood	Leg, pelvis, arm, shoulder, cardiac
Becker	11–25 y	Leg, pelvis, arm, shoulder, cardiac
Limb-girdle	Childhood to adulthood	Shoulder, hip
Facioscapulohumeral	15–40 y	Facial, shoulder, upper arm, leg
Congenital	Childhood	Generalized
Oculopharyngeal	40–50 y	Eyelid, facial, throat, tongue, proximal limbs
Distal (Miyoshi)	40–60 y	Forearm, hand, lower leg, feet
Emery-Dreifuss	10–25 y	Upper arm, lower leg, shoulder, facial, cardiac

Data from Muscular dystrophy: hope through research. Muscular Dystrophy: Hope Through Research. National Institute of Neurological Disorders and Stroke Web site. Available at: http://www.ninds.nih.gov/disorders/md/detail_md.htm. Accessed September 20, 2011.

protein and binds to β-dystroglycan. Mutations in the *LAMA2* gene result in another form of muscular dystrophy.[4]

Mutations in the dystrophin gene that result in a complete loss of dystrophin lead to the Duchenne muscular dystrophy (DMD) phenotype.[5] Mutations that cause reduced amounts of dystrophin or a truncated, dysfunctional form of dystrophin result in the Becker muscular dystrophy (BMD) phenotype. Mutations in components of the DGC complex are thought to lead to a loss of sarcolemmal integrity and render muscle fibers more susceptible to activity- or exercise-induced muscle injury. The mechanisms of muscle injury are relatively well characterized in the dystrophinopathies (ie, DMD/BMD). In others, the genetic basis has only recently been described and the mechanisms of injury are yet to be elucidated (eg, production of the protein DUX4 in facioscapulohumeral muscular dystrophy [FSHD]).[6] Furthermore, even though the genetic basis for a particular muscular dystrophy may be known, in some cases multiple genes or epigenetic modifications may modulate disease expression.

Despite the variation in the pattern and rate of muscular involvement, affected muscles follow a largely similar course of compromise in which the muscles begin to leak creatine kinase and take on excess calcium. The affected muscle fibers lose integrity, resulting in fiber degeneration and weakness. Ultimately, two primary paths result: shortening of the muscle fibers and tendons, leading to muscle atrophy; or replacement of muscle fibers with fat and connective tissue. Less affected or unaffected muscle groups may compensate with hypertrophy. During the course of muscle degeneration, multiple factors may modulate or influence the pathology seen, such as reversible injury, pseudohypertrophy (in which fat has replaced muscle to a degree that the tissue appears hypertrophied by gross examination), atrophy, and fatty replacement over time. These morphologic changes may be readily appreciated with MRI.

PROGRESSION OF MUSCLE CHANGE ASSESSMENT WITH IMAGING

In most forms of muscular dystrophy the muscle cell membrane (sarcolemma) is weakened, making it susceptible to contraction-induced damage and loss of homeostasis. Over time, the muscles become progressively weaker as they are replaced by fat and connective tissue. The rate of progression, severity of changes, and pattern of involvement are related to the type of muscular dystrophy. Considerable phenotypic variation is common in many muscular dystrophies, such as in patients with FSHD (**Fig. 1**). Although evaluation of disease progression can be assessed through muscle strength and function clinically,[7–10] overlapping muscle function and compensatory hypertrophy limit this assessment, particularly in diseases with patterns of selective muscle involvement. Imaging assessment of muscle pathology has the advantage of independent evaluation of individual muscles and potential detection of pathologic changes not appreciable in functional tests. MRI in particular, with its sensitivity to soft tissue contrast and lack of ionizing radiation,[11–13] has become the primary modality in soft tissue imaging and therefore has been increasingly applied to evaluation of muscular dystrophies.[14–16]

Standard MRI is based on the response of hydrogen atoms in a magnetic field to radiofrequency energy deposition (radiofrequency pulse). This radiofrequency pulse causes a perturbation alignment of the hydrogen atom spin. The hydrogen atom then gives off a radiofrequency signal as the spin relaxes back to baseline alignment in the magnetic field. Two types of relaxation behavior describe this return: T1 (longitudinal relaxation) and T2 (transverse relaxation), which are variably altered depending on the particular tissue microenvironment (as described in the later section on Quantitative Assessment of Muscle). The MRI acquisition parameters can be altered to produce T1-weighted or T2-weighted images (**Fig. 2**). Furthermore, although standard MRI images are formed using the relative differences in signal intensity between tissues, imaging sequences can be used that allow calculation of the actual T1 and T2 relaxation rates (quantitative imaging). Finally, signal from fat can be suppressed using particular sequences, such as short-tau inversion recovery (STIR), because of T1 differences between fat and muscle. This fat suppression proves to be particularly useful in identifying excess fluid (edema) in many tissues (see **Fig. 2**). A further point, discussed in more

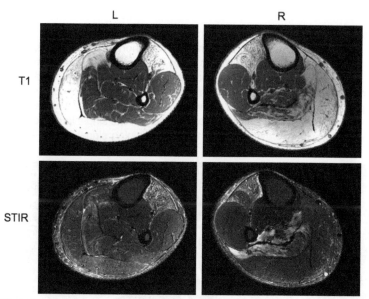

Fig. 1. The left and right legs of this patient with FSHD show marked asymmetry in the T1 and short-tau inversion recovery (STIR) images. The bright muscles in the T1 image indicate replacement of muscle with fat, whereas the bright muscles in the STIR images can be interpreted as edema. Although the pattern of injury appears similar, the difference in hyperintensity suggests a differential time course for each limb.

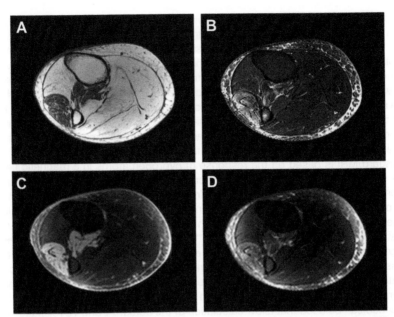

Fig. 2. Examples of: (*A*) T1-weighted image of a lower leg showing extensive fat infiltration (hyperintense muscles). (*B*) STIR image of the lower leg in an FSHD patient showing hyperintensity (edema) in the two muscles that are not fatty replaced: peroneus longus and tibialis posterior. (*C*) T2-weighted image of a lower leg showing hyperintensity of non-fatty replaced muscles in the first echo at 13 ms. (*D*) Later T2-weighted image showing an echo at 110 ms, where most of the tissue has relaxed.

detail later, is that STIR relies on the inversion and nulling of the fat signal, which may be variable in degree, influenced by magnetic field inhomogeneities, and may appear brighter near the margins in acquisitions using surface or phased array coils (**Fig. 3**).

Other fat suppression techniques that rely on radiofrequency pulse tuned to fat signal are also used in some MR imaging sequences. However, adipose tissue may be composed of several types of fat with differing T1 and T2 values. Techniques that rely on fat-suppression pulses typically suppress the single large component (triacylglycerols[17]), with the assumption that the remaining signal will be fairly fat-free.

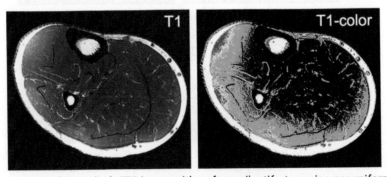

Fig. 3. Example of lower-limb STIR image with surface coil artifact, causing nonuniformity in the signal appearing as a brighter band near the edges of the cross-section. The color T1 displays the extent of the artifact, seen as green, yellow, and red.

Signal from other fat components may remain, which, through interaction, can lead to over- and/or underestimation of the measured signals, thus compromising the quantification of these features of tissue.

MRI can differentiate soft tissues and characterize edema, which is often seen in the course of changes between healthy muscle and the ultimate fatty replacement or atrophy typical of muscular dystrophies. Although the presence of edema is not specific to any one mechanism of muscle degeneration, it is seen at stages, for instance in both DMD and FSHD, and therefore potentially affords the ability to characterize a dynamic stage of injury, thereby serving as a marker of disease earlier in the disease process.

MRI images depend on the uniformity of the magnetic field, and surface coils are often used to enhance signal quality. If the magnetic field is susceptible to inhomogeneities, distortions can appear in the image. In addition, the variation inherent in surface coil sensitivity can produce artifacts near the outer edges of the image. In STIR images, these artifacts can look like edema.

Earlier imaging studies of the muscular dystrophies (DMD, BMD, LGMD) explored muscle involvement using low-field MRI. These typically used a semi-quantitative scale of qualitative images to assess muscle alteration (**Table 2**),[15] such as rating the extent of T1 signal hyperintensity in the muscle reflecting the presence of fat. Results showed that muscles in both the thigh (proximal) and calf (distal) were affected. No association with muscle fiber type (Type I or II muscle fibers) seemed to be predictive of the observed pattern of fat infiltration into the muscle. Observations of hyperintense signal on T2-weighted images led the authors to hypothesize that intramuscular water also increases with disease. A comparable MRI study found similar T1 and T2 changes in myotonic muscular dystrophy (MMD) and FSHD, while also detecting T2 hyperintensities, suggesting an increase in free water fraction.[14]

PATTERNS OF MUSCLE CHANGE IN MUSCULAR DYSTROPHY

DMD, as an example, presents with a pattern of edema and fatty changes in involved muscles similar to other muscular dystrophies. In DMD, a progression of general muscle changes in the legs[11,16] are observed on MRI images:

- Patchy edema/inflammation in the hamstrings and quadriceps and gluteus muscles with sparing of the gracilis (**Fig. 4**). These changes are accompanied by fat infiltration between muscles and a mild infiltration of fat within the gluteus muscles.
- Fatty infiltration that continues in the anterior thigh muscles (adductor magnus, rectus femoris, biceps femoris) with sparing of gracilis and sartorius. Fatty infiltration progresses to the gastrocnemius and soleus muscles, accompanied by edema/inflammation. Pseudohypertrophy is often present in the calf.

Table 2 Semiquantitative muscle grading	
Grade 1	Normal muscle signal intensity (homogeneous, hypointense signal, contrasting sharply with subcutaneous and intermuscular fat)
Grade 2	Slightly hyperintense, patchy intramuscular signal changes
Grade 3	Markedly hyperintense, patchy but widespread intramuscular signal changes
Grade 4	Total, homogeneous hyperintense signal change in whole muscle, equaling the signal intensity of adjacent subcutaneous or paramuscular fat

Data from Lamminen AE. Magnetic resonance imaging of primary skeletal muscle diseases: patterns of distribution and severity of involvement. Br J Radiol 1990;63(756):946–50.

R   L

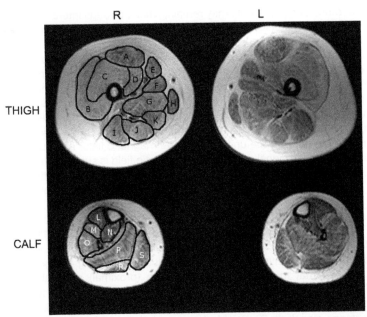

THIGH

CALF

Fig. 4. Thigh and calf cross sections in a muscular dystrophy patient. Muscles in the right thigh are identified: (A) rectus femoris[a]; (B) vastus lateralis[a]; (C) vastus intermedius[a]; (D) vastus medialis[a]; (E) sartorius; (F) adductor longus; (G) adductor magnus; (H) gracilis; (I) biceps femoris (long head)[b]; (J) semitendinosus[b]; (K) semimembranosis[b]. Muscles in the right calf are identified: (L) tibialis anterior; (M) extensor digitorum longus; (N) tibialis posterior; (O) peroneus longus; (P) soleus[c]; (R) lateral gastrocnemius[c]; (S) medial gastrocnemius[c]. [a]muscles of the quadriceps; [b]muscles of the hamstrings; [c]muscles of the calf.

- In fatty-replaced muscle, atrophy can occur, whereas spared muscles may hypertrophy.
- For final stages, edema/inflammation diminishes and fatty replacement with fibrosis occurs in affected muscles.

A similar pattern of change is observed in BMD, although the changes are much milder with a protracted time course. In LGMD, early affected muscles are found in the hamstrings and calf, although subtypes of LGMD can vary greatly in the specific muscles involved. Likewise, in congenital muscular dystrophy (CMD) and Emery-Dreifuss muscular dystrophy (EDMD), distinct patterns of muscle features depend on the subtypes (eg, Ullrich CMD displays distributed involvement of posterior and lateral muscles in the thigh, sparing the gracilis, sartorius, adductor longus, and often rectus femoris; EDMD2 appears as moderate to severe vastus lateralis and intermedius in the thigh and medial gastrocnemius in the calf, whereas the recessive X-linked EDMD has minimal thigh involvement, with the soleus affected in the calf).[11] Although variation in clinical and functional impairment among patients can make the task of pattern definition imprecise, a unifying theme to all types of muscular dystrophy seems to be the presence of edema that likely progresses to fatty replacement,[18] suggesting that, opposed to mere fat/muscle ratios, detailed evaluation of edematous changes might be most useful in characterizing evolving changes.[11]

Although not often the focus of published work, examples of edema are seen in a range of muscular dystrophies. For example, muscle changes in MMD show compartmentation (muscle/edema/fat), with the tibialis anterior, soleus, and gastrocnemii displaying MRI abnormalities (edema-like abnormalities, fatty infiltration, atrophy), whereas the tibialis posterior was least affected.[19] STIR images showed the tibialis anterior, extensor hallucis longus, and flexor hallucis longus to have edema-like abnormalities, whereas the medial gastrocnemius and soleus experienced the most atrophy, with less atrophy apparent in the tibialis anterior, flexor hallucis longus, and extensor hallucis longus. The authors suggested that the edema-like presentation could indicate muscle degeneration, and may serve as a useful biomarker of muscles on the path to degeneration. Likewise, in distal muscular dystrophy, myoedema was observed to occur first, followed by fatty replacement.[10]

A study of changes specific to leg muscles in FSHD showed that posterior leg muscles are infiltrated by fat (hamstrings, gastrocnemii, and soleus) and resemble pseudohypertrophy in these muscles.[20] Not uncommonly, some asymmetry exists in the pattern of affected muscles, as shown in **Fig. 1**. Clinically in patients with FSHD, foot drop is often noted as one of the first functional deficits in the legs, reflecting loss of strength changes in the tibialis anterior, yet these authors noted that in imaging studies, the proximal muscles (hamstrings) were affected before distal muscles. Other imaging studies have noted a similar proximal to distal severity of muscle involvement in the lower extremities.[16] An earlier study noted that fat replacement was more apparent at the myotendon junction than in the muscle belly.[21] Recently investigators suggested that within a muscle, disease progression occurs from distal to proximal,[22] and this is supported in the figures presented in another study.[23] These findings support an overall progression of muscle involvement that generally occurs proximally to distally, although specific muscles clearly can also be affected without such a strict gradient of involvement. Locally within individual muscles, the tissue alterations seem to occur from the distal to the proximal end. Verification of this hypothesis in the lower extremity would require full leg imaging in a longitudinal study, a goal that may be worthwhile to pursue in a range of dystrophies.

A recent review that described the general patterns of disease progression in a range of neuromuscular diseases illustrates the usefulness of MRI in evaluating muscle changes.[24] As a subset of conditions explored, muscular dystrophies were evaluated as discussed later, with T1 and STIR sequences used to identify fat and edema. However, as noted, STIR brightness can be caused not only by muscle edema secondary to necrosis, inflammation, or trauma but also as a result of muscle denervation. Thus, the term *edema-like* is preferred by some, because the cause of the STIR brightness is nonspecific.[24] A growing number of studies have attempted quantitative methods to evaluate edema and fat fractions in muscular dystrophies, discussed in more detail later. The fundamental advantage of focusing on edema is that it may be the earliest indicator of compromised muscle. Although other quantitative methods focused on fat may be useful in evaluating general disease burden,[25] these methods have confounds for detecting edema.

QUANTIFYING CHANGES IN MUSCLE

Several different methods have been developed in an effort to quantify tissue changes on MRI images, from very basic (eg, rating scale) to highly sophisticated, requiring extensive acquisition sequences and analytic customization:

- Rating scale, generally termed as a *semi-quantitative method*
- Dixon method
- Thresholding T1 or T2 images

- Region of interest (ROI) calculation of a mean T1 or T2 value
- Evaluating the T2 decay in multi-echo sequences and calculating the monoexponential fit of the data
- Histogram analysis of gradient-spoiled steady-state free precession (SSFP)
- Evaluating the T2 decay in multi-echo sequences and calculating the biexponential fit of the data
- Non-negative least squares (NNLS) algorithm.

Semiquantitative Assessment of Muscle Changes

Multiple studies have used semi-quantitative scales to rate changes in muscular dystrophy. A recent study that rated fat infiltration used a four-point scale of normal, mild, moderate, or severely involved.[18] Other more defined semi-quantitative grading schemes have also been used (see **Table 2**).[15] Some studies have extended and validated the semi-quantitative approach through using quantitative measurements of T2. For example, a study performed in two patients with BMD, one with FSHD, and three with LGMD showed elevated T2 signal in fatty replaced muscle that corroborated subjective ratings.[26] With the inclusion of STIR imaging, better separation of fat and edema signal has allowed approaches such as a semiquantitative four-point scale of muscle changes, including fat, edema, and atrophy used in a study of FSHD and LGMD.[23] A further study in LGMD evaluated arms and legs with a semi-quantitative score that evaluated muscle, fat, and edema-like appearance.[27] In that study, pelvic girdle and posterior compartments of the thigh were affected by fatty and fibrous replacement, and edema-like changes were found to occur in muscles of the anterior thigh and posterior lower leg. Edema-like changes seemed to occur before fibroadipose replacement. Increasingly, edema has been the focus of muscular dystrophy rating scales, as observed in a study of LGMD.[8] A typical semi-quantitative scale that includes edema is as follows:

- Myoedema absent
- Slight, interfascicular myoedema
- Slight, intrafascicular, segmental myoedema of individual muscle
- Slight, intrafascicular, global myoedema of individual muscle
- Moderate, intrafascicular, segmental myoedema of individual muscle
- Moderate, intrafascicular, global myoedema of individual muscle.

Because edema may be the crucial intermediate state of change between healthy muscle and fatty replacement, methods to further quantify this potential biomarker are likely to prove useful.

Quantitative Assessment of Muscle Changes

Early attempts to move beyond semi-quantitative ratings and quantify the amount of adipose tissue within dystrophic muscles include the Dixon technique.[28] In this technique, two separate images are acquired with a modified spin-echo pulse sequence so that water and fat signals are out of phase by 180°. From these acquisitions, an image containing only water signal and an image containing only fat signal are produced. A two-dimensional (2D) Dixon technique was compared with a SSFP sequence analysis and a monoexponential fit of T2 data for leg muscle changes in oculopharyngeal muscular dystrophy (OPMD).[29] The 2D Dixon technique was found to have value in discriminating between fat and muscle tissue, yet when the amount of fat and muscle was of similar magnitude, the technique was not as effective at differentiating between the tissues. In another study, a three-dimensional (3D) Dixon technique was used to assess total fat content of regions of interest in muscle of patients with DMD, and found that the fat estimate correlated well with the functional test results for those patients.[30] The Dixon method, however, is susceptible to magnetic field inhomogeneity, and may underestimate fat values when fat is dominant and overestimate fat values when muscle is dominant.[29] This technique is also limited in that it cannot be used to identify edema.

Another method of quantifying fat and muscle in dystrophic muscle is to threshold the pixel values in T1 images and identify each pixel as muscle or fat based on the thresholding. This technique was used to evaluate patients with DMD at the whole body level.[31,32] Partial volume, an artifact that occurs when a voxel contains more than one tissue type and causes the signal value to be an average of the two tissue types, was addressed through assignment of the fraction of lean muscle/fat based on the principle that tissue signals add linearly. Edema was not included in the analysis, adding to the challenge in this technique; that is, that the T1 of fat (short; ie, bright) can mix with T1 of edema (long; ie, dark), giving a partial volume value that is close to normal muscle.

An MRI sequence that collects multiple echoes allows for calculation of relaxation time from the decay curve, most simply with a monoexponential approach to fitting the data. This calculation can be performed for longitudinal relaxation (T1) or transverse relaxation (T2). The challenge with the T2 measurement is that the T2 for edema lies intermediate to muscle (short T2; ie, bright) and fat (long T2; ie, dark) values. Depending on how the muscle signal is calculated, edema can be evaluated, but when a large amount of fatty tissue is near normal muscle, this also may appear as edema because of partial volume effects. A study that used these methods in DMD to discriminate between muscle and fat determined that T2 values were found to prolong, whereas T1 values shortened in patients, indicating the transition to fatty infiltration in muscle maps for this patient population[33] (edema was not evaluated in this study). A monoexponential fit of T2 data was also used to evaluate leg muscle changes, with T2 values increasing for patients with OPMD[29] and DMD.[34] This method was also used in patients with DMD treated with steroids, for whom T2 mapping showed that mean T2 values shortened (ie, fat or edema content is decreased) over a 16-month treatment period.[25]

A gradient-spoiled SSFP sequence with a histogram analysis of the free induction decay signal can also be used to determine the fat fraction within skeletal muscle. This method was compared with 2D Dixon and monoexponentially fitted multiecho T2 values in a sample of either patients with OPMD.[29] The authors concluded that the T2 monoexponential fit of the data provided the best analysis to evaluate subtle changes, with the drawback that the data collection time is longer than that for the Dixon or SSFP sequences.

Biexponential fitting has also been used to separately account for the differences in fat and water signal contributions. This method was used to parcel muscle and fat in a study on FSHD.[22] In addition to the biexponential analysis, STIR MRI images were acquired. Comparing these images, two patients had a hyperintense signal on STIR, indicating edema or inflammation that was associated with a prolonged T2 signal.

To further the efforts in quantifying muscle changes as evaluated by MRI, a recent study conducted by the authors' group examined 15 patients with FSHD and 10 controls using T1, STIR, and multiecho T2 sequences.[35] A fat-saturated multiecho T2 sequence was also available for a few subjects. A contrast of a biexponential fit of multiecho T2 data to an NNLS analysis (that accounts for a more physiologic range of tissue relaxation values) showed the ability of each method to identify muscle and edema. Analysis of qualitative information from the T1, STIR, and fat-saturated images showed that the NNLS method could distinguish between muscle and edema better than a biexponential fitting approach, and with a smaller confounding effect from partial volume than analysis of T2 data. However, mild edema was not visible with NNLS analyses, and distinguishing the edema among small tendrils of fat was difficult. With the addition of fat suppression techniques in the multiecho acquisitions, muscle and edema are easier to discriminate because the partial volume effects are minimized.

Imaging sequences using selective fat-suppression with prepulses were used in a study on dogs with DMD, and showed the efficacy of this technique in mapping of muscle compared with edema.[36] The degree of fat suppression achieved in an imaging sequence can be variable, and is related to a variety of factors. More recent work has used methods to account for the signal interactions of multiple fat peaks; these methods, the most tailored approach for removing fat partial volume, will likely prove to be the most efficacious for edema assessment in muscular dystrophy.[37,38]

Now that methods are available for clearer measurement of muscle, edema, and fat, a further goal involves better understanding of the pathology that underlies these edematous changes.

Correlation of Inflammation to MRI Findings

In some muscular dystrophies, inflammation may be a notable feature[39–41] and has been confirmed through quantification of inflammatory cells in muscular dystrophy with lack of dysferlin.[42] A recent study integrating MRI and immunostaining assessed inflammatory markers using flow cytometry on peripheral blood mononuclear cells (PBMC) and immunohistochemistry on biopsy samples from patients with FSHD in muscles that both did not and did show hyperintensities on STIR images.[43] Sequences for T1 and T2-STIR were collected, and muscle biopsies were taken from samples of muscle tissue. Muscle biopsy showed inflammatory infiltrates (cytotoxic and helper T cells) in patients who displayed hyperintensity on T2-STIR images, although those without hyperintensity did not have inflammatory features present. In PBMC, flow cytometry showed cells positive for transcription factors that are involved in regulating specific T cells (T-bet, phosphorylated signal transducers and activators of transcription [pSTAT], pSTAT3) and for the production of pro- and anti-inflammatory cytokines by mononuclear cells (interleukin [IL]-12/IL-23 p40, IL-6, interferon [IFN]-γ, IL-17, tumor necrosis factor [TNF]-γ; IL10, transforming growth factor [TGF]-β). These indicators of inflammatory processes correlated well with hyperintensity on T2-STIR images but were not present when MRI images showed fatty/fibrous replacement of muscle tissue. The hyperintensity of T2-STIR and indicators of inflammatory processes were present only in younger patients with FSHD, suggesting inflammation is present early in the disease.

Exercise

A complicating factor in assessing edema in T2-weighted or STIR images is the fact that T2 values can change with exercise. Muscle edema after physiologic exercise has been studied in detail.[44,45] After an active challenge, STIR hyperintensity can appear within 6 minutes[46] and continue for 20 to 30 minutes after exercise,[47,48] depending on the level of exertion and the condition of the muscle.[49] The time course of recovery, and the type of activity, must be a major consideration in the study design, as does timing of MRI exercise studies. Although patients with muscular dystrophy may have a differential magnitude and time course of edema development related to exercise, this feature does not seem to have biased studies to date, suggesting that the edema seen is pathologic. This idea is supported by prior studies measuring sarcolemmal permeability in dystrophic muscles with and without exercise intervention.[50–54]

Intracellular fluorescent dextran (FDx) was observed in dystrophic muscles, particularly in fibers that appeared pre-necrotic on hematoxylin-eosin (H&E) stained sections, consistent with intracellular edema indicating the start of muscle deterioration.[51–53]

McNeil and Ito[54] were among the first investigators to propose that micro-injuries to the sarcolemma and then subsequent repair may be an important mechanism that regulates muscle atrophy, homeostasis, and hypertrophy. In studies to determine whether plasma membrane injury and rapid repair occurred in skeletal muscles, they examined the medial head of eccentrically exercised rat triceps, using labeled antibodies to show the presence of rat serum albumin within the muscle. Even when no disruption of the sarcolemma was detectable on ordinary light microscopy, the presence of albumin within the muscle was an indication of micro-injury to the sarcolemma.[50] McNeil's group also found that the sarcolemma is so vulnerable to injury that even unexercised caged laboratory rats incur transient sarcolemmal disruptions, as shown by the presence of albumin within their muscles. They proposed that these resealable focal membrane breaks are an early form of exercise-induced injury. Histopathologic studies showing muscle membrane leaks, especially after eccentric exercise, and markedly so in dystrophic muscle, further confirmed this.[51–53] Subsequent studies investigated whether the leaky sarcolemma was part of the dystrophic pathology or a response to exercise. Dystrophin-deficient mdx (a genetically homologous model of DMD) and control C57 mice received intravenous injections of FDx molecules of varying molecular weights as a histologic marker of sarcolemmal injury.[52] Using fluorescent microscopy, uptake of FDx was assessed in sections of quadriceps muscles from three models: non-exercised normal C57 mice, normal mice run downhill (0, 3, and 7 days post-exercise), and non-exercised mdx mice. In non-exercised normal muscles, strong intercellular fluorescence was observed between fibers, with no uptake intracellularly. In normal mice run downhill, only small amounts of intracellular FDx were observed within cells of the quadriceps from days zero and three post-exercise, but not at day seven. On H&E staining, no muscle pathology was observed at day zero, slight pathology was observed at day three, and regeneration was observed at day seven. In contrast, extensive intracellular FDx was observed within the muscles of non-exercised mdx mice, particularly in fibers that appeared pre-necrotic on H&E stained sections. This uptake increased markedly in older (aging) mdx muscles, particularly after eccentric exercise.[53,55] Muscles from control C57 mice that underwent exhaustive eccentric exercise did show significant take up of FDx, indicating sarcolemmal damage.[51] Regenerated (mature) dystrophic muscle also showed significant uptake of the FDx, indicating that regenerated dystrophic muscles still have abnormal membrane permeability.[55]

Using fluorescent dye, muscles from mdx mice were examined after a single bout of downhill running. Seventy-five percent of the fibers of the mdx triceps exhibited transient membrane disruptions, sevenfold greater than control mice.[56] Furthermore, no difference was observed between muscles of control mice after running and those of non-exercised control mice, confirming the finding of previous studies. Several other studies confirmed these findings using other reagents, including Evans blue staining.[57,58]

Comparing MRI with histologic sections of dystrophic muscle also suggests that the myoedema is primarily intracellular, distinguishing it from the intercellular water that may be seen in normal muscle after strenuous exercise.[51] An albumin-targeted contrast agent–enhanced MRI study in mdx and sarcoglycan-deficient mice showed a significant intracellular accumulation of contrast material, indicating an increase in permeability of the sarcolemmal membrane in dystrophic murine muscle.[58] Recent MRI studies have shown a similar relationship of increased signal intensity in dystrophic muscles undergoing necrosis.[59] The leakiness of the muscle membrane in dystrophic muscles clearly can be increased with eccentric exercise, yet the data would indicate that this is a transient phenomenon, peaking roughly 48 to 72 hours post-event, thus timing of MRI evaluation would be critical.

Given that MRI is sensitive at detecting myoedema, which seems to portend preclinical muscle involvement, these studies support the concept of using MRI as a tool for early diagnosis of a dystrophic myopathy. In most dystrophies, creatine kinase elevation is present long before clinical onset. In presymptomatic subjects, MRI is sensitive enough to detect alterations in muscle tissue well before clinical disease onset. The MRI detection of myoedema in a particular compartment of muscles anticipates the topography of subsequent clinical muscle involvement. In symptomatic subjects, MRI changes can noninvasively help detect the pattern and severity of clinical muscle involvement.

Analysis Technique Considerations

For most techniques discussed, limitations exist that restrict the quality of the data and combine with time constraints related to the coverage of anatomy possible in MRI examination of an affected subject. The methods and their restrictions are summarized in **Table 3**.

An issue that has not been described relates to the interpretation of any edema-like abnormalities present in the compartmentation (intra/extracellular, put simply) in tissue. Intra- and extracellular water is thought to be reflected in slow and fast T2 relaxation components, determined using biexponential fitting. These relaxation components can be separated at least to some degree, depending on magnet strength, sequences used to collect data, and methods of analysis. Additional factors, however, complicate the imaging analysis. In a study that evaluated edema in rat muscle, the authors concluded that using a biexponential fitting algorithm to assign specific diffusion components based on water compartments can be compromised by the complexity of water location, environment, and condition (bound vs free) within tissue.[60] In muscular dystrophy, the muscle membranes are often damaged and do not maintain normal gradients and/or water transport, further confounding result interpretation.

Table 3
Analysis limitations

Technique	Limitation
Radiologist rating scale	Subjective; not rigorous; can be influenced by coil effects
Stereologic CT	Radiation; less soft tissue discrimination
Dixon method	Difficulty with contrast when two tissue types have similar magnitude; edema not evaluated
Thresholding T1 or T2 images	Reliant on accurate threshold choice for tissue types
ROI calculation of the mean T1 or T2 value with the ROI	Does not identify specific tissue types
Multiecho T2	Sensitive to B_0 and B_1 inhomogeneities
T2 monoexponential	May be an oversimplification of data
T2 biexponential	Requires a priori assumptions of range of T2 values; no edema characterized
SSFP	Sensitive to B_1 inhomogeneities
NNLS	Requires large number of echoes; insensitive to partial volume near thin tendrils of fat

Considerable work remains for a more complete understanding of normal and patho-logic water compartmentation and its detection.

FUTURE

As technology advances and new MRI sequences are implemented, assessments of disease progression and treatment tracking for muscular dystrophy will also improve. Some techniques on the horizon include assessment of entire muscles instead of a cross-section, use of optimized fat-suppression sequences, and multimodal integra-tion. The advantage to scanning an entire muscle is the ability to appreciate heteroge-neity between distal and proximal changes within a single muscle. These data may be helpful in a longitudinal study to assess where edema and fatty replacement begin in specific muscles. Use of optimized fat suppression, or better modeling the multiple frequency components of fat,[37,38] will allow a more accurate measurement of edema. A more comprehensive method for water relaxation studies combined with diffusion tensor imaging or perfusion studies may help identify water compartmentation. These metrics, combined with the development of rigorous protocols for visualization of muscle fiber architecture,[61,62] may be helpful in differentiating healthy and injured tissue, although caveats remain if assumptions about tissue and image quality are violated.[63]

SUMMARY

Evaluations of muscle affectation patterns in muscular dystrophy have helped to develop a clinical picture of disease progression within the various muscular dystro-phies. Methods to quantify changes within the affected muscles, with a focus on edema, may be useful in the future to assess the effects of targeted treatment strate-gies. Integrating a focus on edema detection within research work may similarly be beneficial to (1) enhance early detection of the disease; (2) reduce error in quantifica-tion of fat content; and (3) guide muscle biopsy to evaluate relevant features.

REFERENCES

1. Hermans MC, Pinto YM, Merkies IS, et al. Hereditary muscular dystrophies and the heart. Neuromuscul Disord 2010;20(8):479–92.
2. Gumerson JD, Michele DE. The dystrophin-glycoprotein complex in the preven-tion of muscle damage. J Biomed Biotechnol 2011;2011:210797.
3. Waite A, Tinsley CL, Locke M, et al. The neurobiology of the dystrophin-associated glycoprotein complex. Ann Med 2009;41(5):344–59.
4. Rajakulendran S, Parton M, Holton JL, et al. Clinical and pathological heteroge-neity in late-onset partial merosin deficiency. Muscle Nerve 2011;44(4):590–3.
5. Morrison LA. Dystrophinopathies. Handb Clin Neurol 2011;101:11–39.
6. Tupler R, Gabellini D. Molecular basis of facioscapulohumeral muscular dystrophy. Cell Mol Life Sci 2004;61(5):557–66.
7. John J. Grading of muscle power: comparison of MRC and analogue scales by physiotherapists. Medical Research Council. Int J Rehabil Res 1984;7(2):173–81.
8. Borsato C, Padoan R, Stramere R, et al. Limb-girdle muscular dystrophies type 2A and 2B: clinical and radiological aspects. Basic Appl Myol 2006;16(1): 17–25.
9. Brooke MH, Griggs RC, Mendell JR, et al. Clinical trial in Duchenne dystrophy. I. The design of the protocol. Muscle Nerve 1981;4(3):186–97.

10. Brummer D, Walter MC, Palmbach M, et al. Long-term MRI and clinical follow-up of symptomatic and presymptomatic carriers of dysferlin gene mutations. Acta Myol 2005;24(1):6–16.
11. Mercuri E, Pichiecchio A, Allsop J, et al. Muscle MRI in inherited neuromuscular disorders: past, present, and future. J Magn Reson Imaging 2007; 25(2):433–40.
12. Schmidt GP, Reiser MF, Baur-Melnyk A. Whole-body imaging of the musculoskeletal system: the value of MR imaging. Skeletal Radiol 2007;36(12):1109–19.
13. Wattjes MP, Kley RA, Fischer D. Neuromuscular imaging in inherited muscle diseases. Eur Radiol 2010;20(10):2447–60.
14. Castillo J, Pumar JM, Rodriguez JR, et al. Magnetic resonance imaging of muscles in myotonic dystrophy. Eur J Radiol 1993;17(3):141–4.
15. Lamminen AE. Magnetic resonance imaging of primary skeletal muscle diseases: patterns of distribution and severity of involvement. Br J Radiol 1990;63(756): 946–50.
16. Marden FA, Connolly AM, Siegel MJ, et al. Compositional analysis of muscle in boys with Duchenne muscular dystrophy using MR imaging. Skeletal Radiol 2005;34(3):140–8.
17. Brix G, Heiland S, Bellemann ME, et al. MR imaging of fat-containing tissues: valuation of two quantitative imaging techniques in comparison with localized proton spectroscopy. Magn Reson Imaging 1993;11(7):977–91.
18. Degardin A, Morillon D, Lacour A, et al. Morphologic imaging in muscular dystrophies and inflammatory myopathies. Skeletal Radiol 2010;39(12):1219–27.
19. Cote C, Hiba B, Hebert LJ, et al. MRI of tibialis anterior skeletal muscle in myotonic dystrophy type 1. Can J Neurol Sci 2011;38(1):112–8.
20. Olsen DB, Gideon P, Jeppesen TD, et al. Leg muscle involvement in facioscapulohumeral muscular dystrophy assessed by MRI. J Neurol 2006;253(11): 1437–41.
21. Hasegawa T, Matsumura K, Hashimoto T, et al. Intramuscular degeneration process in Duchenne muscular dystrophy—investigation by longitudinal MR imaging of the skeletal muscles. Rinsho Shinkeigaku 1992;32(3):333–5 [in Japanese].
22. Kan HE, Scheenen TW, Wohlgemuth M, et al. Quantitative MR imaging of individual muscle involvement in facioscapulohumeral muscular dystrophy. Neuromuscul Disord 2009;19(5):357–62.
23. Schramm N, Born C, Weckbach S, et al. Involvement patterns in myotilinopathy and desminopathy detected by a novel neuromuscular whole-body MRI protocol. Eur Radiol 2008;18(12):2922–36.
24. Fleckenstein JL. MRI of neuromuscular disease: the basics. Semin Musculoskelet Radiol 2000;4(4):393–419.
25. Kim HK, Laor T, Horn PS, et al. Quantitative assessment of the T2 relaxation time of the gluteus muscles in children with Duchenne muscular dystrophy: a comparative study before and after steroid treatment. Korean J Radiol 2010;11(3): 304–11.
26. Phoenix J, Betal D, Roberts N, et al. Objective quantification of muscle and fat in human dystrophic muscle by magnetic resonance image analysis. Muscle Nerve 1996;19(3):302–10.
27. Stramare R, Beltrame V, Dal Borgo R, et al. MRI in the assessment of muscular pathology: a comparison between limb-girdle muscular dystrophies, hyaline body myopathies and myotonic dystrophies. Radiol Med 2010;115(4):585–99.
28. Dixon WT. Simple proton spectroscopic imaging. Radiology 1984;153(1):189–94.

29. Gloor M, Fasler S, Fischmann A, et al. Quantification of fat infiltration in oculopharyngeal muscular dystrophy: comparison of three MR imaging methods. J Magn Reson Imaging 2011;33(1):203–10.

30. Wren TA, Bluml S, Tseng-Ong L, et al. Three-point technique of fat quantification of muscle tissue as a marker of disease progression in Duchenne muscular dystrophy: preliminary study. AJR Am J Roentgenol 2008;190(1):W8–12.

31. Leroy-Willig A, Willig TN, Henry-Feugeas MC, et al. Body composition determined with MR in patients with Duchenne muscular dystrophy, spinal muscular atrophy, and normal subjects. Magn Reson Imaging 1997;15(7):737–44.

32. Pichiecchio A, Uggetti C, Egitto MG, et al. Quantitative MR evaluation of body composition in patients with Duchenne muscular dystrophy. Eur Radiol 2002; 12(11):2704–9.

33. Huang Y, Majumdar S, Genant HK, et al. Quantitative MR relaxometry study of muscle composition and function in Duchenne muscular dystrophy. J Magn Reson Imaging 1994;4(1):59–64.

34. Garrood P, Hollingsworth KG, Eagle M, et al. MR imaging in Duchenne muscular dystrophy: quantification of T1-weighted signal, contrast uptake, and the effects of exercise. J Magn Reson Imaging 2009;30(5):1130–8.

35. Friedman SD, Poliachik SL, Carter GT, et al. The MRI spectrum of fascioscapulohumeral muscular dystrophy (FSHD). Muscle Nerve, in press.

36. Kobayashi M, Nakamura A, Hasegawa D, et al. Evaluation of dystrophic dog pathology by fat-suppressed T2-weighted imaging. Muscle Nerve 2009;40(5):815–26.

37. Vasanawala SS, Yu H, Shimakawa A, et al. Estimation of liver T*(2) in transfusion-related iron overload in patients with weighted least squares T*(2) IDEAL. Magn Reson Med 2011. [Epub ahead of print].

38. Yu H, McKenzie CA, Shimakawa A, et al. Multiecho reconstruction for simultaneous water-fat decomposition and T2* estimation. J Magn Reson Imaging 2007;26(4):1153–61.

39. Deconinck N, Dan B. Pathophysiology of Duchenne muscular dystrophy: current hypotheses. Pediatr Neurol 2007;36(1):1–7.

40. Engvall E, Wewer UM. The new frontier in muscular dystrophy research: booster genes. FASEB J 2003;17(12):1579–84.

41. Gallardo E, Rojas-Garcia R, de Luna N, et al. Inflammation in dysferlin myopathy: immunohistochemical characterization of 13 patients. Neurology 2001;57(11):2136–8.

42. Confalonieri P, Oliva L, Andreetta F, et al. Muscle inflammation and MHC class I up-regulation in muscular dystrophy with lack of dysferlin: an immunopathological study. J Neuroimmunol 2003;142(1-2):130–6.

43. Frisullo G, Frusciante R, Nociti V, et al. CD8(+) T cells in facioscapulohumeral muscular dystrophy patients with inflammatory features at muscle MRI. J Clin Immunol 2011;31(2):155–66.

44. Ogino M, Shiba N, Maeda T, et al. MRI quantification of muscle activity after volitional exercise and neuromuscular electrical stimulation. Am J Phys Med Rehabil 2002;81(6):446–51.

45. Sesto ME, Radwin RG, Block WF, et al. Anatomical and mechanical changes following repetitive eccentric exertions. Clin Biomech (Bristol, Avon) 2005;20(1):41–9.

46. Ploutz-Snyder LL, Nyren S, Cooper TG, et al. Different effects of exercise and edema on T2 relaxation in skeletal muscle. Magn Reson Med 1997;37(5):676–82.

47. Fisher MJ, Meyer RA, Adams GR, et al. Direct relationship between proton T2 and exercise intensity in skeletal muscle MR images. Invest Radiol 1990;25(5):480–5.

48. Summers RM, Brune AM, Choyke PL, et al. Juvenile idiopathic inflammatory myopathy: exercise-induced changes in muscle at short inversion time inversion-recovery MR imaging. Radiology 1998;209(1):191–6.

49. Patten C, Meyer RA, Fleckenstein JL. T2 mapping of muscle. Semin Musculoskelet Radiol 2003;7(4):297–305.

50. McNeil PL, Khakee R. Disruptions of muscle fiber plasma membranes. Role in exercise-induced damage. Am J Pathol 1992;140(5):1097–109.

51. Carter GT, Kikuchi N, Abresch RT, et al. Effects of exhaustive concentric and eccentric exercise on murine skeletal muscle. Arch Phys Med Rehabil 1994; 75(5):555–9.

52. Carter GT, Kikuchi N, Horasek SJ, et al. The use of fluorescent dextrans as a marker of sarcolemmal injury. Histol Histopathol 1994;9(3):443–7.

53. Carter GT, Wineinger MA, Walsh SA, et al. Effect of voluntary wheel-running exercise on muscles of the mdx mouse. Neuromuscul Disord 1995;5(4):323–32.

54. McNeil PL, Ito S. Molecular traffic through plasma membrane disruptions of cells in vivo. J Cell Sci 1990;96(Pt 3):549–56.

55. Wineinger MA, Abresch RT, Walsh SA, et al. Effects of aging and voluntary exercise on the function of dystrophic muscle from mdx mice. Am J Phys Med Rehabil 1998;77(1):20–7.

56. Brussee V, Tardif F, Tremblay JP. Muscle fibers of mdx mice are more vulnerable to exercise than those of normal mice. Neuromuscul Disord 1997;7(8):487–92.

57. Vilquin JT, Brussee V, Asselin I, et al. Evidence of mdx mouse skeletal muscle fragility in vivo by eccentric running exercise. Muscle Nerve 1998;21(5):567–76.

58. Straub V, Donahue KM, Allamand V, et al. Contrast agent-enhanced magnetic resonance imaging of skeletal muscle damage in animal models of muscular dystrophy. Magn Reson Med 2000;44(4):655–9.

59. Kinali M, Arechavala-Gomeza V, Cirak S, et al. Muscle histology vs MRI in Duchenne muscular dystrophy. Neurology 2011;76(4):346–53.

60. Ababneh Z, Beloeil H, Berde CB, et al. Biexponential parameterization of diffusion and T2 relaxation decay curves in a rat muscle edema model: decay curve components and water compartments. Magn Reson Med 2005;54(3):524–31.

61. Budzik JF, Le Thuc V, Demondion X, et al. In vivo MR tractography of thigh muscles using diffusion imaging: initial results. Eur Radiol 2007;17(12):3079–85.

62. Kermarrec E, Budzik JF, Khalil C, et al. In vivo diffusion tensor imaging and tractography of human thigh muscles in healthy subjects. AJR Am J Roentgenol 2010;195(5):W352–6.

63. Zaraiskaya T, Kumbhare D, Noseworthy MD. Diffusion tensor imaging in evaluation of human skeletal muscle injury. J Magn Reson Imaging 2006;24(2):402–8.

Cardiac MRI in Muscular Dystrophy: An Overview and Future Directions

Randolph K. Otto, MD[a],*, Mark R. Ferguson, MD[a],
Seth D. Friedman, PhD[b]

KEYWORDS

- MRI • Muscular dystrophy • Cardiac
- Duchenne muscular dystrophy • Becker muscular dystrophy
- X-linked dilated cardiomyopathy

Cardiac complications are present in most muscular dystrophies.[1,2] Although the range of injurious mechanisms is extremely varied, including defined modulating factors (eg, putative genes, signaling, and maintenance),[3] age (or disease progression) at diagnosis and initial treatment,[4] and treatment dosing,[5] the need to characterize disease features with high accuracy is paramount. Because MRI can provide precise chamber volumes from three-dimensional images, and a wide range of other functional metrics, it is considered the measurement gold standard. Paterson and colleagues[6] describe methods other than MRI (eg, CT, positron emission tomography, single photon emission CT). Because dystrophinopathies (eg, Duchenne muscular dystrophy, Becker muscular dystrophy, X-linked dilated cardiomyopathy) represent most of the published work incorporating MRI strain investigation, this literature is summarized to emphasize the current and future role of MRI in disease management.

MRI images focused on anatomy are typically acquired during the diastolic portion of the cardiac cycle to eliminate cardiac motion, with breath-holding generally used to eliminate respiratory artifacts. Multiple averaged acquisitions are another approach to ameliorating respiratory artifacts in patients who cannot perform breath-holds, as is often the case with advanced stages of muscular dystrophy. Specific modification of the sequence parameters produces longitudinal (T1) or transverse relaxation (T2) weighting, which is helpful for characterizing the myocardial tissues. Black blood sequences have been used traditionally for anatomic analysis and generally use

[a] Department of Radiology, Seattle Children's Hospital, 4800 Sandpoint Way, Room R4488, Seattle, WA 98105, USA
[b] Department of Radiology, Center for Clinical and Translational Research, Seattle Children's Hospital, Seattle, WA, USA
* Corresponding author.
E-mail address: Randolph.Otto@seattlechildrens.org

Phys Med Rehabil Clin N Am 23 (2012) 123–132
doi:10.1016/j.pmr.2011.11.008
1047-9651/12/$ – see front matter © 2012 Published by Elsevier Inc.

electrocardiogram-gated spin echo techniques with successive nonselective and slice-selective inversion pulses, allowing suppression of the blood pool signal with restoration of myocardial signal before image acquisition.

The current workhorse for functional cardiac MRI is the balanced steady-state free precession (SSFP) gradient echo technique, which mainly replaced spoiled gradient echo imaging. SSFP sequences have bright-blood characteristics from T2/T1 effects, and image acquisition is segmented and spread over multiple heartbeats with the resulting cine allowing assessment of the entire cardiac cycle. Myocardial motion is easily depicted with cine sequences typically yielding a temporal resolution in the range of 50 ms (ie, 20 frames per cardiac cycle at a heart rate of 60 beats per minute), which provides a method for subjective assessment of myocardial contractility and wall motion abnormalities. Higher temporal resolutions can be used for valve information. Ventricular contours are traced on individual end systolic and end diastolic images to calculate ventricular volumes using the modified Simpson's method (**Fig. 1**). These volumes are used to derive the following usual parameters of ventricular function:

ESV: end systolic volume
EDV: end diastolic volume
SV: stroke volume = EDV – ESV
EF: ejection fraction = (SV/EDV) × 100
Cardiac output; SV × heart rate

Phase contrast techniques use gradient echo techniques to derive quantitative velocity and flow results from the blood pool within the vessel of interest. Various permutations of this technique are helpful in identifying flow disturbances, such as with stenosis, valvular pathology, and intracardiac shunts.

Administration of gadolinium-based contrast agents has efficacy in identifying and characterizing myocardial pathology. Typical gadolinium chelates accumulate within the extracellular space where they shorten T1 and T2 relaxation, with delayed clearance in areas of fibrosis or impaired vascularity. This detail forms the basis of late (delayed) gadolinium enhancement (LGE) techniques now widely used for detecting myocardial infarction and various cardiomyopathies. An example of LGE in a patient with Duchenne muscular dystrophy is shown in **Fig. 2**.

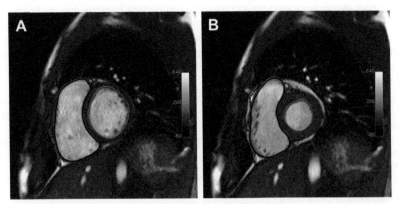

Fig. 1. End diastolic (*A*) and end systolic (*B*) short-axis SSFP images with endocardial contour tracings depicting right (*blue*) and left (*red*) ventricles.

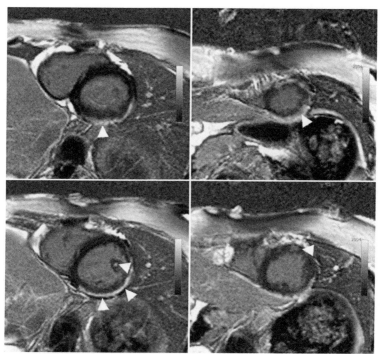

Fig. 2. Postcontrast phase-sensitive inversion-recovery (PSIR) true fast imaging with steady-state free precession (FISP) short-axis images showing subepicardial, transmural, and papillary muscle delayed myocardial enhancement in a 17-year-old patient with Duchenne muscular dystrophy (*white arrows*).

Various methods of strain imaging provide an alternate way to quantify myocardial tissue and wall deformation. Most commonly, several slices are sampled in the short-axis plane. The most reported metric derived from these methods is circumferential strain (ε_{cc}), which is the shortening/wringing motion during systole, whereas other strain parameters, such as radial and longitudinal deformation, are also used. Furthermore, some studies focus on diastolic strain metrics.[7] MRI parameters are principally in units of magnitude, although they can be reformatted to look at coherent changes in time, which is discussed in more detail.

Since its development approximately 20 years ago,[8] strain assessment has been applied to a range of conditions and questions, such as patients with thalassemia[9]; a healthy cohort to determine relationship between cardiac parameters (eg, volumes) and strain metrics[10]; and patients after heart transplant.[7] Widespread application has not been realized, however, probably because of the extra time required for examination (making it difficult in ill patients) and the limited availability of free or low-cost post-processing methods.

Three main analysis methods are described in the literature: harmonic phase tagging (HARP), which is the most common; fast cine displacement-encoded (DENSE); and cine sequence-based feature tracking (FT[11]). Processed data then evaluate directional changes over time in cross-hatched "tags," whereas in DENSE, the information is contained in opposing field gradients. **Fig. 3** provides an example of a tagged image. Although HARP/DENSE methods are more similar than different,[12] DENSE is often used for applications focused on greater in-plane resolution, at the

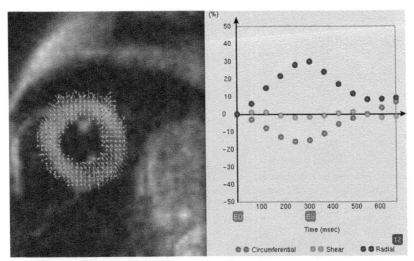

Fig. 3. Example tags and strain metrics in a pediatric patient using fast cine displacement-encoded (DENSE). (Software *Courtesy of* Auckland MRI Research Group; with permission.)

expense of signal-to-noise per unit time. FT uses standard cine magnitude images plus segmentation to generate a strain map of the heart walls, with the caveat that this approach excludes a within-tissue component.[11]

Duchenne muscular dystrophy, the most frequent (6/100,000 live births[13]) and severe of the dystrophinopathies, has been the focus of most articles using cardiac MRI, and strain specifically. Hermans and colleagues[1] provide an excellent survey of broadly focused muscular dystrophy genetics, with attention to cardiac findings. Dystrophin is a large protein that composes part of the normal muscle membrane. In Duchenne muscular dystrophy, the entire reading frame is absent, resulting in complete protein absence, whereas in Becker muscular dystrophy (affecting 2.4/100,000 live births[13]) the reading frame remains, resulting in abnormally low or variable protein levels.[14] In contrast, X-linked dilated cardiomyopathy does not result in skeletal muscle symptoms, although a rapidly progressive fatal cardiomyopathy occurs in the second decade of life.[1]

The functional consequence of these membrane gaps is that muscle becomes highly vulnerable to injury during normal function. Because of the dramatic injury progression over time in these diseases, research investigation has focused on the early detection of subclinical vulnerabilities in the heart, with the hope that treatment can be initiated to delay or forestall life-threatening consequences.

STRAIN AS AN EARLY INDICATOR OF HEART PROBLEMS

The Cincinnati group has completed several investigations related to the early use of MRI strain metrics in Duchenne muscular dystrophy.[11,15,16] Hor and colleagues[15] focused on a sample of 70 children with Duchenne muscular dystrophy spanning a wide age and range of functional impairment (from normal to impaired EF and LGE) compared with control subjects. Importantly, in the youngest most unaffected (<10 years of age, with no changes in EF or LGE), strain metrics (ε_{cc}) were abnormal relative to the control group. In older and more symptomatic subjects (eg, EF decreases and positive LGE), strain values were further decreased. These results were replicated in a follow-up study in an expanded sample (N = 191).[15] That study also compared strain metrics from HARP with those generated from postprocessing of the routine cine images (FT). Methods were highly concordant in measuring ε_{cc} in the patient sample (R = 0.854), and when combining the patient group with controls (N = 0.899), supporting the validity of measuring strain from this conventionally acquired sequence. However, a companion letter stated[17] that HARP analyses outperformed feature-based tagging on discriminating young versus old subjects and in terms of accuracy (eg, FT showed a relative underestimation of circumferential strain because the heart wall does not get labeled and tracked). Although these stated concerns are valid, easy implementation of strain with MRI has largely been hampered by the need to acquire and analyze additional specialized sequences. Although the software to perform FT is not freely available, the ability to turn a routine cine sequence into strain metrics hints at the tremendous caches of historical data that could be explored for research purposes.

A follow-up study in an expanded sample (N = 236) included a measure of cross-correlation delay (XCD).[16] XCD is computed from the timing of the ε_{cc} parameters across paired cardiac segments. The analysis then divides the anatomic distribution of XCD into clustered segments (several contiguous segments) or dispersed segments (variable segments around the ring). Results suggested that XCD changes were not common in the sample as a whole, but more frequent (31.2%) in the most affected sample of older boys (N = 16) with EF less than 55% and LGE. The pattern of result was found to be dispersed, a distribution that is noted to have a poor response to resynchronization therapy. Although these methods await further work to evaluate efficacy in other cohorts, the study illustrates the range of metrics that can be achieved with strain analyses.

COMPLEXITY OF INTERPRETING STRAIN METRICS

Strain metrics are not, however, without substantial complexity of interpretation. Ashford and colleagues[18] illustrated this in a small sample of patients with Duchenne muscular dystrophy (N = 13; 11/13 treated with routine long-term corticosteroids), whose circumferential strain (ε_{cc}, HARP), measured at the heart base, mid-ventricle, and apex, was abnormal in a range of cardiac segments (global, septum, anterior, lateral). Older patients had a greater burden of abnormalities, including regional wall changes, ventricular dilation, and decreased left ventricular function. Although anatomic features, such as areas of fibrosis as assessed with LGE, offer one parsimonious explanation for strain differences, diastolic increases compared with normative values were also seen. The authors note that the role of these pre-load effects on heart deformation, perhaps related to corticosteroid use in most patients (11/13), might be an important factor to consider when examining group differences.

STRAIN ACROSS THE LONGITUDINAL COURSE

Few studies have evaluated strain metrics as indices of change across the developmental course of muscular dystrophy. A recent study[19] evaluated 57 patients with Duchenne muscular dystrophy across a range of severities ranging from younger than 10 years plus normal ejection fraction, to older than 10 years plus low ejection fraction plus positive LGE. Across 6 to 28 months, subjects within all categories showed a consistent decline in ε_{cc} (~13%, HARP, mid-ventricle slice), whereas no consistent changes were observed in EF (it fluctuated in change score around zero). Although preliminary, and requiring replication in larger cohorts, this study provides provocative support for the role of strain metrics as sensitive measures for following disease progression and, by extension, modulation of evolution with treatment intervention.

STRAIN AS A TREATMENT INDEX

Duchenne muscular dystrophy is often managed with corticosteroids early, then angiotensin enzyme inhibitors, and later with receptor blockers (with the progression of cardiomyopathy).[20–22] Although no data describe the effects of treatment on strain in muscular dystrophy, studies in other diseases provide variable evidence for strain metrics being sensitive to therapeutic intervention. For example, a study in eight patients undergoing stem cell implantation (LV scar and border) showed strain improvements (at 3 months, which foreshadowed EDV changes at 6 months[23]). By contrast, another study examining strain metric changes in a sample of 15 patients treated with intracoronary stem cell injection versus controls (no injection) showed more marked strain improvement in the control treatment, leading to the conclusion that stem cell therapy did not improve strain.[24]

TREATMENT INDEXES: STRAIN IN OTHER METHODS

Although this review focuses on MRI, methods such as echocardiography (eg, ultrasound and Doppler as the two main varieties) and electrical measures (electrocardiogram) represent the most frequently used clinical management tools (because of cost, availability, and patient tolerance). Although this article does not reflect an exhaustive review, it seemed useful to describe the relative concordance between strain magnitude measured with MRI compared with strain rate measured with alternative methods (eg, Doppler).

In a study evaluating 16 patients with Duchenne muscular dystrophy over a broader age range[8–23] with EF impairment (median, 0.52), significant association ($P = .02$) between velocity vector echocardiography strain rates and MRI strain magnitudes (summary from systolic strain in six myocardial regions at both basal and mid-cavity myocardium) were observed, although the r value was low (r = 0.26), supporting only partial overlap in sensitivity.[25] Tissue strain reductions resulting from scarring (seen on LGE) were most prevalent in free wall segments (inferolateral, anterolateral, and lateral). Changes were also seen in other regions without scarring (inferoseptal, anteroseptal, and anterior segments), illustrating the amount and complexity of data that can be generated with these methods.

In patients with Becker muscular dystrophy with echocardiography, 8 of 15 were found to have EF reduction.[26] Using MRI, 12 of 15 patients were shown to have EF reductions, with 11 of 15 showing LGE. From a treatment perspective, only four subjects entering the study were on medication for cardiac dysfunction, whereas 10 were considered in need of treatment from MRI results. Despite the formidable strengths/availability/cost benefits to non-MRI echo approaches, the ability to detect, diagnose, and follow small changes over time is best accomplished by MRI.

T2 MEASUREMENT

Several studies have explored using transverse relaxation metrics to evaluate disease features in Duchenne muscular dystrophy. T2 measured using a spin-echo or gradient echo (yielding T2*) acquisition provides information about the local environment being experienced by water protons. Inflammation will increase T2 relaxation rate, whereas conditions such as fibrosis will shorten the T2 relaxation rate. An examination in 17 patients and matched controls showed reduction in T2 within heart and sternocleidomastoid muscle, with the authors concluding that this biomarker may have substantial efficacy for measuring abnormal tissue features.[27] Although this idea has theoretical validity, a letter in response to this study described the substantial difficulties in study interpretation without the collection of complete cardiac metrics, most specifically LGE, that would confirm the presence of structural abnormalities.[28] In keeping with the complexity of interpretation, a study of 20 patients with Duchenne muscular dystrophy (15–18 years of age) having a constellation of structural abnormalities (ESV increases, EF decreases, LGE areas in 6 of 20, and healing myocarditis from biopsy in 3) did not show consistent cardiac/muscle T2 differences.[29]

A more recent study by Wansapura and colleagues[30] sought to refine this biomarker through evaluating the distribution of T2s present in the myocardium using a measure of T2 distribution (full width half maximum [FWHM]) in 26 patients with Duchenne muscular dystrophy. This measure was selected because the pattern of abnormalities in Duchenne muscular dystrophy may involve both fibrosis and inflammation, which will broaden the width of distribution without a potential change in the central tendency (eg, mean, median). Although FWHM of T2 was not different in a youngest sample studied (5–10 years of age [n = 8] having normal EF and LGE), width increases were observed as age and injury severity increased (>12 years of age, with and without EF changes). Furthermore, FWHM was related to the degree of strain abnormality (HARP, ε_{cc}), with the suggestion that T2 might be more sensitive to detecting micro-structural features than LGE. This conclusion awaits further confirmation. Also noted in the literature is the clear difficulty in accurately measuring T2 from only two echoes.[31] This area requires methodological improvement, and could be a component of future work.

LGE

LGE is a powerful technique for assessing structural changes in heart. This point is illustrated in a study by Puchalski and colleagues,[32] who evaluated LGE features in 74 patients with Duchenne muscular dystrophy (13.7 ± 4.1 years of age). For 30 of 74 (mostly younger patients), no LGE was observed. Of the 44 with LGE, 88% had normal function as measured through routine cardiac function assessment, whereas 6 showed a decline in left ventricular ejection fraction. Dilation of the left ventricle was seen in 15 of the former and all 6 of the latter patients. In patients with LGE, a common pattern included involvement of the basolateral free wall, with sparing of the septum and right ventricle, a pattern also seen at necropsy.[32] Wall motion abnormalities were suggested to be related to decreased wall thickness, another factor that should be considered when interpreting strain metrics (and may be different depending on whether HARP or FT is used).

Another small study in 10 patients (8 with Duchenne muscular dystrophy, 2 with Becker muscular dystrophy) showed the challenges with interpretation of LGE, with one rater finding 33 (19.4%) segments affected, whereas the other rater found 23 affected segments (13.5%).[33] Perhaps less variable was the finding that 89% of the segments identified with fibrosis showed LGE. These findings were present in patients with preserved left ventricular and right ventricular function, supporting (as found in the other studies) that these pathologic changes precede functional symptoms.

DUCHENNE MUSCULAR DYSTROPHY (FEMALE CARRIERS)

MRI changes have also been shown in female carriers of Duchenne muscular dystrophy, as Politano and colleagues[34] describe in a large longitudinal cohort. An MRI example[35] reports on a 27-year-old woman presenting with dilated cardiomyopathy on echocardiogram and MR-measured ventricle dilation, diffuse hypokinesia, and LGE indicative of fibrosis. Perhaps most importantly, treatment with carvedilol was effective at slowing progression at 2-year follow-up, a testament to matching and monitoring of treatment response.

Several other female patients with similar LGE features have been reported in the literature,[35–37] including one who had no cardiac symptoms.[38] As discussed by the investigators, subthreshold features in the absence of symptoms may be an indicator for therapy initiation, an idea that can be generalized to other X-linked diseases.

THE FULL PICTURE IN MUSCULAR DYSTROPHY: CARDIAC MAGNETIC RESONANCE + STRAIN + LGE + T2: WHAT, WHEN, AND WHERE?

Although strain methods alone may be most efficacious for characterizing cardiac function in young unaffected patients, in older or more affected patients, both strain and LGE results may be necessary to accurately ascribe causality to any measured differences. Although this is a gross oversimplification of the complicated factors related to heart function, a multivariate model is probably needed to best ascribe causality in patients with later-stage disease who have a wide range of abnormal features (eg, systolic pressure, wall-thickness changes, myopathy, LGE). The future explanatory role of other variables (eg, T2) clearly requires more study to adequately determine incremental benefit to prediction, with the downside being a more extended MRI examination in already challenged individuals. Also in question is the real benefit of tagging methods that include the heart wall (eg, vector- vs cine sequence–based [FT]), and the necessity of and variance explained from having many more slices to define strain.

Although of substantial research interest, the fact that strain metrics have not been used much over the past 20 years[17] is potentially changing with these collective findings in muscular dystrophy. At the most basic level, strain indices have the ability to reveal pathology in the youngest of patients who do not yet have changes in EF or LGE. They appear sufficiently robust to reliably assess longitudinal changes over time, and appear sensitive to measure changes with treatment. Although treatment changes in humans remain focused on slowing functional decline and on symptom amelioration for the near term (eg, with drugs such as corticosteroids), the ability to test and refine biomarkers in animal models[39] and novel treatments[40] is preparing the field for more curative approaches.

Should a critical metric or metrics obtain consensus, rapid MRI examinations could be designed and implemented for more frequent serial monitoring and to help serve all but the most severely affected of patients. In the meantime, further work is needed to evaluate the generalizability of these metrics to other cohorts, and make accessible analytic methods that can be easily applied to further patient care and research in muscular dystrophy.

REFERENCES

1. Hermans MC, Pinto YM, Merkies IS, et al. Hereditary muscular dystrophies and the heart. Neuromuscul Disord 2010;20:479–92.
2. Hsu DT. Cardiac manifestations of neuromuscular disorders in children. Paediatr Respir Rev 2010;11:35–8.
3. Shathasivam T, Kislinger T, Gramolini AO. Genes, proteins and complexes: the multifaceted nature of FHL family proteins in diverse tissues. J Cell Mol Med 2010;14:2702–20.
4. Markham LW, Kinnett K, Wong BL, et al. Corticosteroid treatment retards development of ventricular dysfunction in Duchenne muscular dystrophy. Neuromuscul Disord 2008;18:365–70.

5. Matsumura T, Tamura T, Kuru S, et al. Carvedilol can prevent cardiac events in Duchenne muscular dystrophy. Intern Med 2010;49:1357–63.
6. Paterson DI, OMeara E, Chow BJ, et al. Recent advances in cardiac imaging for patients with heart failure. Curr Opin Cardiol 2011;26:132–43.
7. Korosoglou G, Osman NF, Dengler TJ, et al. Strain-encoded cardiac magnetic resonance for the evaluation of chronic allograft vasculopathy in transplant recipients. Am J Transplant 2009;9:2587–96.
8. Zerhouni EA, Parish DM, Rogers WJ, et al. Human heart: tagging with MR imaging—a method for noninvasive assessment of myocardial motion. Radiology 1988;169:59–63.
9. Magri D, Sciomer S, Fedele F, et al. Early impairment of myocardial function in young patients with beta-thalassemia major. Eur J Haematol 2008;80:515–22.
10. Fernandes VR, Edvardsen T, Rosen BD, et al. The influence of left ventricular size and global function on regional myocardial contraction and relaxation in an adult population free of cardiovascular disease: a tagged CMR study of the MESA cohort. J Cardiovasc Magn Reson 2007;9:921–30.
11. Hor KN, Gottliebson WM, Carson C, et al. Comparison of magnetic resonance feature tracking for strain calculation with harmonic phase imaging analysis. JACC Cardiovasc Imaging 2010;3:144–51.
12. Kuijer JP, Hofman MB, Zwanenburg JJ, et al. DENSE and HARP: two views on the same technique of phase-based strain imaging. J Magn Reson Imaging 2006;24:1432–8.
13. Emery AE. Population frequencies of inherited neuromuscular diseases—a world survey. Neuromuscul Disord 1991;1:19–29.
14. Laing NG, Davis MR, Bayley K, et al. Molecular diagnosis of Duchenne muscular dystrophy: past, present and future in relation to implementing therapies. Clin Biochem Rev 2011;32:129–34.
15. Hor KN, Wansapura J, Markham LW, et al. Circumferential strain analysis identifies strata of cardiomyopathy in Duchenne muscular dystrophy: a cardiac magnetic resonance tagging study. J Am Coll Cardiol 2009;53:1204–10.
16. Hor KN, Wansapura JP, Al-Khalidi HR, et al. Presence of mechanical dyssynchrony in Duchenne muscular dystrophy. J Cardiovasc Magn Reson 2011;13:12.
17. Simonetti OP, Raman SV. Straining to justify strain measurement. JACC Cardiovasc Imaging 2010;3:152–4.
18. Ashford MW Jr, Liu W, Lin SJ, et al. Occult cardiac contractile dysfunction in dystrophin-deficient children revealed by cardiac magnetic resonance strain imaging. Circulation 2005;112:2462–7.
19. Hagenbuch SC, Gottliebson WM, Wansapura J, et al. Detection of progressive cardiac dysfunction by serial evaluation of circumferential strain in patients with Duchenne muscular dystrophy. Am J Cardiol 2010;105:1451–5.
20. McNally EM. New approaches in the therapy of cardiomyopathy in muscular dystrophy. Annu Rev Med 2007;58:75–88.
21. McNally EM. Duchenne muscular dystrophy: how bad is the heart? Heart 2008;94:976–7.
22. McNally EM, MacLeod H. Therapy insight: cardiovascular complications associated with muscular dystrophies. Nat Clin Pract Cardiovasc Med 2005;2:301–8.
23. Williams AR, Trachtenberg B, Velazquez DL, et al. Intramyocardial stem cell injection in patients with ischemic cardiomyopathy: functional recovery and reverse remodeling. Circ Res 2011;108:792–6.

24. Hopp E, Lunde K, Solheim S, et al. Regional myocardial function after intracoronary bone marrow cell injection in reperfused anterior wall infarction: a cardiovascular magnetic resonance tagging study. J Cardiovasc Magn Reson 2011;13:22.
25. Bilchick KC, Salerno M, Plitt D, et al. Prevalence and distribution of regional scar in dysfunctional myocardial segments in Duchenne muscular dystrophy. J Cardiovasc Magn Reson 2011;13:20.
26. Yilmaz A, Gdynia HJ, Baccouche H, et al. Cardiac involvement in patients with Becker muscular dystrophy: new diagnostic and pathophysiological insights by a CMR approach. J Cardiovasc Magn Reson 2008;10:50.
27. Mavrogeni S, Tzelepis GE, Athanasopoulos G, et al. Cardiac and sternocleidomastoid muscle involvement in Duchenne muscular dystrophy: an MRI study. Chest 2005;127:143–8.
28. Finsterer J, Stollberger C. Clinical implications of MRI to assess cardiac and pulmonary function in patients with Duchenne muscular dystrophy. Chest 2010; 138:756–7 [author reply: 757].
29. Mavrogeni S, Papavasiliou A, Spargias K, et al. Myocardial inflammation in Duchenne Muscular Dystrophy as a precipitating factor for heart failure: a prospective study. BMC Neurol 2010;10:33.
30. Wansapura JP, Hor KN, Mazur W, et al. Left ventricular T2 distribution in Duchenne muscular dystrophy. J Cardiovasc Magn Reson 2010;12:14.
31. Ghugre NR, Enriquez CM, Coates TD, et al. Improved R2* measurements in myocardial iron overload. J Magn Reson Imaging 2006;23:9–16.
32. Puchalski MD, Williams RV, Askovich B, et al. Late gadolinium enhancement: precursor to cardiomyopathy in Duchenne muscular dystrophy? Int J Cardiovasc Imaging 2009;25:57–63.
33. Silva MC, Meira ZM, Gurgel Giannetti J, et al. Myocardial delayed enhancement by magnetic resonance imaging in patients with muscular dystrophy. J Am Coll Cardiol 2007;49:1874–9.
34. Politano L, Nigro V, Nigro G, et al. Development of cardiomyopathy in female carriers of Duchenne and Becker muscular dystrophies. JAMA 1996;275:1335–8.
35. Barison A, Aquaro GD, Passino C, et al. Cardiac magnetic resonance imaging and management of dilated cardiomyopathy in a Duchenne muscular dystrophy manifesting carrier. J Neurol 2009;256:283–4.
36. Walcher T, Kunze M, Steinbach P, et al. Cardiac involvement in a female carrier of Duchenne muscular dystrophy. Int J Cardiol 2010;138:302–5.
37. Yilmaz A, Gdynia HJ, Ludolph AC, et al. Images in cardiovascular medicine. Cardiomyopathy in a Duchenne muscular dystrophy carrier and her diseased son: similar pattern revealed by cardiovascular MRI. Circulation 2010;121: e237–9.
38. Finsterer J, Stollberger C, Avanzini M, et al. Late gadolinium enhancement as subclinical myocardial involvement in a manifesting Duchenne carrier. Int J Cardiol 2011;146:231–2.
39. Dubowitz V. Therapeutic efforts in Duchenne muscular dystrophy; the need for a common language between basic scientists and clinicians. Neuromuscul Disord 2004;14:451–5.
40. Yokota T, Pistilli E, Duddy W, et al. Potential of oligonucleotide-mediated exon-skipping therapy for Duchenne muscular dystrophy. Expert Opin Biol Ther 2007;7:831–42.

Neuromuscular Ultrasonography: Quantifying Muscle and Nerve Measurements

David Mayans, MD, Michael S. Cartwright, MD,
Francis O. Walker, MD*

KEYWORDS

- Neuromuscular ultrasound • Amyotrophic lateral sclerosis
- Muscle hypertrophy • Muscle atrophy • Nerve enlargement
- Carpal tunnel syndrome • Leprosy

There is an inherent conflict between interpreting ultrasound imaging, which generates rich, highly textured complex representations of 3-dimensional space, and the rendering of these images into discrete measures for statistical analysis Reducing images to a small set of numbers, by necessity, ignores vast amounts of useful data, but the process is a prerequisite for generating objective information that can be shared by the clinical community. This article illustrates how ultrasound imaging is used in quantitative ways. The goal is not to supplant or diminish the importance of descriptive findings but to make the field amenable to statistical methods and standards for making diagnoses and designing therapeutic trials of new interventions. The discussion focuses first on muscle ultrasonography, a technique that was developed more than a decade earlier than nerve ultrasound, to illustrate key elements in determining how to best extract quantitative information from complex images. The discussion then applies some of these same principles to the study of 2 common nerve disorders.

Dr Cartwright has funding from the NIH/NINDS (1K23NS062892) to study neuromuscular ultrasound.
Disclosures: None.
Department of Neurology, Wake Forest School of Medicine, Medical Center Boulevard, Winston-Salem, NC 27157-1078, USA
* Corresponding author.
E-mail address: fwalker@wfubmc.edu

Phys Med Rehabil Clin N Am 23 (2012) 133–148
doi:10.1016/j.pmr.2011.11.009

MUSCLE ULTRASONOGRAPHY
Size Measurements

Conceptually, the simplest way to identify muscle is to measure its size. All ultrasound instruments are equipped with electronic calipers so that once a muscle is imaged, its boundaries can be identified and measured. However, there are several caveats[1–6]:

(1) In the relaxed state, the muscle is compressible and even slight pressure on the transducer can lead to significant changes in measured thickness. A commonly used effective strategy is to place the transducer on the muscle with ample gel, optimize the image, and then use the minimal pressure required to not lose transducer contact with the skin surface.

(2) Muscle dimensions vary with location, so selecting a reliable and consistent site for measurement is a prerequisite for obtaining normative data or for performing serial measurements over time. Bony landmarks, and fixed or proportional distances from them, are commonly used.

(3) Careful transducer management is required to ensure that the probe is held precisely in a parallel or transverse manner toward the muscle of interest so as for optimal size measurements and to ensure that the angle of insonation is perpendicular to the long dimensions of the muscle to ensure optimal echogenicity measurements.

(4) Muscle dimensions change with contraction/relaxation, so it is critical to ensure that the subject is cooperating for either full relaxation or contraction.

(5) Muscle blood flow increases significantly with even low levels of exertion, and this can influence measured size of the muscle[5]; typically patients are imaged after a brief period of rest.[2] Muscle mass is largely composed of water (75%),[6] and, because muscle represents a large portion of the body water reserve (30%), it may change with dehydration or fluid overload.

Several clinical studies, discussed later, have shown that the technical issues of muscle size measurements can be managed and that the technique is capable of providing useful information about muscle function and dysfunction. Using a series of simple questions, the following sections address the evidence that supports the value of ultrasound measurements of muscle size.

Are ultrasound measurements of muscle size reliable?

The studies that have looked at the test-retest reliability of muscle thickness and cross-sectional area show that there is a correlation coefficient of 0.98 to 0.99 and a correlation of 0.99 with magnetic resonance imaging (MRI) measurements of muscle.[7–11] Because of the way ultrasonography processes speed of sound, which is slightly faster in muscle than average human tissue, the technique may consistently underestimate muscle thickness by a few percentage points, but, because this underestimate is invariant and directly related to measures obtained by MRI, its significance is moot.[12]

Can ultrasonography accurately quantify changes in muscle thickness with activation?

There are several simple ways to evaluate the ability of ultrasonography to measure variations in muscle thickness. The simplest is to show that it can measure changes in muscle size and shape in response to muscle contraction. This has been well documented[13–16] in published studies and is easily demonstrated by imaging any muscle in the relaxed and contracted state (**Fig. 1**).

Is ultrasonography capable of demonstrating an increase in muscle size with exercise?

A somewhat greater test of the utility of ultrasonography as a tool for measuring muscle size derives from studies that evaluate the effect of exercise. Ultrasonography

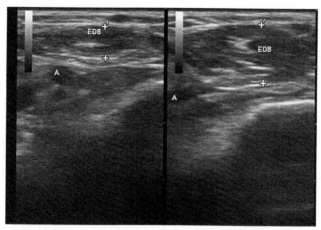

Fig. 1. Two identical cross-sectional images of the extensor digitorum brevis (EDB). On the left, the muscle (EDB), which is just above a small artery (A), is fully relaxed, and the crosses show the thickness at 2.8 mm. On the right, the muscle is fully contracted, displacing the artery, with a thickness of 5.1 mm.

proves to be a reliable and valid method for measuring the hypertrophy of muscles in the extremities, pelvic floor, and diaphragm that results from formal exercise programs.[17–27] Four illustrative studies (**Fig. 2**) are worth reviewing in more depth. Downey and colleagues[24] studied the response of diaphragm thickness to inspiratory muscle training exercises in healthy young adults. After 8 weeks of training, which involved deep breathing against large inspiratory loads, diaphragm thickness increased by 10% and inspiratory muscle strength increased 25%. Enright and

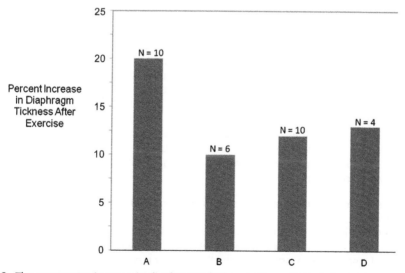

Fig. 2. The percentage increase in diaphragm thickness after a dedicated exercise program in (A) 10 patients with cystic fibrosis,[25] (B) 6 healthy controls,[24] (C) 10 healthy controls,[26] and (D) 4 healthy controls.[27] Although the N is small, the results from different studies show good concordance.

colleagues[25,26] showed a similar improvement in diaphragm thickness in healthy controls and also showed an almost 20% increase in diaphragm thickness in adults with cystic fibrosis after this same type of training. In healthy controls, even an exercise program of biceps curls and sit-ups can lead to significant increases in diaphragm thickness.[27] In all studies, there was improvement in a variety of other measured parameters of pulmonary function in tandem with the changes seen on ultrasonography.

Fujiwara and colleagues[18] showed that heel-raising exercises in elderly women significantly increased gastrocnemius (6%) and soleus (12%) thickness, and McNee[21] showed that strength training in children with cerebral palsy increased the volume of the medial and lateral gastrocnemius muscles by about 15%. As such, it is clear that exercise training, in healthy young and old controls and diseased individuals, leads to increased muscle thickness and improves measures of strength and function. However, studies have yet to confirm significant effects of exercise on neuromuscular disease outcomes. So, although ultrasonography is a valid way to measure direct effects of exercise on muscle size, establishing this measure as a marker of clinical benefit requires additional studies. The link seems likely, and, given its ease of use and availability, confirmatory studies can be performed without undue expense or delay.

Can muscle ultrasonography measure loss of muscle size with disuse?
Another way to evaluate the usefulness of muscle ultrasonography is its ability to assess loss of muscle mass in nonneuromuscular conditions commonly associated with atrophy.[19,23,28] Kawakami and colleagues[19] used ultrasonography to show that muscle mass in the lower extremities decreased significantly (3%–4%) after 20 days of strict bed rest in healthy controls. Reid and colleagues[23] showed that muscle thickness decreases even more rapidly in critically ill patients, 1.6% per day. Triandafilou and Kamper[28] showed that ultrasonography sensitively detects the loss of muscle mass in the affected hands of patients who have had a stroke and that this loss significantly exceeds the difference of muscle sizes expected between dominant and nondominant hands.

Is ultrasonography capable of measuring the size differences of muscles between populations of children, seniors, and adult men and women?
Another test of the utility of muscle ultrasonography measures involves how well it assesses differences in muscle size in large populations of individuals. As adults grow older, there is an age-specific decline in muscle size, particularly in the quadriceps. This effect is muted in those who remain physically active in old age.[8,29–32] Ultrasonography has proven to be a robust tool for demonstrating this effect in a more cost-effective manner than MRI. Similarly, ultrasonography confirms differences in the thickness of the dominant versus nondominant upper extremity and between men and women. Ultrasonography also shows the increase in muscle mass in children that occurs with maturation.

Is it possible to track progressive loss of muscle mass in chronic neuromuscular disorders?
A more direct test of the clinical relevance of muscle ultrasonography is its ability to track changes in muscle size in progressive neuromuscular diseases. Studies in large groups of patients with adult and childhood motor neuron disease and muscular dystrophy have used ultrasound to show that those with longer duration or severity of symptoms have smaller muscle size.[11,33–40] Pseudohypertrophy of muscles occurs in some disorders such as Duchenne muscular dystrophy, a finding ultrasonography also readily quantifies.[10] In addition to cross-sectional disease population studies,

there are 2 recent smaller studies that show ultrasonography can be used to serially measure muscle size changes over time in patients with amyotrophic lateral sclerosis (ALS).[33,34] Lee and colleagues[33] showed that there was a statistically significant progression of muscle atrophy over time in patients with motor neuron disease in a sample of 3 muscles; however, in a larger sample of muscles in a greater number of patients, Arts and colleagues[34] were unable to show a significant progression of atrophy in patients with ALS. Taken together, these studies provide evidence that ultrasonography has the potential for being a useful biomarker in neuromuscular disease, but, in ALS at least, further studies are needed to determine if this technique can be used as a surrogate end point for treatment outcomes. Ultrasonography can measure muscle size and its change over time, but the question remains if muscle loss in ALS is sufficiently distributed in multiple muscles and linearly progressive to be amenable to standard statistical calculations for estimating functional disability and disease severity.

Can ultrasonography measure the effect of drugs on causing either loss or enhancement of muscle thickness?

A final test of the usefulness of ultrasound measurements of muscle size is to assess its responsiveness to drug treatment. Hamjian and Walker,[41] in a series of healthy controls, showed that muscle ultrasonography of the extensor digitorum brevis was a sensitive indicator of atrophy after small doses of botulinum toxin. In hemiplegic patients admitted to an intensive care unit, Moukas and colleagues[42] showed that serial ultrasound measurements of muscle size could demonstrate an enhanced rate of atrophy in those treated with steroids and neuromuscular junction blockers. Candow and colleagues,[43] in healthy exercising adults, showed that creatine supplementation significantly enhanced muscle thickness. Cardiac ultrasonography, a technique of considerable similarity to skeletal muscle ultrasonography, has been used to detect changes in heart muscle size in health and disease for many years.[44] This technique is responsive to reductions in cardiac wall thickness in heart transplant recipients treated with sirolimus and to increases in wall thickness in patients undergoing hemodialysis treated with growth hormone.[45] These findings show that ultrasonography is a measure that can detect bidirectional changes in muscle size in response to a variety of pharmacologic interventions in even fairly small samples of patients.

How promising are ultrasound measurements of muscle size as potential surrogate end points of disease severity?

It seems clear that ultrasonography is a useful technique for measuring muscle size and that this property has immediate diagnostic implications and the potential to be a useful tool for clinical decision making. This technique meets the requirements of a useful surrogate end point of neuromuscular disease as listed, in a simplified form, in **Box 1**. Of 5 key variables that characterize an ideal surrogate end point, the cost and convenience of ultrasonography is self-evident in that it is noninvasive, painless, safe, and routinely available with just a modest amount of training. It is clearly valid from both a technical and clinical perspective. The technique is simple, reliable, and well standardized as a measure of tissue size. From a clinical perspective, atrophy is a robust manifestation of most neuromuscular diseases. Muscle size is known to correlate strongly with strength, a variable of clinical significance. Furthermore, normalization of atrophied muscles is almost a necessity for therapeutic intervention to work in a neuromuscular disorder; put another way, it would be difficult to envision a mechanism of action that would not involve increase in muscle size. Although not discussed in detail, the measurement precision of ultrasonography is quite good, with known standards of biological variation in the populations studied and

---

Box 1
Characteristic of surrogate markers

1. Validity (technical/clinical)
2. Responsiveness to disease and treatment
3. Measurement precision
   a. Biological variation
   b. Acquisition process
4. Convenience; for example speed of use, portability, patient tolerance
5. Cost

An ideal surrogate marker should identify a physiologic process on a direct pathway between treatment and outcome.

---

straightforward image acquisition and measurement techniques. These are objective and amenable to central oversight if needed. Perhaps of greatest significance is that the studies demonstrate bidirectional responsiveness and sensitivity of ultrasound measurements of muscle size to a variety of diseases and the outcomes of diverse therapeutic interventions. However, to become fully acceptable as a surrogate end point, muscle ultrasonographic measurements of muscle size need to be validated in a pivotal clinical trial of therapeutic benefit. Because there are few currently meaningful therapies for progressive neuromuscular disorders, such validation likely will have to await the emergence of newer interventions.

Echogenicity Measurements of Muscle

Another useful parameter to study muscle is ultrasound echogenicity.[2,3,46] Healthy muscle tissue is normally echolucent or dark. Given the highly organized structure of muscle, sound mostly is transmitted through the tissue with reflections occurring primarily at sites of fibrous structures in the muscle, such as the vasculature, perimysium, and epimysium. However, in myopathies and neurogenic disorders, muscle tissue undergoes atrophy, necrosis, inflammation, fatty infiltration, and fibrosis. These changes set up multiple new planes of sound reflection in muscle, and, as a result, diseased muscle becomes progressively more echogenic, with loss of the normal heterogeneity of healthy muscle and its supporting fibrous stroma.

Measuring muscle echo intensity, however, is technically more complex than measuring muscle size. There is no set convention among ultrasound instrument manufacturers as to how to best display brightness, so the relationship between the brightness displayed on a screen and the actual intensity of reflected echoes varies somewhat from instrument to instrument, depending on proprietary software used by each manufacturer.[2,3] In fact, there is no set standard for image contrast or brightness in the field. Sonographers may differ in their opinions on optimal brightness settings for performing certain types of diagnostic studies.[12] The subjectivity of brightness settings is further limited by the absence of any good correlative measurement, other than microscopic anatomy, which, at best, provides an indirect correlation.[46] Although muscle size as measured by ultrasonography is subject to comparisons of size as measured by other techniques, echo intensity measurements are only directly apparent by ultrasonography.

Further complicating the display of echogenicity is the nature of human visual perception.[12] In general, the brightness of most objects depends largely on the extent of ambient illumination and fairly little with respect to the object perceived. An object's perceived size, in contrast, is constant regardless of illumination. Studies of human perception have shown that size is cognitively coded in a linear manner. As such, even if a subject cannot tell the relative height in inches of 2 adjacent objects, they can give accurate estimates of their relative size. In contrast, brightness is coded cognitively in an exponential manner[47]; as such, the relative brightness of 2 objects is nonlinear and not easily appreciated in a quantitative manner. Using a standard oscilloscope display, amplitude mode (A-mode) ultrasonography can display the amplitude of an ultrasound signal precisely but only for the display of a single element from the multiple elements in a linear array transducer.[12] Such 1-dimensional displays are of limited use and are impractical in modern imaging. Although necessary for tissue imaging, the use of brightness mode (B-mode) ultrasonography requires mapping amplitude as brightness. However, something is lost in translation because this conversion, from a perceptual perspective, involves displaying amplitude information on a log scale instead of a linear scale. Although difficult to characterize the impact of this translational shift, **Fig. 3** helps to show the difference of expressing something on a linear versus a log scale. This subject is discussed in more detail elsewhere.[12]

Further complicating the interpretation of ultrasound brightness is the number of operator-controlled parameters that alter echogenicity of a tissue. These parameters include time gain compensation, the angle of incidence of the transducer, and power and gain settings. Fortunately, these are manageable through careful technique, which includes standardized instrument settings, transducer positioning, and using the same instrument. However, such settings may be not be equivalent on different instruments, given the differences in proprietary display parameters.[2,11,29,34,36] Alternatively, a somewhat more complex process involving backscatter analysis[48–51] allows for comparison of data from different instruments. In either case, technical factors can be managed effectively to obtain useful data on echogenicity. One factor, however, which is a patient variable that is more difficult to control, is the variability of the sound-absorbing characteristics of superficial layers of tissue on the echogenicity of deeper layers. In practice, this variability does not seem to be particularly problematic in that most muscle imaging involves muscles fairly close to the surface and the variation present in most superficial tissue is minimal. However, excess subcutaneous edema, superficial fat, or hypertrophic skin disorders can distort echogenicity measurements and may play a significant role in the evaluation of certain groups of patients (eg, critically ill patients with pronounced edema).

As would be expected, there are fewer studies that have measured echogenicity in neuromuscular diseases than studies that have measured muscle thickness.

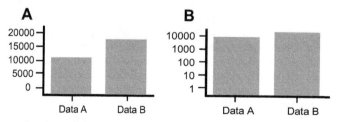

Fig. 3. Bar graph using a (A) standard size scale and (B) a log scale. Note that the log scale adjustment significantly diminishes the apparent magnitude of the difference. Use of B-mode imaging, by displaying amplitude as brightness, tends to reduce perceived echo intensity differences because of the different way the human brain processes size versus illumination.

Nonetheless, increased echogenicity was recognized early as a key parameter in the diagnosis of chronic neuromuscular disease (**Fig. 4**). The finding has been validated numerically using digital technology, descriptively and by qualitative rating scales scored by blinded investigators.[8,10,11,29,34–37,51–59] At least as a diagnostic parameter, ultrasound echogenicity measurements of muscle provide added value.

Does increased echogenicity serve as a useful measure of disease severity?

In cross-sectional studies of groups of patients, there is some evidence to suggest that greater echogenicity is seen in more advanced forms of motor neuron disease or at least in disease of longer duration.[34–36] The change of echogenicity over time has not been as well studied in human muscular dystrophy. However, in dystrophic mice, there is evidence to suggest that it might be a useful progressive disease biomarker.[60,61] There is also evidence that increased echogenicity of muscle inversely correlates with survival in ALS. This effect is most pronounced when estimating the rate of change of echogenicity from baseline based on normal values and the known duration of symptoms.[36] When looked at serially over 6 months in a group of 31 patients with ALS, however, the change in echo-intensity over time was too variable and inconsistent to track disease severity. As a marker of the presence of muscle disease, echogenicity is quite useful; however, as a marker of disease evolution or regression, the limited data available are unconvincing.

One potential problem with ultrasound echogenicity is its predicted responsiveness to disease therapy. There are concerns that changes in echogenicity may not be reversible even should patients improve from their underlying disorder.[36] Because increased echogenicity results from fibrosis and fatty changes in muscle, it may be that changes in echogenicity are chronic and may not necessarily repair with clinical improvement. For example, old polio patients may have markedly asymmetric recovery from paraplegia. Ultrasound images from affected limbs, one that is flaccid and one that shows normal strength, may show virtually equal echogenicity.[62] Further

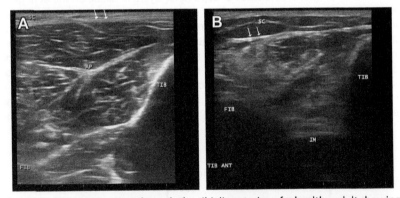

Fig. 4. (*A*) Normal cross section through the tibialis anterior of a healthy adult showing the tibia (TIB), a faint outline of the fibula (FIB), and a prominent central aponeurosis (AP) in the muscle. At the top of the image is a very thin layer of subcutaneous tissue (SC) with arrows pointing to the upper edge of the muscle. (*B*) Cross section of the tibialis anterior from a young adult with hereditary motor and sensory neuropathy. The subcutaneous tissue (SC) layer is thicker with the muscle edge deeper (*arrows*), the fibula (FIB) and interosseous membrane (IM) that connects the fibula and tibia (TIB) show markedly reduced depth of the muscle. The muscle is distinctly more echogenic, which tends to obscure the bone edge of the tibia, with a sort of moth-eaten appearance more typical of neurogenic than myopathic change.

improvements in techniques for quantifying echogenicity may help in determining if ultrasonography can detect a reduction in preexisting echogenicity or forestall the progression of echogenicity in neuromuscular disorders undergoing effective therapy.

Muscle Dynamics

By its very nature, measuring movement is typically more complex than measuring findings on a still image, because movement involves measurements across multiple images. However, certain techniques can simplify such measurements. Motion mode (M-mode) imaging can capture movement on a single still image, such as the duration of a compound muscle action potential or fasciculation (**Fig. 5**).[4] Ultrasonography records the duration of a mechanical event, such as muscle contraction, whereas electromyography records the duration of a compound surface membrane potential, an electrical event that is far shorter.[4,12]

Perhaps the simplest measure of muscle movement is the degree of thickening on contraction of muscle. This has been measured in the diaphragm[24–27] and is easily measured in other muscles. To date, it has not been proven that this measurement adds value to the measurement of muscle thickness alone, but it has not been looked at rigorously. Another common muscle movement of interest is fasciculations. Benign

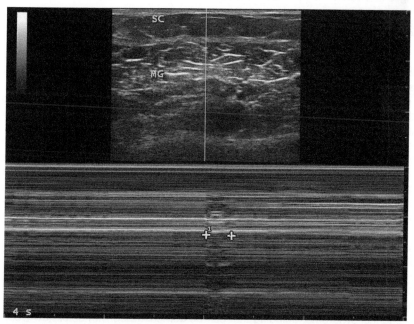

Fig. 5. Cross-sectional image of the median gastrocnemius muscle (MG) with a thin layer of subcutaneous tissue (SC) above it. The vertical line through the center of the muscle is displayed below, using M-mode (motion mode) ultrasonography. The 1 line of ultrasound data, from a single transducer element from a linear array of multiple elements, is displayed below as it changes over 4 seconds. At about half way during this 4-second epoch, a fasciculation occurs in the muscle, marked by a focal perturbation that lasts 253 milliseconds. Both contraction (thickening) and relaxation is seen during this transient motor unit discharge. The duration exceeds that of electrically recorded fasciculations because ultrasonography captures the mechanical behavior of muscle, whereas electrodiagnostic measurements only capture the brief change in muscle membrane potential.

fasciculations are quite common, and a recent study by Daube and Kumar[63] suggests that, at least after vigorous exercise, these fasciculations occur in virtually 100% of normal individuals in the abductor hallucis muscle. Ultrasonography can also be used to count fasciculations in a given area of muscles.[64] Such findings can be of considerable diagnostic use in early forms of the disease,[65,66] but they do not seem to be particularly useful in quantifying severity of disease in ALS.[34] This is not surprising in that one would anticipate that fasciculation frequency would have a U-shaped relationship with severity of symptoms in motor neuron disease, with a gradual increase in frequency as the disease goes through early stages and a gradual decrease in frequency in later stages of the disorder concomitant with significant lower motor neuron loss.

Another area of potential interest in quantification is muscle blood flow. Muscle blood flow is known to increase dramatically after even small amounts of exercise, and this effect can contribute to measured muscle volume.[67] Little, however, is known about muscle blood flow in primary neuromuscular disorders other than that increased blood flow is seen in inflammatory myopathies.[68] In animal models of muscular dystrophy, abnormal blood flow regulation is seen in relation to changes in nitric oxide function,[69] but the significance of this finding in human disease is unknown. Access to ultrasonography may make it possible for clinicians to more actively study blood flow changes in a variety of pathologic states.

QUANTIFICATION OF NERVE ULTRASONOGRAPHY

The most common types of nerve disorders, entrapment neuropathies, tend to show changes that are the inverse of the changes seen on muscle imaging of chronic neuromuscular disease. Although chronically diseased muscles become atrophic and hyperechoic, chronically compressed nerves tend to become enlarged and hypoechoic. In both cases, the changes are clearly of diagnostic usefulness. For example, currently, there are more than 250 published studies of nerve ultrasonography in carpal tunnel syndrome showing that measured nerve enlargement and loss of echogenicity are hallmark diagnostic features of the disorder. However, it is unclear if these changes are useful as surrogate markers in nerve disease. This is because there is a structural limit to how much a compressed nerve can enlarge; with increasingly severe compression and axonal loss, nerves may have less swelling than in less pronounced cases, and there is a floor effect of how much echogenicity a nerve can lose. This suggests that there may be an inverted U-shaped relationship between nerve enlargement and severity of compression neuropathy and possibly a similar relationship with loss of echogenicity; as such, they may have some limitations as surrogate markers of severity of compression.

The cause of increased size and loss of echogenicity of compressed nerves is not well understood, but, in part, this may result from increased vascularity of the nerve in carpal tunnel syndrome, a finding that can be demonstrated with color flow Doppler (**Fig. 6**). Excess blood flow would tend to engorge the nerve and, because blood is much less echoic than tissue, would reduce nerve echogenicity.[70–73] Both ultrasound-guided steroid injections and surgical treatment of carpal tunnel syndrome lead to prompt and sustained reductions in nerve size as measured by cross-sectional area.[70–72,74,75] When Cartwright and colleagues[70] looked at median nerve vascularity in conjunction with nerve size, both decreased in tandem in patients with carpal tunnel syndrome after ultrasound-guided steroid injections around the median nerve. Nerve echogenicity, measured by examiner rating, showed a similar time course of improvement. As such, there may be a role of ultrasound in gauging treatment effects in carpal

A

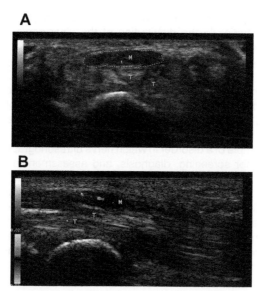

B

Fig. 6. (*A*) Cross-sectional image of the wrist showing a markedly enlarged and somewhat flattened median nerve. The cross-sectional area of the nerve (*green tracing*) is 31 mm^2, which is about 4 times the normal size. Note that the nerve is hypoechoic, particularly when compared with the tendons immediately below it that are much brighter. (*B*) Sagittal view of the median nerve using color flow Doppler. Note the linear blue elements within the nerve, which demonstrate a stable pulsating blood flow within it, a finding not seen in normal healthy nerves. There is random transient noise in nearby structures such as the tendons (T).

tunnel syndrome because several measures demonstrate responsiveness to therapeutic intervention in these studies.

Is Quantitative Ultrasonography Useful in Infectious Neuropathy?

If carpal tunnel syndrome is the most common treatable focal neuropathy, it seems likely that leprosy may be the most common curable generalized polyneuropathy, at least from a global perspective.[76] Leprosy's worldwide prevalence and the potential for ultrasonography to significantly affect its management warrant its inclusion in this review. Two major categories of leprosy include lepromatous, which is a diffuse infection of skin and nerves caused by reduced cell-mediated immunity in the disorder, and tuberculoid, in which there is an active immunologic response to the disease, restricting its distribution to relatively few areas of skin and nerve.[76] In up to 25% of patients undergoing antibiotic therapy, there are treatment reactions, usually in lepromatous forms of the disease.[76] These reactions can be mild but can also be associated with significant inflammatory impairment of nerve function. Increased blood flow in nerves, detected by color Doppler ultrasonography, provides evidence of such treatment reactions.[77]

Ultrasound measurements showing increased nerve size are a sensitive indicator of the presence of neuropathy in leprosy.[78,79] This is not surprising because it is well known that nerves are often palpably enlarged in leprosy, particularly in areas where they are superficial and in tissues that are typically cooler than core body temperature, for example, the ulnar nerve at the elbow, the tibial nerve at the ankle, the fibular nerve at the fibular head, and the greater auricular nerve.[76]

Another study of leprosy, at least one of semiquantitative impact, is the use of vaso-motor blood flow studies in the distribution of the ulnar nerve. Wilder-Smith and colleagues[80] showed that color Doppler measurements of blood flow in the ulnar artery by ultrasonography were sensitive and specific in identifying small fiber auto-nomic dysfunction in 12 patients with leprosy compared with 20 healthy controls. The study is of interest because it demonstrates not only the diagnostic utility of ultra-sound in this disorder, in which small fiber dysfunction is significant in terms of tissue injury and digit loss, but also the potential of ultrasound to diagnose other disorders of small fibers controlling the autonomic nervous system.

Leprosy is an example of a disorder in which nerve ultrasonography may prove to be a useful technique for screening, diagnosis, and assessment of the extent of the disease. However, of even greater importance, leprosy is treatable, and, as such, it can help establish the responsiveness of ultrasound measures of nerve disease in this disorder to antibiotic therapy. Because a percentage of treated patients develop treatment reactions, it is also likely that ultrasonography can contribute to their recog-nition and management. In this context, leprosy could prove to be a model disease for studying how a low-cost portable imaging technology can alter the diagnosis, treat-ment, and management of nerve disease prevalent in populations with limited access to sophisticated electrophysiologic testing.

SUMMARY

Ultrasonography, first used to study muscle in 1980 and nerve in 1991, has evolved into a valid technique for the diagnosis of nerve and muscle disease.[56,81] Recent studies have suggested an additional role for neuromuscular ultrasonography as a measure of disease severity and distribution. Improved understanding of how to analyze and quantitate the complex findings provided by ultrasound imaging is helping to build a case for the use of ultrasound measurements as potential surrogate end points of neuromuscular disease and its response to treatment. By including ultra-sound assessment in ongoing and future clinical trials of therapeutic interventions in neuromuscular disease, it will be possible to determine how the technique can be used to facilitate clinical trials and the evaluation of new promising therapies.

REFERENCES

1. Walker FO, Cartwright MS, Weisler ER, et al. Ultrasound of nerve and muscle. Clin Neurophysiol 2004;115:495–507.
2. Pillen S, van Alfen N, Zwarts M. Ultrasound of muscle. In: Walker FO, Cartwright MS, editors. Neuromuscular ultrasound. Philadelphia: Elsevier; 2011. p. 37–57.
3. Zaidman CM. Ultrasound of muscular dystrophies, myopathies, and muscle pathology. In: Walker FO, Cartwright MS, editors. Neuromuscular ultrasound. Phil-adelphia: Elsevier; 2011. p. 131–50.
4. Walker FO. Neuromuscular ultrasound as a complement to the electrodiagnostic evaluation. In: Aminoff MJ, editor. Aminoff's Electrodiagnosis in Clinical Neurology. 6th edition. Elsevier; 2012.
5. Walker FO. Normal neuromuscular sonography. In: Tegeler CH, Babikian VL, Gomez CR, editors. Neurosonology. New York: Mosby-Year-Book; 1996. p. 397–405.
6. Sarvazyan A, Sarvazyan A. Acoustical assessment of body water balance. J Acoust Soc Am 2011;130(4):2539.
7. Reeves ND, Maganaris CN, Narici MV. Ultrasonographic assessment of human skeletal muscle size. Eur J Appl Physiol 2004;91:116–8.

8. Reimers CD, Harder T, Saxe H. Age-related muscle atrophy does not affect all muscles and can partly be compensated by physical activity: an ultrasound study. J Neurol Sci 1998;59:60–6.
9. Sanada K, Kearns CF, Midorikawa T, et al. Prediction and validation of total and regional skeletal muscle mass by ultrasound in Japanese adults. Eur J Appl Physiol 2006;96:24–31.
10. Reimers CD, Schlotter B, Eicke BM, et al. Calf enlargement in neuromuscular diseases: a quantitative ultrasound study in 350 patients and review of the literature. J Neurol Sci 1996;143:46–56.
11. Pillen S, Arts IM, Zwarts MJ. Muscle ultrasound in neuromuscular disorders. Muscle Nerve 2008;37(6):679–93.
12. Walker FO. Basic principles of ultrasound. In: Walker FO, Cartwright MS, editors. Neuromuscular ultrasound. Philadelphia: Elsevier; 2011. p. 1–23.
13. Pinto RZ, Ferreira PH, Franco MR, et al. Effect of two lumbar spine postures on transversus abdominis muscle thickness during a voluntary contraction in people with and without low back pain. J Manipulative Physiol Ther 2011;34:164–72.
14. Jhu JL, Chai HM, Jan MH, et al. Reliability and relationship between 2 measurements of transversus abdominis dimension taken during an abdominal drawing-in maneuver using a novel approach of ultrasound imaging. J Orthop Sports Phys Ther 2010;40:826–32.
15. Delaney S, Worsley P, Warner M, et al. Assessing contractile ability of the quadriceps muscle using ultrasound imaging. Muscle Nerve 2010;42:530–8.
16. Kubo K, Kawata T, Ogawa T, et al. Outer shape changes of human masseter with contraction by ultrasound morphometry. Arch Oral Biol 2006;51:146–53.
17. Ronei PS, Gomes N, Radaelli R, et al. Effect of range of motion on muscle strength and thickness. J Strength Cond Res 2011. [Epub ahead of print].
18. Fujiwara K, Toyama H, Asai H, et al. Effects of regular heel-raise training aimed at the soleus muscle on dynamic balance associated with arm movement in elderly women. J Strength Cond Res 2011;25:2605–15.
19. Kawakami Y, Akima H, Kubo K, et al. Changes in muscle size, architecture, and neural activation after 20 days of bed rest with and without resistance exercise. Eur J Appl Physiol 2001;84:7–12.
20. Krentz JR, Farthing JP. Neural and morphological changes in response to a 20-day intense eccentric training protocol. Eur J Appl Physiol 2010;110:333–40.
21. McNee AE, Gough M, Morrissey MC, et al. Increases in muscle volume after plantarflexor strength training in children with spastic cerebral palsy. Dev Med Child Neurol 2009;51:429–35.
22. Braekken IH, Majida M, Engh ME, et al. Morphological changes after pelvic floor muscle training measured by 3-dimensional ultrasonography: a randomized controlled trial. Obstet Gynecol 2010;115:317–24.
23. Reid CL, Campbell IT, Little RA. Muscle wasting and energy balance in critical illness. Clin Nutr 2004;23(2):273–80.
24. Downey AE, Chenoweth LM, Townsend DK, et al. Effects of inspiratory muscle training on exercise responses in normoxia and hypoxia. Respir Physiol Neurobiol 2007;156:137–46.
25. Enright S, Chatham K, Ionescu AA, et al. Inspiratory muscle training improves lung function and exercise capacity in adults with cystic fibrosis. Chest 2004;126:405–11.
26. Enright SJ, Unnithan VB, Heward C, et al. Effect of high-intensity inspiratory muscle training on lung volumes, diaphragm thickness, and exercise capacity in subjects who are healthy. Phys Ther 2006;86(3):345–54.

27. DePalo VA, Parker AL, Al-Bilbeisi F, et al. Respiratory muscle strength training with non-respiratory maneuvers. J Appl Physiol 2004;96(2):731–4.

28. Triandafilou KM, Kamper DG. Investigation of hand muscle atrophy in stroke survivors. Clin Biomech 2011. [Epub ahead of print].

29. Arts IM, Pillen S, Schelhaas HJ, et al. Normal values for quantitative muscle ultrasonography in adults. Muscle Nerve 2010;41(1):32–41.

30. Ikezoe T, Mori N, Nakamura M, et al. Atrophy of the lower limbs in elderly women: is it related to walking ability? Eur J Appl Physiol 2011;111(6):989–95.

31. Scholten RR, Pillen S, Verrips A, et al. Quantitative ultrasonography of skeletal muscles in children: normal values. Muscle Nerve 2003;27:693–8.

32. Trappe TA, Lindquist DM, Carrithers JA. Muscle-specific atrophy of the quadriceps femoris with aging. J Appl Physiol 2001;90:2070–4.

33. Lee CD, Song Y, Peltier AC, et al. Muscle ultrasound quantifies the rate of reduction of muscle thickness in amyotrophic lateral sclerosis. Muscle Nerve 2010;42(5):814–9.

34. Arts IM, Overeem S, Pillen S, et al. Muscle changes in amyotrophic lateral sclerosis: a longitudinal ultrasonography study. Clin Neurophysiol 2011;122:623–8.

35. Wu JS, Darras BT, Rutkove SB. Assessing spinal muscular atrophy with quantitative ultrasound. Neurology 2010;75:526–31.

36. Arts IM, Overeem S, Pillen S, et al. Muscle ultrasonography to predict survival in amyotrophic lateral sclerosis. J Neurol Neurosurg Psychiatry 2011;82(5):552–4.

37. Arts IM, van Rooij FG, Overeem S, et al. Quantitative muscle ultrasonography in amyotrophic lateral sclerosis. Ultrasound Med Biol 2008;34:354–61.

38. Yoshioka Y, Ohwada A, Sekiya M, et al. Ultrasonographic evaluation of the diaphragm in patients with amyotrophic lateral sclerosis. Respirology 2007;12:304–7.

39. Cartwright MS, Walker FO, Griffin LP, et al. Peripheral nerve and muscle ultrasound in amyotrophic lateral sclerosis. Muscle Nerve 2011;44:346–51.

40. Schedel H, Reimers CD, Nägele M, et al. Imaging techniques in myotonic dystrophy. A comparative study of ultrasound, computed tomography and magnetic resonance imaging of skeletal muscles. Eur J Radiol 1992;15(3):230–8.

41. Hamjian JA, Walker FO. Serial neurophysiological studies of intramuscular botulinum-A-toxin in humans. Muscle Nerve 1994;17:1385–92.

42. Moukas M, Vassiliou MP, Amygdalou A, et al. Muscular mass assessed by ultrasonography after administration of low-dose corticosteroids and muscle relaxants in critically ill hemiplegic patients. Clin Nutr 2002;21:297–302.

43. Candow DG, Chilibeck PD, Burke DG, et al. Effect of different frequencies of creatine supplementation on muscle size and strength in young adults. J Strength Cond Res 2011;25:1831–8.

44. Kushwaha SS, Raichlin E, Sheinin Y, et al. Sirolimus affects cardiomyocytes to reduce left ventricular mass in heart transplant recipients. Eur Heart J 2008;29:2742–50.

45. Jensen PB, Ekelund B, Nielsen FT, et al. Changes in cardiac muscle mass and function in hemodialysis patients during growth hormone treatment. Clin Nephrol 2000;53:25–32.

46. Reimers K, Reimers CD, Wagner S, et al. Skeletal muscle sonography: a correlative study of echogenicity and morphology. J Ultrasound Med 1993;12:73–7.

47. Stevens SS. To honor Feschner and to repeal his law: a power function, not a log function, describes the operating characteristic of a sensory system. Science 1961;133:80–6.

48. Zaidman CM, Holland MR, Anderson CC, et al. Calibrated quantitative ultrasound imaging of skeletal muscle using backscatter analysis. Muscle Nerve 2008;38: 893–8.
49. Zaidman CM, Connolly AM, Malkus EC, et al. Quantitative ultrasound using backscatter analysis in Duchenne and Becker muscular dystrophy. Neuromuscul Disord 2010;20:805–9.
50. Zaidman CM, Malkus EC, Siener C, et al. Qualitative and quantitative skeletal muscle ultrasound in late-onset acid maltase deficiency. Muscle Nerve 2011; 44:418–23.
51. Heckmatt JZ, Pier N, Dubowitz V. Assessment of quadriceps femoris muscle atrophy and hypertrophy in neuromuscular disease in children. J Clin Ultrasound 1988;16:177–81.
52. Heckmatt JZ, Pier N, Dubowitz V. Measurement of quadriceps muscle thickness and subcutaneous tissue thickness in normal children by real-time ultrasound imaging. J Clin Ultrasound 1988;16(3):171–6.
53. Heckmatt JZ, Dubowitz V. Ultrasound imaging and directed needle biopsy in the diagnosis of selective involvement in muscle disease. J Child Neurol 1987;2: 205–13.
54. Heckmatt JZ, Dubowitz V. Detecting the Duchenne carrier by ultrasound and computerized tomography. Lancet 1983;2:1364.
55. Heckmatt JZ, Leeman S, Dubowitz V. Ultrasound imaging in the diagnosis of muscle disease. J Pediatr 1982;101:656–60.
56. Heckmatt JZ, Dubowitz V, Leeman S. Detection of pathological change in dystrophic muscle with B-scan ultrasound imaging. Lancet 1980;1:1389–90.
57. Brockmann K, Becker P, Schreiber G, et al. Sensitivity and specificity of qualitative muscle ultrasound in assessment of suspected neuromuscular disease in childhood. Neuromuscul Disord 2007;17:517–23.
58. Pillen S, Verrips A, van Alfen N, et al. Quantitative skeletal muscle ultrasound: diagnostic value in childhood neuromuscular disease. Neuromuscul Disord 2007;17:509–16.
59. Zuberi SM, Matta N, Nawaz S, et al. Muscle ultrasound in the assessment of suspected neuromuscular disease in childhood. Neuromuscul Disord 1999;9:203–7.
60. Ahmad N, Bygrave M, Chhem R, et al. High-frequency ultrasound to grade disease progression in murine models of Duchenne muscular dystrophy. J Ultrasound Med 2009;28:707–16.
61. Laux D, Blasco H, Ferrandis JY, et al. In vitro mouse model in Duchenne muscular dystrophy diagnosis using 50-MHz ultrasound waves. Ultrasonics 2010;50: 741–3.
62. Walker FO. Diagnostic ultrasound in neuromuscular disease. In: Shefner J, Dashe JF, editors. Available at: http://www.uptodate.com/contents/diagnostic-ultrasound-in-neuromuscular-disease?source=search_result&search=neuromuscular+ultrasound&selectedTitle=1%7E150. Accessed November 28, 2011.
63. Daube JR, Kumar N. Surface recorded fasciculation potential characteristics. Muscle Nerve 2011;44:688.
64. Walker FO, Harpold JG, Donofrio PD, et al. Sonographic imaging of muscle contraction and fasciculations: a comparison with electromyography. Muscle Nerve 1990;13:33–9.
65. Misawa S, Noto Y, Shibuya K, et al. Ultrasonographic detection of fasciculations markedly increases diagnostic sensitivity of ALS. Neurology 2011;77:1532–7.
66. Swash M, Carvalho M. Muscle ultrasound detects fasciculations and facilitates diagnosis in ALS. Neurology 2011;77:1508–9.

67. van Holsbeeck MT, Joseph HI. Sonography of muscle. In: van Holsbeeck MT, Joseph HI, editors. Musculoskeletal ultrasound. St Louis (MO): Mosby; 2001. p. 23–9.
68. Shook SJ. Ultrasound of inflammatory myopathies. In: Walker FO, Cartwright MS, editors. Neuromuscular ultrasound. Philadelphia: Elsevier; 2011. p. 125–31.
69. Stamler JS, Meissner G. Physiology of nitric oxide in skeletal muscle. Physiol Rev 2001;81:209–37.
70. Cartwright MS, White DL, Demar S, et al. Median nerve changes following steroid injection for carpal tunnel syndrome. Muscle Nerve 2011;44:25–9.
71. Mallouhi A, Pulzl P, Trieb T, et al. Predictors of carpal tunnel syndrome: accuracy of gray-scale and color Doppler sonography. AJR Am J Roentgenol 2006;186: 1240–5.
72. Joy V, Therimadasamy AK, Chan YC, et al. Combined Doppler and B-mode sonography in carpal tunnel syndrome. J Neurol Sci 2011;308:16–20.
73. Yayama T, Kobayashi S, Awara K, et al. Intraneural blood flow analysis during an intraoperative Phalen's test in carpal tunnel syndrome. J Orthop Res 2010;28: 1022–5.
74. El-Karabaty H, Hetzel A, Galla TJ, et al. The effect of carpal tunnel release on median nerve flattening and nerve conduction. Electromyogr Clin Neurophysiol 2005;45:223–7.
75. Vögelin E, Nüesch E, Jüni P, et al. Sonographic follow-up of patients with carpal tunnel syndrome undergoing surgical or nonsurgical treatment: prospective cohort study. J Hand Surg Am 2010;35:1401–9.
76. Rodrigues LC, Lockwood DNj. Leprosy now: epidemiology, progress, challenges, and research gaps [review]. Lancet Infect Dis 2011;11(6):464–70.
77. Martinoli C, Derchi LE, Bertolotto M, et al. US and MR imaging of peripheral nerves in leprosy. Skeletal Radiol 2000;29:142–50.
78. Lolge SJ, Morani AC, Chaubal NG, et al. Sonographically guided nerve biopsy. J Ultrasound Med 2005;24:1427–30.
79. Elias J Jr, Nogueira-Barbosa MH, Feltrin LT, et al. Role of ulnar nerve sonography in leprosy neuropathy with electrophysiologic correlation. J Ultrasound Med 2009; 28:1201–9.
80. Wilder-Smith EP, Wilder-Smith AJ, Nirkko AC. Skin and muscle vasomotor reflexes in detecting autonomic dysfunction in leprosy. Muscle Nerve 2000;23:1105–12.
81. Buchberger W, Schön G, Strasser K, et al. High-resolution ultrasonography of the carpal tunnel. J Ultrasound Med 1991;10:531–7.

The Paradox of Muscle Hypertrophy in Muscular Dystrophy

Joe N. Kornegay, DVM, PhD[a,b,c,d,]*, Martin K. Childers, DO, PhD[e],
Daniel J. Bogan, BA[a,c,d], Janet R. Bogan, BS[a,c,d], Peter Nghiem, DVM[f],
Jiahui Wang, PhD[g], Zheng Fan, MD[b,d], James F. Howard Jr, MD[b,d],
Scott J. Schatzberg, DVM, PhD[h], Jennifer L. Dow, BS[a,c,d], Robert W. Grange, PhD[i],
Martin A. Styner, PhD[g,j], Eric P. Hoffman, PhD[f], Kathryn R. Wagner, MD, PhD[k,l]

KEYWORDS

• Muscular dystrophy • DMD • GRMD • Muscle hypertrophy

By the age of 3 years, his mother noted that his lower extremities grew in volume. Her attention was first drawn to this enlargement of his calves which entered his stockings with difficulty.
  —Duchenne's description of his first patient, Joseph Sarrazin, as cited by Tyler[1]

[a] Department of Pathology and Laboratory Medicine, School of Medicine, University of North Carolina-Chapel Hill, Chapel Hill, NC 27599, USA
[b] Department of Neurology, School of Medicine, University of North Carolina-Chapel Hill, Chapel Hill, NC 27599, USA
[c] Gene Therapy Center, School of Medicine, University of North Carolina-Chapel Hill, Chapel Hill, NC 27599, USA
[d] Senator Paul D. Wellstone Muscular Dystrophy Cooperative Research Center, University of North Carolina-Chapel Hill, Chapel Hill, NC 27599, USA
[e] Section of PM&R, Department of Neurology, School of Medicine, Wake Forest University Health Sciences, Room 258, Dean Biomedical Research Building, 391 Technology Way, Winston-Salem, NC 27101, USA
[f] Department of Integrative Systems Biology, George Washington University School of Medicine and Research Center for Genetic Medicine, Children's National Medical Center, 111 Michigan Avenue, NW, Washington, DC 20010, USA
[g] Department of Psychiatry, University of North Carolina-Chapel Hill, Chapel Hill, NC 27599, USA
[h] Veterinary Emergency and Specialty Center of Santa Fe, 2001 Vivigen Way, Santa Fe, NM 87505, USA
[i] Department of Human Nutrition, Foods, and Exercise, Virginia Tech University, 321 Wallace Hall, Blacksburg, VA 24061, USA
[j] Department of Computer Science, University of North Carolina-Chapel Hill, Chapel Hill, NC 27599, USA
[k] Center for Genetic Muscle Disorders, Kennedy Krieger Institute, 801 North Broadway, Baltimore, MD 21205, USA
[l] Departments of Neurology and Neuroscience, The Johns Hopkins School of Medicine, 707 Broadway, Baltimore, MD 21205, USA
* Corresponding author. School of Medicine, Campus Box 7525, University of North Carolina-Chapel Hill, Chapel Hill, NC 27599.
E-mail address: joe_kornegay@med.unc.edu

Phys Med Rehabil Clin N Am 23 (2012) 149–172
doi:10.1016/j.pmr.2011.11.014
1047-9651/12/$ – see front matter © 2012 Elsevier Inc. All rights reserved.

Mutations in the human dystrophin gene cause 2 clinical phenotypes, Duchenne muscular dystrophy (DMD) and Becker muscular dystrophy (BMD), distinguished principally based on the age at which patients lose the ability to ambulate.[2,3] Boys with DMD become wheelchair users before 14 years of age, whereas those with BMD walk beyond age 16 years.[4] The basis for this clinical distinction can largely be traced to the fact that DMD mutations result in the loss of the mRNA reading frame, virtually eliminating dystrophin protein production, and BMD mutations preserve the reading frame, allowing production of a partially functional protein.[5] Muscles of patients with both forms express variable pathologic changes that generally lead to profound muscle atrophy. In contrast, some muscles, most notably the gastrocnemius, enlarge. Although hypertrophy has typically been attributed to deposition of fat and connective tissue, so-called pseudohypertrophy,[6,7] imaging studies have shown true hypertrophy in some individuals.

There are 3 mammalian models in which spontaneous dystrophin gene mutations lead to distinct phenotypes of muscular dystrophy: the mdx mouse,[8,9] golden retriever muscular dystrophy (GRMD) dog,[10,11] and feline hypertrophic muscular dystrophy (FHMD) cat.[12,13] The GRMD model most closely mirrors DMD at multiple levels, including progressive disease that leads primarily to muscle atrophy. The mdx mouse progresses through an initial phase of muscle hypertrophy followed in old age by atrophy. In contrast, the FHMD cat has persistent muscle hypertrophy. The role of true hypertrophy has been more broadly accepted in these models, with less attention paid to contributions made by fat and connective tissue in muscle enlargement.

In principle, relative muscle sparing or hypertrophy could be either beneficial or detrimental. The benefits are obvious because preservation of strength should enhance motor function in activities ranging from ambulation to breathing. Harmful effects are less clear and relate to the potential for muscle hypertrophy to exacerbate contractures and postural instability. Additional deleterious consequences occur due to difficulties in eating because of glossal hypertrophy and regurgitation resulting from either esophageal hypomotility or obstruction at the level of the hypertrophied diaphragm. Whether the hypertrophy results from an actual increase in muscle mass or fat and connective tissue, studies directed at defining underlying mechanisms could provide insight into the pathogenesis of dystrophin deficiency and inform treatment development.

VARIABLE MUSCLE INVOLVEMENT AND HYPERTROPHY

Effects of dystrophin deficiency vary among species, individuals, and muscles. Reasons for phenotypic variation are poorly understood and raise questions about primary versus secondary effects of dystrophin deficiency.[14]

DMD and BMD

Extensor muscles that undergo eccentric muscle contraction, such as the quadriceps femoris, are particularly vulnerable in DMD.[15] In contrast, the extraocular muscles[16] are largely spared, and other muscles undergo striking paradoxical hypertrophy. Although attention has focused on gastrocnemius (calf) enlargement (**Fig. 1**), hypertrophy occurs in many other muscles. Presumptive cases of DMD characterized by hypertrophy of the calves, deltoid, and infraspinatus muscles were seen in Italy and England as early as the 1830s well before Duchenne's classic account.[1] In a 1995 review of 84 patients with DMD from India, 94% had calf enlargement, followed by the infraspinatus (88%), deltoid (52%), and tibialis anterior (40%).[17] The selective muscular involvement extended to different heads of the deltoid and quadriceps, which showed concomitant atrophy and hypertrophy. Calf hypertrophy was evident on physical examination in 20 of 26 (77%) BMD cases in another study.[18] These

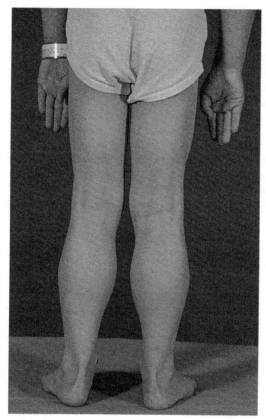

Fig. 1. Nine-year-old boy with DMD demonstrating characteristic calf hypertrophy. (*Courtesy of* James F. Howard Jr.)

patients were further studied with computed tomography to determine the pattern and course of muscle involvement. Hypertrophy was seen in the calves (42%), sartorius (42%), gracilis (42%), adductor longus (38%), semitendinosus (19%), and rectus femoris (11%). Patients with DMD and/or BMD have also been shown to have hypertrophy of the tongue (macroglossia),[19] diaphragm,[20] and hypothenar (palm)[21] muscles, among others.

Dating to Duchenne's monograph, muscle hypertrophy in DMD and BMD has been attributed to deposition of fat and connective tissue, giving rise to the term pseudohypertrophic muscular paralysis.[1] Indeed, histopathologic studies have documented fibrosis and fatty change in the calves and other hypertrophied muscles.[6,7] Walton[22] speculated that true hypertrophy also contributes to muscle enlargement, perhaps occurring early in the disease course, followed by pseudohypertrophy. However, because of inherent limitations of sequential muscle sampling in human patients, the time course and relative roles of true hypertrophy and pseudohypertrophy have remained unsettled. Specialized imaging techniques have complemented and, in some cases, essentially replaced histopathologic evaluation of muscle biopsy samples. Increasingly, use of these techniques has documented features consistent with a true increase in contractile mass. In one such study, 10 of 16 patients with BMD had calf enlargement on ultrasonography, and 9 of them were judged to have true hypertrophy.[23] Another study, cited earlier, found that enlarged muscles visualized with computed tomography were often rounded and had normal densities, suggesting true hypertrophy.[18] A further paper, in which magnetic resonance imaging (MRI) was evaluated, showed that the gracilis and sartorius muscles were relatively spared and/or hypertrophied in 10 patients with DMD.[24] We are particularly intrigued by the relative sparing of the sartorius muscle (**Fig. 2**) because of our own studies of cranial sartorius hypertrophy in GRMD (see later).[25]

Ideally, imaging and histopathologic results should be correlated to define the relative contributions that fat, fibrous connective tissue, and myofiber hyperplasia or hypertrophy make to muscle enlargement. Few such studies have been completed in DMD. In one paper that correlated computed tomography and histochemistry findings, apparent true hypertrophy of the gastrocnemius in a 7-year-old boy with DMD was judged to be caused by myofiber hyperplasia rather than hypertrophy.[6] With this said, hypertrophied myofibers are also seen early in the disease and persist throughout life.[7]

The mdx Mouse

More extensive pathologic studies can be done with animal models, potentially allowing better definition of mechanisms contributing to differential muscle involvement. Just as in DMD, muscles are variably affected in the mdx mouse, ranging from the unaffected extraocular muscles[26] to the severely involved diaphragm.[27] Limb muscles undergo dramatic necrosis at 3 to 4 weeks of age followed by robust regeneration and muscle hypertrophy.[28–31] Changes vary among muscles, with the predominantly slow twitch soleus being more involved at 3 to 4 weeks[29,32,33] and the fast twitch extensor digitorum longus at 32 weeks and beyond.[29,33] Muscle hypertrophy causes mdx mice to be larger than normal between about 10 and 40 weeks of age, after which they lose weight in concert with a loss of muscle mass.[28,29,33] Reflecting the early strong

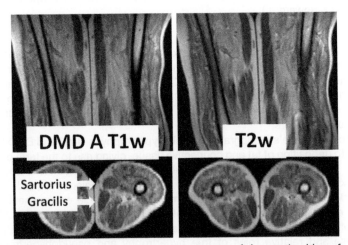

Fig. 2. T1- and T2-weighted magnetic resonance images of the proximal leg of a boy with DMD in the anteroposterior (*top*) and transverse (*bottom*) planes. The transverse image is at the level of the midfemur. Most muscles have been partially to near totally replaced with signal-intense material compatible with fat. Note that the subcutaneous fat has comparable signal intensity in both T1- and T2-weighted images. In contrast to the properties of most muscles seen, the sartorius and gracilis muscles (*arrows*) are largely unaffected.

regenerative response, mdx mice have increased numbers of small regenerating fibers with central nuclei at 3 weeks of age.[28,32,34] The percentage of larger regenerated myofibers increases with age, approaching 70% and 90% in the soleus and extensor digitorum longus, respectively, by 26 weeks.[32] Because populations of both small and large fibers occur concomitantly, mean fiber diameter of mdx mice typically is normal.[28,35] The concomitant occurrence of large and small fibers suggests that both hyperplasia and hypertrophy contribute to muscle hypertrophy.[31]

Unlike DMD, mdx mice have minimal fatty change and fibrosis,[33] indirectly implicating true hypertrophy as the cause for muscle enlargement.[31] The time course of pathologic lesions in the mdx mouse leads to corresponding functional changes, with affected mice being weaker at 2 to 4 weeks and then recovering.[36–38] Absolute tension generated by mdx muscles is typically higher by 8 to 16 weeks of age.[31,36,39] When corrected for cross-sectional area, isomeric soleus muscle force of younger ($\leq$100 days) mdx mice was lower than normal, whereas values for older ($\geq$100 days) mdx mice were higher.[39] Coulton and colleagues[39] commented that, "when mdx mice lose muscle fibers by necrosis, they do not just replace them with equally efficient new muscle, but with heavier, stronger, muscles than the wild-type." Typical of this pattern and consistent with our own findings in the GRMD dog (see later), isometric tension generated by the tibialis anterior is considerably lower in mdx mice at 3 to 4 weeks[36] but exceeds normal values by 8 to 16 weeks.[31,36] Pathologic changes in the tibialis anterior also occur earlier than those in the soleus and gastrocnemius muscles.[36] Taken together, these mdx mouse data show clear evidence that early necrosis leads to a dramatic regenerative response that can lead to functional hypertrophy.

Contraction kinetics in mdx mice also differ from normal. Relaxation times were increased in the soleus, independent of age,[40] and in the tibialis anterior at 3 to 4 weeks[36] but not at later ages.[36,37] Although twitch-tetany ratios were decreased compared with normal in the soleus of variably aged mdx mice,[40] a reverse relationship was seen in the tibialis anterior at 7 to 8 weeks.[37] Relaxation times of the mdx tibialis anterior were also increased at 3 to 4 weeks,[36] but values normalized in older mice.[36,37]

FHMD

Male cats with weakness, histologic features typical of muscular dystrophy, and gross and histologic evidence of muscle hypertrophy were characterized before the discovery of dystrophin.[41] Subsequently, an analogous syndrome was reported in cats with dystrophin deficiency.[12,13,42] One of these FHMD cats was shown to have a dystrophin gene deletion that included the skeletal muscle and neuronal Purkinje cell promoters and first exons.[42] The most striking clinical feature in all these cats was gross hypertrophy of their axial and appendicular muscles, as well as the tongue, diaphragm, and esophageal muscularis. In one study, 4 muscles (biceps brachii, cranial tibialis, gastrocnemius, and diaphragm) from 2 FHMD cats weighed twice as much as those from comparably sized normal cats.[12] Physical evidence of hypertrophy has been noted as early as 3 months[13] and seems to become more pronounced with age. As an example, the circumference of the neck in one cat increased from 28 to 33 cm between 14 and 25 months of age.[12] On microscopic examination, FHMD cats have myofiber size variation, with increased populations of both small regenerating and hypertrophied myofibers and an overall mean myofiber diameter in the normal range.[43] In keeping with progressive hypertrophy, the mean myofiber diameter of FHMD cats increased more so than that of normal cats between 3 to 4 and 6 to 9 months of age. In addition, there was myofiber necrosis and splitting and both gross and individual myofiber mineralization. The relative absence of fibrosis in FHMD cats up to 2 years of age suggests that the muscle enlargement is most likely because of true hypertrophy.[12]

GRMD Dog

As with DMD and the mdx mouse, the extraocular muscles are largely spared in GRMD.[44,45] Other muscles become involved as a function of age and usage. Muscles that are used heavily in utero and early in life, such as the tongue, diaphragm, and limb flexors, are acutely necrotic during the neonatal period.[44,45] Extensor muscles demonstrate a more delayed pattern of involvement, reflecting their greater use in weight bearing. As with the mdx mouse, muscles that undergo early necrosis may then regenerate and even hypertrophy. In one of the original GRMD dogs studied by our group, the hamstrings, tongue, diaphragmatic crura, and esophageal muscularis were enlarged.[10]

A further study in our laboratory showed that most GRMD pelvic limb muscles atrophy, whereas the caudal and cranial sartorius and popliteus hypertrophy.[25] Cranial sartorius muscle weights were corrected for body weight and endomysial space to determine true muscle weights (g/kg) in 3 GRMD age groups (4–10, 13–26, and 33–66 months) and grouped normal dogs (6–20 months) (**Table 1**). Corrected GRMD weights in the younger dogs were greater than those of normal dogs, indicating that the cranial sartorius undergoes initial true muscle hypertrophy. Values of both older groups were less than those of the younger dogs, suggesting that the cranial sartorius muscle atrophies over time, with an associated increase in the endomysial space because of deposition of fat and connective tissue.

Our studies of force/torque generated by individual and grouped GRMD muscles are in keeping with these pathologic data and findings from mdx mice. We initially evaluated tension generated by the peroneus longus muscle.[46] Absolute twitch tension and both muscle- and body-weight-corrected twitch tension in GRMD dogs were low compared with normal littermates at 3 months of age. Tetanic tension was affected similarly. However, although absolute values were still reduced at 6 months,

Table 1
Morphometric GRMD vs. normal canine cranial sartorius histopathologic data (mean ± SD)

Pathologic Lesion	Normal (6–20 mo; n = 12)	GRMD		
		Group 1 4–10 mo; n = 15	Group 2 13–26 mo; n = 4	Group 3 33–66 mo; n = 4
Corrected muscle weight (g/kg)[a]	1.3075 ± 0.2079	3.0573 ± 0.7635	2.4725 ± 0.7556	1.4650 ± 0.6575
Percentage of endomysial space[b]	2.8083 ± 1.3468	27.1857 ± 15.3869	44.1275 ± 14.6462	58.9100 ± 14.2060
True muscle weight (g/kg)[c]	1.2699 ± 0.1966	2.2063 ± 0.6884	1.3758 ± 0.5078	0.5720 ± 0.2423
Mean fiber diameter (μm)[d]	42.1658 ± 4.3542	57.4980 ± 11.7419	63.1295 ± 13.3033	47.0850 ± 17.7029

[a] Normal<GRMD, Group 1 ($P<.05$); GRMD Group 1>GRMD Group 3 ($P<.05$).
[b] Normal<GRMD Groups 1–3 (all $P<.05$).
[c] Normal<GRMD, Group 1 ($P<.001$); GRMD Group 1>GRMD Groups 2 ($P<.05$) and 3 ($P<.001$).
[d] Normal<GRMD Groups 1 and 2; $P<.01$ for Group 1 and $P<.05$ for Group 2.
Data from Kornegay JN, Cundiff DD, Bogan DJ, et al. The cranial sartorius muscle undergoes true hypertrophy in dogs with golden retriever muscular dystrophy. Neuromuscul Disord 2003;13:493–500.

twitch and tetanic tension corrected for either muscle or body weight was not statistically different (**Fig. 3**), suggesting that the peroneus longus recovers from an initial period of necrosis. Moving forward, we have primarily evaluated force/torque generated by tarsal joint flexors (including the cranial tibialis and peroneus longus) and extensors (including the gastrocnemius and superficial digital flexor that is analogous to the soleus).[47] For these measurements, the peroneal and tibial nerves are stimulated percutaneously so that the paw pulls (peroneal nerve, flexion) or pushes against (tibial nerve, extension) a lever interfaced with a force transducer. In our initial study, force values were measured at 3, 4.5, 6, and 12 months of age. While absolute and body-weight-corrected GRMD twitch and tetanic force values were lower than normal at all ages, tarsal flexion and extension were differentially affected (**Fig. 4**). Flexion values were especially low at 3 months, whereas extension was affected more at later ages.

We have used tetanic tarsal joint force measurements to evaluate effects of prednisone (2 mg/kg) given to GRMD dogs for a 4-month period beginning at 2 months of age.[48] Tarsal extension force increased in treated versus control GRMD dogs, whereas flexion paradoxically decreased. In light of our force studies, we assumed that the paradoxical decline in flexion occurred because prednisone attenuated early necrosis in muscles such as the peroneus longus and cranial tibialis that would have otherwise led to functional hypertrophy.

Contraction kinetics in GRMD dogs for both the peroneus longus[46] and grouped tarsal joint flexors and extensors[47] also differed from normal. Post-tetanic potentiation for the peroneus longus was more pronounced in GRMD versus normal dogs at both 3 and 6 months. Twitch contraction and relaxation times were dramatically prolonged, and there was concomitant sustained electrical activity at or before 6 months of age in some severely affected dogs. For the grouped muscles, the twitch-tetany ratio was generally lower, post-tetanic potentiation for flexion values was less marked, and extension relaxation and contraction times were longer. As discussed further

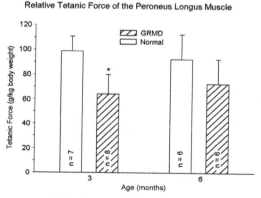

Fig. 3. Tetanic force corrected for body weight (g/kg) generated by the peroneus longus muscle of normal and GRMD dogs at 3 and 6 months of age. Values for the GRMD dogs are lower (*P*<.05)* at 3 months. However, although body-weight-corrected force is proportionally lower in normal dogs at 6 months, it has increased in GRMD dogs, such that values for the 2 groups are no longer significantly different. (*Data from* Kornegay JN, Sharp NJ, Bogan DJ, et al. Contraction tension and kinetics of the peroneus longus muscle in golden retriever muscular dystrophy. J Neurol Sci 1994;123:100–7.)

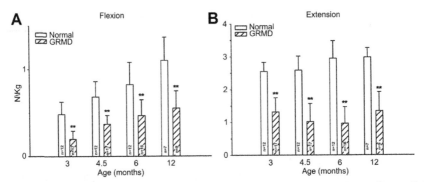

Fig. 4. Tetanic force, corrected for body weight (N/kg), generated by tarsal joint flexors (*left*) and extensors (*right*) from normal dogs and GRMD dogs at 3, 4.5, 6, and 12 months of age. Values for GRMD dogs are lower (*P*<.01 for all) than those of normal dogs at all ages. However, the differential between GRMD and normal dogs differs. Flexion values are especially low at 3 months, whereas extension is affected more at later ages. (*From* Kornegay JN, Bogan DJ, Bogan JR, et al. Contraction force generated by tibiotarsal joint flexion and extension in dogs with golden retriever muscular dystrophy. J Neurol Sci 1999;166:119; with permission.)

later, prolonged relaxation times with underlying sustained electrical activity and more generalized complex repetitive discharges could play a role in muscle hypertrophy.

POSTURAL INSTABILITY AND CONTRACTURES

Comparative aspects of gait abnormalities, postural changes, and joint contractures in humans and animal models must be interpreted in light of fundamental differences in conformation, some of which arise because of quadrupedal versus bipedal locomotion. As an example, the line of the pelvis from the tuber ischium to the wing of the ilium extends in a vertical plane, perpendicular to the walking surface, in humans but is oriented more horizontally, largely parallel to the ground, in quadrupeds. Thus, changes in pelvic orientation innately differ among patients with DMD, mdx mice, and GRMD dogs. In some cases, muscle weakness in DMD causes the posture to shift toward one normally assumed by quadrupeds and vice versa. The pelvis tilts anteriorly toward a more horizontal position to maintain postural stability in DMD[49] but shifts toward a vertical plane in GRMD dogs[50] (see later). Another factor relates to whether the leg/limb stance is plantigrade (humans and mice) or digitigrade (dogs).[51,52] Humans and mice walk on their phalanges, carpal, and tarsal bones, whereas dogs normally walk only on their distal and intermediate phalanges (digits). With neuromuscular diseases, in general, dogs become more plantigrade in the pelvic limbs,[53,54] adopting a stance more in keeping with that normally used by humans. A third stance, termed unguligrade, involves walking only on the tip of the distal digit.[52,55] The fact that horses have this posture explains use of the term equinus in DMD patients who toe walk.

DMD and BMD

Most DMD natural history studies include measurements of muscle strength, joint contractures, and timed function tests. Results from these tests are used to track disease progression and offer insight on clinical milestones, such as the loss of ambulation and the need for ventilatory support. Contracture and muscle strength scores generally correlate, deteriorate synchronously over time, and contribute mutually to postural instability.[56,57] As discussed later, unequal muscle weakness in DMD precipitates a vicious cycle that can lead to debilitating contractures and loss of ambulation (**Fig. 5**).[58]

Generally, contractures are caused by inactivity and restricted motion of the affected joint,[59,60] with a subsequent increase of collagen cross-links in periarticular connective tissue.[61] Major causes include forced joint immobilization to stabilize fractures,[60] spasticity associated with upper motor neuron lesions,[62] and primary neuromuscular diseases.[63] Joint contractures occur more commonly in DMD than other neuromuscular diseases[63] and have long been recognized as a major factor in disease morbidity. In one review that included 43 patients with DMD, the ankle (34/43), knee (29/43), hip (29/43), and elbow (28/43) were affected most frequently.[63] The ankle was also most commonly affected in BMD, occurring in 4 of 7 patients. Despite the prominent role that joint contractures play in these dystrophies, causative mechanisms are not fully understood. Underlying abnormal positioning presumably occurs because of an imbalance of forces acting on the joint, because diseased muscles are either disproportionately weakened or shortened by fibrosis. Relevant to this review, several studies have assessed the proportional strength of agonist and antagonist muscles operating at joints of patients with DMD. Some studies have concluded that muscular imbalance contributes to contractures,[57,64–66] whereas another found no such association.[67] Those finding a relationship noted a strong negative correlation between extensor muscle weakness and flexor contracture severity in DMD. As opposing extensor muscles weakened, flexor contractures worsened. Disproportionate flexor muscle hypertrophy would logically exaggerate this process. In a somewhat similar vein, contractures occurring because of spasticity also are magnified by enhanced flexor muscle activity.[62]

Postural instability and leg contractures are of special interest in DMD because of their role in the loss of ambulation. The relative sequence and proportional involvement of flexor and extensor muscles is critical. Early weakness of the hip (gluteus

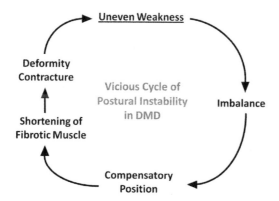

Fig. 5. Vicious cycle of postural instability that leads to loss of ambulation in patients with DMD. Uneven weakness leads to imbalance and compensatory postural changes that ultimately result in shortening of muscles and contractures. The process is self-perpetuating. (*Modified from* Roy L, Gibson DA. Pseudohypertrophic muscular dystrophy and its surgical management: review of 30 patients. Can J Surg 1970;13:14; with permission.)

maximus) and knee (quadriceps femoris) extensors necessitates postural changes to maintain ambulation. Increased anterior pelvic tilt and lumbar lordosis are adopted to shift the center of gravity forward of the knee and behind the hip, respectively.[49] Johnson[68] suggested that this posture allows passive ligamentous stabilization of these joints. Of comparative interest, a somewhat analogous system of ligamentous support (stay apparatus) allows horses to remain standing while sleeping.[69] Relative preservation of hip (including the sartorius) and knee (hamstrings) flexors in DMD creates destabilizing torque forces and also contributes to contractures at both levels.[70] Toe walking is adopted to stabilize the knee and later plays a role in the development of ankle equinus.[71] Plantar flexor contractures associated with equinus are aggravated by unbalanced muscle activity at the ankle, with selective weakening of the tibialis anterior and peroneus longus muscles and relative sparing of the triceps surae (collectively, the 2 heads of the gastrocnemius and soleus).[57,71] One investigator characterized this as a return to the infantile digitigrade pattern of walking, perhaps in an effort to put less stress on the weakened tibialis anterior muscle.[72] These contractures may initially have beneficial effects because tension in the gastrocnemius muscles pulls on the femoral condyles, extending the knee.[73] Iliotibial band (hip) contractures also extend the knee, providing additional stability. However, in advanced stages, heel cord and iliotibial band tightening destabilize gait, prompting the development of various corrective surgical procedures.[65,74] Scoliosis is typically a late complication of DMD, occurring in boys after they have gone into wheelchairs, with the side of convexity almost always toward the dominant hand.[75] The developing spine is thought to become deformed by excessive unbalanced forces from the dominant extremity. Scoliosis restricts expansion of the chest and tracks closely with respiratory disease.[76] Importantly, this biomechanical interplay in scoliosis shows that application of disproportionate (asymmetric) muscle force to the developing skeleton can cause bony maldevelopment with clinical consequences.

As discussed earlier, mechanisms contributing to preferential calf and other flexor muscle sparing or hypertrophy, starting with whether there is an actual increase in contractile tissue, are especially intriguing. If one accepts that these muscles undergo true hypertrophy in at least some patients, the timing and functionality of the muscle enlargement and whether it is playing a beneficial or detrimental role become critical. This would be particularly relevant with treatments, such as myostatin inhibition, that are intended to increase muscle mass (see later).

The mdx Mouse

Kyphosis analogous to scoliosis in DMD has been characterized in the mdx mouse. Just as with DMD, there is an association between spinal deformity and respiratory compromise. Mechanisms to account for kyphosis have not been defined, although Laws and Hoey[77] speculated that muscle hypertrophy could contribute. In a separate proof-of-concept study, this same group evaluated the potential for intramuscular injection of antisense oligonucleotides into paraspinal muscles to ameliorate kyphosis.[78] The treated group had less thoracic deformity than controls, but other outcome parameters did not differ between the groups. Weights of the latissimus dorsi, diaphragm, and intercostals muscles were increased in mdx mice in both treated and control mice. Force generation by these muscles was not increased, and histologic features were more in keeping with muscle degeneration and fibrosis than true hypertrophy. Thus, although not the central focus of this study, there was not a definite link between muscle hypertrophy and kyphosis.

Contractures of the tarsal (talocrural, ankle) joint have recently been characterized in the mdx mouse.[79] As discussed earlier, both mice and humans have a plantigrade stance, so there could be analogous operative forces. In keeping with findings from DMD, mdx mice had plantar flexor contractures, evidenced by decreased dorsiflexion and range of motion. There was an associated increase in gastrocnemius wet muscle weight, and torque generated by the dorsiflexors was proportionally lower than that of the gastrocnemius muscles.

FHMD

Because of their muscle hypertrophy, FHMD cats have a stiff stilted gait with their hocks adducted.[12,13] They adopt a "falling down technique" to move into lateral recumbency and are unable to turn their heads and groom.[12] FHMD cats also do not close their mouths completely, presumably because of glossal hypertrophy,[12,13] which interferes with eating and swallowing, ultimately causing dehydration and azotemia.[13] The esophagus may have decreased contractility[13] and can be constricted by the hypertrophied diaphragm,[12,13] resulting in regurgitation. A syndrome similar to malignant hyperthermia has been characterized in several cats that died during stress or anesthesia (see discussion linking calcium homeostasis in this condition and muscle hypertrophy).[42,80]

GRMD Dog

Gait and postural changes in GRMD must be considered in the context of marked phenotypic variation among affected dogs.[81,82] Severely affected dogs may die within the first 10 days of life,[81] whereas others live well into adulthood.[83] By 6 weeks of age, GRMD dogs advance their pelvic limbs simultaneously (*bunny hopping*) and subsequently exhibit a progressively more stilted gait.[81] Those with a severe phenotype develop a characteristic plantigrade stance between 3 and 6 months, as evidenced by hyperextension of the carpus and hyperflexion of the tarsus.[81,84] Over this same period, the elbows become abducted and the hocks are adducted. Concomitantly, the pelvic limbs shift forward, as the tuber ischium of the pelvis moves ventrally and cranially. In severe cases, the line of the pelvis may be oriented in an essentially vertical plane, perpendicular to the walking surface (**Fig. 6**).[50] Some of these dogs lose the ability to walk and must be euthanized.

Beyond the initial 6 months of life, clinical signs in GRMD dogs tend to stabilize and further adaptive changes help to maintain postural stability. With both video gait analysis[85] and accelerometry,[86] GRMD dogs walk more slowly and their stride length is decreased. Accelerometry demonstrated a redistribution of power at gait, with a decrease in the craniocaudal plane and a compensatory increase mediolaterally to maintain balance.[86] On video gait analysis, older, generally mildly affected dogs had a more upright stance, with relatively greater extension of the stifle and lesser flexion of the tarsus.[85] This posture presumably is adopted in an effort to stabilize their stance in the face of quadriceps weakness. In our experience, GRMD dogs rarely become nonambulatory after the initial critical period of destabilization at 3 to 6 months of age. Some have a normal life span; we currently have a 12-year-old GRMD dog with a remarkably mild phenotype in our colony.

One of our earlier studies showed that 6-month-old GRMD dogs positioned in dorsal recumbency for force measurements have abnormally acute (contracted) tarsal joint angles.[46,84] Other investigators have subsequently described methods to measure joint angles at maximal flexion and extension in normal dogs.[87,88] We

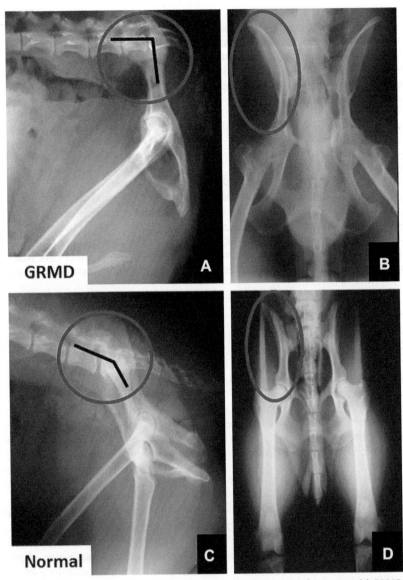

Fig. 6. Lateral (A) and ventrodorsal (B) radiographs of the pelvis of a 4-year-old GRMD dog and a normal dog (C and D) for comparison. Note the marked vertical tilt of the pelvis in the GRMD dog (A), so that the angle formed by the wing of the ilium and lumbar spine is much more acute at approximately 90° (angle marked by lines within the red circle). The wings of the ilia flare laterally in the GRMD dog (*red circle* in B). (*From* Brumitt JW, Essman SC, Kornegay JN, et al. Radiographic features of Golden Retriever muscular dystrophy. Vet Radiol Ultrasound 2006;47:578; with permission.)

now use the method suggested by Jaegger and colleagues[87] to measure pelvic limb joint angles and range of motion. By 6 months of age, GRMD dogs tend to have more restricted maximal flexion of the hip joint, increased maximal stifle extension, and more acute maximal tarsal flexion. To objectively characterize the cranioventral shift of the pelvis, we also measure the angle formed by 2 lines extending cranially from the tuber ischium, one drawn parallel to the lumbar spine and the other extending to the midpoint of the tuber coxae. This angle is larger in dogs with GRMD than in normal dogs at 6 months of age.

Mechanisms contributing to postural and joint angle changes in GRMD dogs have not been defined. The cranioventral pelvic shift may be an adaptive response, as affected dogs move their pelvic limbs under the torso to maintain balance. The resultant posture is similar to that achieved by boys with DMD when they shift their pelvis forward.[49] Alternatively, unbalanced hip flexor and extensor strength might play a role. Relative preservation of the hamstring muscles in GRMD dogs could pull the tuber ischium ventrally and also contribute to decreased maximal hip flexion values. As discussed earlier, considering the role that the sartorius and iliotibial band play in hip flexor contractures in DMD,[74] true hypertrophy of the cranial sartorius could be playing an analogous role in GRMD. In support of a relationship, we have previously shown that cranial sartorius circumference correlates negatively with tarsal joint angle in affected dogs.[25] Still, it is unclear whether there is truly a cause-and-effect relationship. The hypertrophied cranial sartorius could actively pull the stifle joint forward, with the tarsus passively following to assume a plantigrade position. On the other hand, cranial sartorius hypertrophy and plantigrade stance might have common root causes but no direct functional relationship. In any case, cranial sartorius hypertrophy or contracture does seem to affect the developing pelvis in young GRMD dogs, as the ilial wings from which it originates flare laterally (see Fig. 6),[50] presumably in response to unopposed torque. This is somewhat analogous to scoliosis resulting from unbalanced force applied by the dominant arm in boys with DMD[75] and emphasizes the potential for disproportionate muscle size and strength to cause skeletal deformity.

Local imbalance of agonist and antagonist muscles could also be playing a role in postural changes at the tarsal and carpal joints of GRMD dogs. Consistent with findings in DMD, we have shown that GRMD extensor and flexor muscles operating at the tarsal joint are differentially affected. Flexion values are especially low at 3 months, whereas extension is affected more at later ages (see Fig. 4).[47] At 6 months of age, the tarsal extension-flexion force ratio correlates positively with tarsal joint angle, which is to say that dogs with stronger extensors have larger joint angles and a less severe phenotype.[89] We have not systematically studied joint angles in the thoracic limb and can only speculate on mechanisms involved in carpal hyperextension. It seems unlikely that a reverse pattern of muscle involvement, whereby extensor muscles are relatively preserved, is responsible. Importantly, plantigrade stance is a nonspecific clinical sign in dogs and cats with neuromuscular disease,[53,54] independent of underlying cranial sartorius hypertrophy. This suggests that the pelvic limb plantigrade posture, coupled with hyperextension of the carpus (so-called palmigrade stance),[53] may simply reflect distal muscle weakness. The pivot point would logically differ between the carpus (hyperextension) and tarsus (hyperflexion) to keep the footpads in contact with the walking surface.

Spinal curvature is not a major feature of GRMD. Lumbar kyphosis may occur in tandem with the cranioventral shift of the pelvis; lordosis can be seen more chronically.[81] The lordotic posture could occur because of unequal application of force on the developing spine, with relative restriction of vertebral growth dorsally (posteriorly) or exaggerated growth ventrally (anteriorly).[90,91] Relative preservation of the psoas major muscle in GRMD dogs[25] might exert disproportionate force on the ventral lumbar spine, contributing to both hip flexor contractures and lordosis.

MECHANISMS CONTRIBUTING TO MUSCLE HYPERTROPHY

Differences in the severity, distribution, and nature of pathologic lesions leading to muscle enlargement in DMD and the 3 animal models should offer clues on mechanisms contributing to muscle hypertrophy in dystrophin deficiency. In the mdx mouse and GRMD cranial sartorius, muscle hypertrophy follows early necrosis. We believe that a convergence of factors driving muscle regeneration and differentiation leads to a disordered or overly robust proliferative response in GRMD. Although it is tempting to speculate on a similar mechanism in DMD and FHMD, no direct evidence links early necrosis and hypertrophy in these diseases. The relative lack of fatty infiltration in muscles of the mammalian models raises additional mechanistic questions relating to the efficiency of muscle regeneration among species and their propensity for fatty change secondary to muscle injury. These questions are generally beyond the scope of this article. Here, we review central concepts and suggest potential drivers for muscle hypertrophy in light of findings in affected animals.

Muscle mass can expand through either increased cell number (hyperplasia) or size (hypertrophy), with proliferation playing a greater role in developing muscle[92] and hypertrophy being more important in maturity.[93] Both myofiber hyperplasia and hypertrophy are thought to contribute to increased muscle size in DMD and the animal models.[6,7,25,31,43] Muscle size is regulated by a complex set of genes that establish a balance between forces that would otherwise lead to either atrophy or hypertrophy.[94] With regard to muscle mass in DMD, much attention has focused on insulin-like growth factor 1, which is known to promote muscle hypertrophy by activating the phosphatidylinositol 3 kinase/Akt pathway and, in turn, mTOR and further downstream targets.[95] Activation of the Akt-mTOR pathway is associated with muscle hypertrophy in the mdx mouse, and Akt expression is increased in DMD muscles.[96] These findings led the investigators to conclude that "vigorous activation of hypertrophic processes during prenecrotic stages of disease might reduce the severity of pathology or extend the prenecrotic stage of disease."[96]

Many other factors could be driving or supporting muscle hypertrophy. Anderson and colleagues[97] found increased binding activity of basic fibroblast growth factor (bFGF) in mdx mouse versus DMD and GRMD muscle, suggesting that its expression might augment the regenerative response by recruiting more muscle precursor cells. However, in a subsequent study, administration of bFGF did not enhance muscle regeneration in mdx mice.[98] Transforming growth factor β_2 (TGF-β_2) levels are increased in both newly formed myotubes of regenerating muscle[99] and in muscle samples from patients with DMD.[100] The glycoprotein osteopontin (OPN; secreted phosphoprotein 1) functions as a proinflammatory/fibrotic cytokine in mdx mice[101] and serves as a genetic modifier in DMD.[102] Importantly, OPN also promotes myogenesis[103] and so could play a dual role in transitioning muscle from an inflamed to regenerative state. We have found increased levels of both TGF-β_2 and OPN in GRMD muscles; moreover, TGF-β_2 tends to track positively with the degree of cranial sartorius hypertrophy (Nghiem and colleagues, unpublished data, 2011).

The complex repetitive discharges seen on electromyography in the 3 dystrophin-deficient animal models[10,13,104] and, to a lesser extent, in DMD[105] offer an additional mechanism to account for muscle hypertrophy. Sustained electrical activity (myotonia) and muscle contractions associated with chloride and sodium channelopathies can lead to dramatic muscle hypertrophy in the nondystrophic myotonias.[106,107] Spontaneous discharges in dystrophin-deficient muscle may occur because of altered ion currents across the damaged muscle cell membrane, with an associated shift in the resting membrane potential. Sustained muscle contraction would presumably augment muscle size, just as it does in myotonia. A positive correlation was observed between Akt pathway activity and muscle hypertrophy in a group of patients with myotonic dystrophy.[108]

While correlative data are largely circumstantial, abnormal calcium homeostasis could predispose to both muscle hypertrophy and susceptibility to malignant hyperthermia–like syndromes. Myofiber calcium levels are increased in DMD[109] and each of the 3 mammalian models.[13,110,111] Increased cytosolic levels of calcium also occur in malignant hyperthermia caused by mutations in the ryanodine receptor gene.[112] Myofiber hypertrophy is a predictor of susceptibility to malignant hyperthermia in humans[113] and occurs in susceptible dogs.[114] Although patients with DMD are not at increased risk for malignant hyperthermia itself, they do occasionally develop a similar syndrome when anesthetized with volatile gases.[115] Among the dystrophin-deficient animal models, cats are particularly prone to a malignant hyperthermia–like syndrome[80] and demonstrate the most striking muscle hypertrophy.[12,13] We have seen a similar metabolic syndrome in GRMD dogs anesthetized with isoflurane and sevoflurane. In addition, changes in contraction kinetics of the GRMD peroneus longus muscle occur as it is increasing in size and are compatible with those seen with a delay in calcium sequestration.[46]

MYOSTATIN INHIBITION IN MUSCLE DISEASE

Beyond the incalculable emotional trauma for patients with DMD and their families, society pays a huge price. Yearly health care costs exceed $30,000 per patient with DMD, 10 to 20 times those of other hospitalized groups.[116] In Australia, overall annual costs for each patient, including personal care and lost productivity, have been estimated to be $126,000 and yearly costs due to muscular dystrophy have been placed at approximately $1.5 billion.[117] These figures offer a window into the broader societal impact of more common degenerative muscle disorders such as sarcopenia and cancer cachexia. Sarcopenia incidence increases over life, with approximately 15% of women and 30% of men affected at age 80 years.[118] Direct health care costs attributable to sarcopenia in the United States approached $20 billion in 2000.[119]

The collective incidence and cost of health care for the muscular dystrophies and other muscle wasting disorders is a major driver for the pharmaceutical industry.[120,121] One strategy for promoting muscle regeneration involves inhibiting myostatin (Mstn; growth/differentiation factor 8), a negative regulator of muscle growth. Humans,[122] cattle,[123] sheep,[124] and dogs[125] with myostatin mutations have dramatic muscle hypertrophy. Dystrophin-deficient mdx mice in which myostatin is knocked out $(Mstn^{-/-})$[126] or inhibited postnatally[127] also have a less severe phenotype. Conversely, results from other dystrophic murine models in which myostatin was knocked out have varied,[128,129] with some mice showing increased morbidity.[130] There are questions about potential senescence of myostatin-deficient cells that have undergone multiple divisions.[129] Moreover, abnormalities have been identified in muscle tendons from $Mstn^{-/-}$ mice.[131]

Although genetically engineered mice have provided an extremely powerful tool to study the molecular pathogenesis of disease, results do not necessarily extrapolate to humans, presumably because of differences between murine and human size and physiology.[132] These shortcomings are partially obviated with canine models, which have been used extensively to study disease pathogenesis and treatment efficacy.[133,134] This trend toward the use of canine genetic models such as GRMD to study human disease will likely accelerate with the recent sequencing of the canine genome.[135] Thus, ideally, results from myostatin-deficient mdx mice should be corroborated in dystrophic dogs in which the gene has been knocked out. Unfortunately, transgenic technology in the dog is very cumbersome and inefficient, essentially precluding use of this approach.[136] With this in mind, we have developed a canine (*GRippet*) model by crossbreeding dystrophin-deficient GRMD dogs with myostatin-heterozygous (*Mstn*$^{+/-}$) whippets.

A total of 4 dystrophic *Mstn*$^{+/-}$ GRippets and 3 dystrophic *Mstn* wild-type (*Mstn*$^{+/+}$) dogs from 2 litters have been evaluated using various phenotypic tests at 6 to 8 months of age. Rather than showing improvement, the dystrophic *Mstn*$^{+/-}$ GRippets were more clinically affected than their dystrophic *Mstn*$^{+/+}$ littermates, apparently because of disproportionate enlargement of certain muscles. In particular, unequal hypertrophy of proximal pelvic limb muscles, as determined by MRI (**Fig. 7** and **Table 2**) and necropsy, seemed to exaggerate postural abnormalities. Gross cranial sartorius muscle hypertrophy was particularly prominent. In general, atrophy or hypertrophy of individual muscles in dystrophic *Mstn*$^{+/+}$ dogs was exaggerated in the dystrophic *Mstn*$^{+/-}$ GRippets. Some dystrophic *Mstn*$^{+/-}$ GRippets had commensurate, more pronounced atrophy/hypoplasia of the quadriceps femoris muscle.

Data from these *GRippet* dogs indicate that mechanisms contributing to selective muscle hypertrophy or atrophy/hypoplasia in dystrophin-deficient muscle may be exaggerated by partial loss of myostatin. Clearly, findings from a genetic model in which myostatin is inhibited from conception will not necessarily predict the outcome of staged postnatal treatments. However, at the very least, our results imply that differential effects of myostatin inhibition on muscle could have

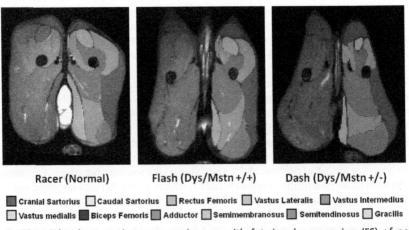

Racer (Normal)   Flash (Dys/Mstn +/+)   Dash (Dys/Mstn +/-)

■ Cranial Sartorius □ Caudal Sartorius ■ Rectus Femoris ■ Vastus Lateralis ■ Vastus Intermedius
□ Vastus medialis ■ Biceps Femoris ■ Adductor □ Semimembranosus ■ Semitendinosus □ Gracilis

Fig. 7. T2-weighted magnetic resonance images with fat signal suppression (FS) of pelvic limb muscles at midthigh from 3 crossbred GRMD and myostatin-heterozygous (*Mstn*$^{+/-}$) dogs from the first litter. Note the proportional enlargement of the sartorius and hamstring muscles and the associated atrophy/hypoplasia of the quadriceps of the dystrophic *Mstn*$^{+/+}$ dog, *Flash*, relative to the normal dog, *Racer*, and the even more dramatic differential size of these muscles in the dystrophic *Mstn*$^{+/-}$ dog, *Dash* (also see volumetric measurements from these sections in **Table 2**). Segmentation was done using ITK-SNAP (http://www.itksnap.org/pmwiki/pmwiki.php).[137]

Table 2
MRI volumetric measurements of proximal pelvic limb muscles in crossbred GRMD and Mstn$^{+/-}$ dogs[a]

Muscle	Racer (Normal/Mstn$^{+/+}$)			Flash (Dys/Mstn$^{+/+}$)			Dash (Dys/Mstn$^{+/-}$)		
	Volume (mm³)	Volume (mm³/kg)	Percent of Section	Volume (mm³)	Volume (mm³/kg)	Percent of Section	Volume (mm³)	Volume (mm³/kg)	Percent of Section
Cranial sartorius	101	5.87	1.77	168	16.15	4.25	309	30.00	8.01
Caudal sartorius	29	1.69	0.51	52	5.0	1.32	109	10.78	2.83
Sartorius total	*130*	*7.56*	*2.28*	*220*	*21.15*	*5.57*	*418*	*40.78*	*10.84*
Rectus femoris	279	16.22	4.89	181	17.40	4.58	69	6.70	1.79
Vastus lateralis	635	36.91	11.13	419	40.29	10.60	232	22.52	6.01
Vastus medialis	351	20.41	6.16	127	12.21	3.21	132	12.82	3.42
Vastus intermedius	480	27.91	8.42	207	19.90	5.23	130	12.62	3.37
Quadriceps total	*1745*	*101.45*	*30.60*	*934*	*89.80*	*23.62*	*563*	*54.66*	*14.59*
Semimembranosus	807	46.92	14.16	578	55.58	14.62	807	78.35	20.92
Semitendinosus	284	16.51	4.98	509	48.94	12.88	680	66.02	17.63
Hamstring total	*1091*	*63.43*	*19.14*	*1087*	*104.52*	*27.50*	*1487*	*144.37*	*38.55*
Biceps femoris	1156	67.21	20.28	643	61.83	16.27	612	59.42	15.86
Gracilis	634	36.86	11.12	214	20.58	5.41	176	17.09	4.56
Adductor	945	54.94	16.57	855	82.11	21.63	602	58.45	15.60
Total	*5701*	*331.45*	*99.99*	*3953*	*380.10*	*100*	*3858*	*374.77*	*100*

[a] Measurements were made on 1-mm slices illustrated in **Fig. 7** using the software program, ITK-SNAP.[137]

deleterious consequences, in keeping with various other findings reviewed in this article.

SUMMARY

Mutations in the dystrophin gene cause Duchenne and Becker muscular dystrophy in humans and syndromes in mice (mdx mouse), dogs (golden retriever muscular dystrophy and other canine mutations), and cats (feline hypertrophic muscular dystrophy). While affected humans and dogs have progressive disease that leads primarily to muscle atrophy, certain muscles undergo paradoxical hypertrophy. Mdx mice progress through an initial phase of muscle hypertrophy followed by atrophy. Cats have persistent muscle hypertrophy. In both humans and animals, muscles are not uniformly affected, with some atrophying as others enlarge. Disproportionate involvement of flexor and extensor muscles acting at joints can exaggerate contractures. Muscle hypertrophy in humans has generally been attributed to deposition of fat and connective tissue (pseudohypertrophy), but recent Imaging studies suggest that increased muscle mass (true hypertrophy) also occurs. True hypertrophy plays a more prominent role than fibrosis and fatty deposition in the animal models. Various mechanisms could potentially account for increased muscle mass and, thereby, be manipulated therapeutically. However, for maximal benefit, treatments should uniformly increase mass or preferentially improve strength of clinically-important muscles. Treatments that result in disproportionate muscle enlargement may exaggerate postural instability and joint contractures. These deleterious consequences of muscle hypertrophy should be considered when developing treatments for muscular dystrophy and other muscle wasting disorders.

REFERENCES

1. Tyler KL. Origins and early descriptions of "Duchenne muscular dystrophy". Muscle Nerve 2003;28:402–22.
2. Hoffman EP, Brown RH, Kunkel LM. Dystrophin: the protein product of the Duchenne muscular dystrophy locus. Cell 1998;51:919–28.
3. Prior TW, Bridgeman SJ. Experience and strategy for the molecular testing of Duchenne muscular dystrophy. J Mol Diagn 2005;7:317–26.
4. Malhotra S, Hart K, Klamut H, et al. Frame-shift deletions in patients with Duchenne and Becker muscular dystrophy. Science 1988;242:755–9.
5. Koenig M, Beggs AH, Moyer M, et al. The molecular basis for Duchenne versus Becker muscular dystrophy: correlation of severity with type of deletion. Am J Hum Genet 1989;45:498–506.
6. Jones DA, Round JM, Edwards RH, et al. Size and composition of the calf and quadriceps muscles in Duchenne muscular dystrophy. A tomographic and histochemical study. J Neurol Sci 1983;60:307–22.
7. Cros D, Harnden P, Pellissier JF, et al. Muscle hypertrophy in Duchenne muscular dystrophy. A pathological and morphometric study. J Neurol 1989; 236:43–7.
8. Bulfield G, Siller WG, Wight PA, et al. X chromosome-linked muscular dystrophy (mdx) in the mouse. Proc Natl Acad Sci U S A 1984;81:1189–92.
9. Gillis JM. Understanding dystrophinopathies: an inventory of the structural and functional consequences of the absence of dystrophin in muscles of the mdx mouse. J Muscle Res Cell Motil 1999;20:605–25.
10. Kornegay JN, Tuler SM, Miller DM, et al. Muscular dystrophy in a litter of golden retriever dogs. Muscle Nerve 1988;11:1056–64.

11. Cooper BJ, Winand WN, Stedman H, et al. The homologue of the Duchenne locus is defective in X-linked muscular dystrophy of dogs. Nature 1988;334: 154–6.

12. Carpenter JL, Hoffman EP, Romanul FC, et al. Feline muscular dystrophy with dystrophin deficiency. Am J Pathol 1989;135:909–19.

13. Gaschen FP, Hoffman EP, Gorospe JR, et al. Dystrophin deficiency causes lethal muscle hypertrophy in cats. J Neurol Sci 1992;110:149–59.

14. Hoffman EP, Gorospe RM. The animal models of Duchenne muscular dystrophy: windows on the pathophysiological consequences of dystrophin deficiency. Curr Top Membr 1991;38:113–55.

15. Edwards RH, Jones DA, Newham DJ, et al. Role of mechanical damage in the pathogenesis of proximal myopathy in man. Lancet 1984;1:548–52.

16. Karpati G, Carpenter S. Small-caliber skeletal muscle fibers do not suffer deleterious consequences of dystrophic gene expression. Am J Med Genet 1986; 25:653–8.

17. Pradhan S, Mittal B. Infraspinatus muscle hypertrophy and wasting of axillary folds important signs in Duchenne muscular dystrophy. Clin Neurol Neurosurg 1995;97:134–8.

18. de Visser M, Verbeeten B Jr. Computed tomography of the skeletal musculature in Becker-type muscular dystrophy and benign infantile spinal muscular atrophy. Muscle Nerve 1985;8:435–44.

19. Ardran GM, Hamilton A, Kemp FH. Enlargement of the tongue and changes in the jaws with muscular dystrophy. Clin Radiol 1973;24:359–64.

20. De Bruin PF, Ueki J, Bush A, et al. Diaphragm thickness and inspiratory strength in patients with Duchenne muscular dystrophy. Thorax 1997;52:472–5.

21. Renard D, Labauge P. Thenar and hypothenar muscle hypertrophy in Becker muscular dystrophy. Neuromuscul Disord 2010;20:281.

22. Walton JN. Clinical examination of the neuromuscular system. In: Walton JN, editor. Disorders of voluntary muscle. London: Churchill Livingstone; 1981. p. 448–80.

23. Reimers CD, Schlotter B, Eicke BM, et al. Calf enlargement in neuromuscular diseases: a quantitative ultrasound study in 350 patients and review of the literature. J Neurol Sci 1996;143:46–56.

24. Marden FA, Connolly AM, Siegel MJ, et al. Compositional analysis of muscle in boys with Duchenne muscular dystrophy using MR imaging. Skeletal Radiol 2005;34:140–8.

25. Kornegay JN, Cundiff DD, Bogan DJ, et al. The cranial sartorius muscle undergoes true hypertrophy in dogs with golden retriever muscular dystrophy. Neuromuscul Disord 2003;13:493–500.

26. Karpati G, Carpenter S, Prescott S. Small-caliber skeletal muscle fibers do not suffer necrosis in mdx mouse dystrophy. Muscle Nerve 1988;11:795–803.

27. Stedman HH, Sweeney HL, Shrager JB, et al. The mdx mouse diaphragm reproduces the degenerative changes of Duchenne muscular dystrophy. Nature 1991;352:536–9.

28. Coulton GR, Morgan JE, Partridge TA, et al. The mdx mouse skeletal muscle myopathy: 1. A histological, morphometric, and biochemical investigation. Neuropathol Appl Neurobiol 1988;14:53–70.

29. Pastoret C, Sebille A. Mdx mice show progressive weakness and muscle deterioration with age. J Neurol Sci 1995;129:97–105.

30. DiMario JX, Uzman A, Strohman RC. Fiber regeneration is not persistent in dystrophic (MDX) mouse skeletal muscle. Dev Biol 1991;148:314–21.

31. Sacco P, Jones DA, Dick JR, et al. Contractile properties and susceptibility to exercise-induced damage of normal and mdx mouse tibialis anterior muscle. Clin Sci 1992;82:227–36.

32. Carnwath JW, Shotton DM. Muscular dystrophy in the mdx mouse: histopathology of the soleus and extensor digitorum longus muscles. J Neurol Sci 1987;80:39–54.

33. Anderson JE, Bressler BH, Ovalle WK. Functional regeneration in the hindlimb skeletal muscle of the mdx mouse. J Muscle Res Cell Motil 1988;9:499–515.

34. Torres LF, Duchen LW. The mutant mdx: inherited myopathy in the mouse. Morphological studies of nerves, muscles and end-plates. Brain 1987;110:269–99.

35. Tanabe Y, Esaki K, Nomura T. Skeletal muscle pathology in X chromosome-linked muscular dystrophy (mdx) mouse. Acta Neuropathol 1986;69:91–5.

36. Dangain J, Vrbova G. Muscle development in mdx mutant mice. Muscle Nerve 1984;7:700–4.

37. Quinlan JG, Johnson SR, McKee MK, et al. Twitch and tetanus in mdx mouse muscle. Muscle Nerve 1992;15:837–42.

38. Muntoni F, Mateddu A, Marchei F, et al. Muscular weakness in the mdx mouse. J Neurol Sci 1993;120:71–7.

39. Coulton GR, Curtin NA, Morgan JE, et al. The mdx mouse skeletal muscle myopathy: II. Contractile properties. Neuropathol Appl Neurobiol 1988;14:299–314.

40. Dupont-Versteegden EE, McCarter RJ. Differential expression of muscular dystrophy in diaphragm versus hindlimb muscles of mdx mice. Muscle Nerve 1992;15:1105–10.

41. Vos JH, van der Linde-Sipman JS, Goedegebuure SA. Dystrophy-like myopathy in the cat. J Comp Pathol 1986;96:335–41.

42. Winand NJ, Edwards M, Pradhan D, et al. Deletion of the dystrophin muscle promoter in feline muscular dystrophy. Neuromuscul Disord 1984;4:433–45.

43. Gaschen F, Burgunder JM. Changes of skeletal muscle in young dystrophin-deficient cats: a morphological and morphometric study. Acta Neuropathol 2001;101:591–600.

44. Valentine BA, Cooper BJ, Cummings JF, et al. Canine X-linked muscular dystrophy: morphologic lesions. J Neurol Sci 1990;97:1–23.

45. Nguyen F, Cherel Y, Guigand L, et al. Muscle lesions associated with dystrophin deficiency in neonatal golden retriever puppies. J Comp Pathol 2002;126:100–8.

46. Kornegay JN, Sharp NJ, Bogan DJ, et al. Contraction tension and kinetics of the peroneus longus muscle in golden retriever muscular dystrophy. J Neurol Sci 1994;123:100–7.

47. Kornegay JN, Bogan DJ, Bogan JR, et al. Contraction force generated by tibiotarsal joint flexion and extension in dogs with golden retriever muscular dystrophy. J Neurol Sci 1999;166:115–21.

48. Liu JM, Okamura CS, Bogan DJ, et al. Effects of prednisone in canine muscular dystrophy. Muscle Nerve 2004;30:767–73.

49. Sutherland DH, Olshen R, Cooper L, et al. The pathomechanics of gait in Duchenne muscular dystrophy. Dev Med Child Neurol 1991;23:3–22.

50. Brumitt JW, Essman SC, Kornegay JN, et al. Radiographic features of Golden Retriever muscular dystrophy. Vet Radiol Ultrasound 2006;47:574–80.

51. Charteris J, Leach D, Taves C. Comparative kinematic analysis of bipedal and quadrupedal locomotion: a cyclographic technique. J Anat 1979;128:803–19.

52. Polly PD. Limbs in mammalian evolution. In: Hall BK, editor. Fins into limbs: evolution, development, and transformation. Chicago: University of Chicago Press; 2007. p. 245–68.

53. Hanson SM, Smith MO, Walker TL, et al. Juvenile-onset distal myopathy in Rottweiler dogs. J Vet Intern Med 1998;12:103–8.
54. Bensfield AC, Evans J, Pesayco JP, et al. Recurrent demyelination and remyelination in 37 young Bengal cats with polyneuropathy. J Vet Intern Med 2011;25: 882–9.
55. Wentink GH. Dynamics of the hind limb at walk in horse and dog. Anat Embryol 1979;155:179–90.
56. Vignos PJ Jr, Spencer GE Jr, Archibald JC. Management of muscular dystrophy of childhood. JAMA 1963;184:89–96.
57. Brooke MH, Fenichel GM, Griggs RC, et al. Clinical investigation in Duchenne dystrophy: 2. Determination of the "power" of therapeutic trials based on the natural history. Muscle Nerve 1983;6:91–103.
58. Roy L, Gibson DA. Pseudohypertrophic muscular dystrophy and its surgical management: review of 30 patients. Can J Surg 1970;13:13–21.
59. Kottke FJ. The effects of limitation of activity upon the human body. JAMA 1966; 196:825–30.
60. Akeson WH, Amiel D, Abel MF, et al. Effects of immobilization on joints. Clin Orthop Relat Res 1987;219:28–37.
61. Akeson WH, Amiel D, Mechanic GL, et al. Collagen cross-linking alterations in joint contractures: changes in the reducible cross-links in periarticular connective tissue collagen after nine weeks of immobilization. Connect Tissue Res 1977;5:15–9.
62. Young RR, Wiegner AW. Spasticity. Clin Orthop Relat Res 1987;219:50–62.
63. Johnson ER, Fowler WM Jr, Lieberman JS. Contractures in neuromuscular disease. Arch Phys Med Rehabil 1992;73:807–10.
64. Archibald KC, Vignos PJ Jr. A study of contractures in muscular dystrophy. Arch Phys Med Rehabil 1959;40:150–7.
65. Siegel IM. Equinocavovarus in muscular dystrophy. Its treatment by percutaneous tarsal medullostomy and soft tissue release. Arch Surg 1972;104:644–6.
66. Wagner MB, Vignos PJ Jr, Carlozzi C. Duchenne muscular dystrophy: a study of wrist and hand function. Muscle Nerve 1989;12:236–44.
67. McDonald CM, Abresch RT, Carter GT, et al. Profiles of neuromuscular diseases. Duchenne muscular dystrophy. Am J Phys Med Rehabil 1995;74:S70–92.
68. Johnson EW. Walter J. Zeiter Lecture: pathokinesiology of Duchenne muscular dystrophy: implications for management. Arch Phys Med Rehabil 1977;58:4–7.
69. Schuurman SO, Kersten W, Weijs WA. The equine hind limb is actively stabilized during standing. J Anat 2003;202:355–62.
70. Hsu JD. Orthopedic approaches for the treatment of lower extremity contractures in the Duchenne muscular dystrophy patient in the United States and Canada. Semin Neurol 1995;15:6–8.
71. Hsu JD, Furumasu J. Gait and posture changes in the Duchenne muscular dystrophy child. Clin Orthop Relat Res 1993;288:122–5.
72. Trias D, Gioux M, Cid M, et al. Gait analysis of myopathic children in relation to impairment level and energy cost. J Electromyogr Kinesiol 1994;4:67–81.
73. Mukherjee AK, Mokashi MG. Epidemiology. The incidence and management of joint contracture in India. Clin Orthop Relat Res 1987;219:87–92.
74. Rideau Y. Treatment of orthopedic deformity during the ambulatory stage of Duchenne muscular dystrophy. In: Serratrice G, Cros D, Desnuelle C, editors. Neuromuscular disease. New York: Raven; 1984. p. 557–64.
75. Johnson EW, Yarnell SK. Hand dominance and scoliosis in Duchenne muscular dystrophy. Arch Phys Med Rehabil 1976;57:462–4.

76. Rideau Y, Jankowski LW, Grellet J. Respiratory function in the muscular dystrophies. Muscle Nerve 1981;4:155–64.
77. Laws N, Hoey A. Progression of kyphosis in mdx mice. J Appl Physiol 2004;97: 1970–7.
78. Laws N, Cornford-Nairn RA, Irwin N, et al. Long-term administration of antisense oligonucleotides into the paraspinal muscles of mdx mice reduces kyphosis. J Appl Physiol 2008;105:662–8.
79. Garlich MW, Baltgalvis KA, Call JA, et al. Plantarflexion contracture in the mdx mouse. Am J Phys Med Rehabil 2010;89:976–85.
80. Gaschen F, Gaschen L, Seiler G, et al. Lethal peracute rhabdomyolysis associated with stress and general anesthesia in three dystrophin-deficient cats. Vet Pathol 1998;35:117–23.
81. Valentine BA, Cooper BJ, de Lahunta A, et al. Canine X-linked muscular dystrophy. An animal model of Duchenne muscular dystrophy: clinical studies. J Neurol Sci 1988;88:69–81.
82. Ambrósio CE, Fadel L, Gaiad TP, et al. Identification of three distinguishable phenotypes in golden retriever muscular dystrophy. Genet Mol Res 2009;8: 389–96.
83. Ambrósio CE, Valadares MC, Zucconi E, et al. Ringo, a Golden Retriever Muscular Dystrophy (GRMD) dog with absent dystrophin but normal strength. Neuromuscul Disord 2008;18:892–3.
84. Kornegay JN, Sharp NJ, Schueler RO, et al. Tibiotarsal joint contracture in dogs with golden retriever muscular dystrophy. Lab Anim Sci 1994;44:331–3.
85. Marsh AP, Eggebeen JD, Kornegay JN, et al. Kinematics of gait in golden retriever muscular dystrophy. Neuromuscul Disord 2010;20:16–20.
86. Barthélémy I, Barrey E, Thibaud JL, et al. Gait analysis using accelerometry in dystrophin-deficient dogs. Neuromuscul Disord 2009;19:788–96.
87. Jaegger G, Marcellin-Little DJ, Levine D. Reliability of goniometry in Labrador retrievers. Am J Vet Res 2002;63:979–86.
88. Nicholson HL, Osmotherly PG, Smith BA, et al. Determinants of passive hip range of motion in adult Greyhounds. Aust Vet J 2007;85:217–21.
89. Kornegay JN, Bogan JR, Bogan DJ, et al. Golden retriever muscular dystrophy (GRMD): developing and maintaining a colony and physiological functional measurements. In: Duan D, editor. Muscle gene therapy: methods and protocols, Methods in molecular biology, vol. 709. New York: Humana Press; 2011. p. 105–23.
90. Coleman SS. The effect of posterior spine fusion on vertebral growth in dogs. J Bone Joint Surg Am 1968;50:879–96.
91. Kioschos HC, Asher MA, Lark RG, et al. Overpowering the crankshaft mechanism. The effect of posterior spinal fusion with and without stiff transpedicular fixation on anterior spinal column growth in immature canines. Spine 1996;21:1168–73.
92. Moss FP, Leblond CP. Satellite cells as the source of nuclei in muscles of growing rats. Anat Rec 1971;170:421–35.
93. McCarthy JJ, Mula J, Miyazaki M, et al. Effective fiber hypertrophy in satellite cell-depleted skeletal muscle. Development 2011;138:3657–66.
94. Sandri M. Signaling in muscle atrophy and hypertrophy. Physiology 2008;23: 160–70.
95. Shavlakadze T, Chai J, Maley K, et al. A growth stimulus is needed for IGF-1 to induce skeletal muscle hypertrophy in vivo. J Cell Sci 2010;123:960–71.
96. Peter AK, Crosbie RH. Hypertrophic response of Duchenne and limb-girdle muscular dystrophies is associated with activation of Akt pathway. Exp Cell Res 2006;312:2580–91.

97. Anderson JE, Kakulas BA, Jacobsen PF, et al. Comparison of basic fibroblast growth factor in X-linked dystrophin-deficient myopathies of human, dog and mouse. Growth Factors 1993;9:107–21.
98. Mitchell CA, McGeachie JK, Grounds MD. The exogenous administration of basic fibroblast growth factor to regenerating skeletal muscle in mice does not enhance the process of regeneration. Growth Factors 1996;13:37–55.
99. McLennan IS, Koishi K. Cellular localisation of transforming growth factor-beta 2 and -beta 3 (TGF-beta2, TGF-beta3) in damaged and regenerating skeletal muscles. Dev Dyn 1997;208:278–89.
100. Murakami N, McLennan IS, Nonaka I, et al. Transforming growth factor-beta2 is elevated in skeletal muscle disorders. Muscle Nerve 1999;22:889–98.
101. Vetrone SV, Montecino-Rodriguez E, Kudryashova E, et al. Osteopontin promotes fibrosis in dystrophic mouse muscle by modulating immune cell subsets and intramuscular TGF-β. J Clin Invest 2009;119:1583–94.
102. Pegoraro E, Hoffman EP, Piva L, et al. SPP1 genotype is a determinant of disease severity in Duchenne muscular dystrophy. Neurology 2011;76: 219–26.
103. Uaesoontrachoon K, Yoo HJ, Tudor EM, et al. Osteopontin and skeletal muscle myoblasts: association with muscle regeneration and regulation of myoblast function in vitro. Int J Biochem Cell Biol 2008;40:2303–14.
104. Kurihara T, Kishi M, Saito N, et al. Electrical myotonia and cataract in X-linked muscular dystrophy (mdx) mouse. J Neurol Sci 1990;99:83–92.
105. Hausmanowa-Petrusewicz I, Jedrzejowska H. Correlation between electromyographic findings and muscle biopsy in cases of neuromuscular disease. J Neurol Sci 1971;13:85–106.
106. Trip J, Pillen S, Faber CG, et al. Muscle ultrasound measurements and functional muscle parameters in non-dystrophic myotonias suggest structural muscle changes. Neuromuscul Disord 2009;19:462–7.
107. Sinha MK, Chaurasia RN, Verma R. A family with autosomal recessive generalised myotonia with Herculean appearance. J Assoc Physicians India 2011;59: 120–2.
108. Li X, Zhang W, Lv H, et al. Activities of Akt pathway and their correlation with pathological changes in myotonic dystrophy. Beijing Da Xue Xue Bao 2010; 42:526–9 [in Chinese].
109. Bodensteiner JB, Engel AG. Intracellular calcium accumulation in Duchenne dystrophy and other myopathies: a study of 567,000 muscle fibers in 114 biopsies. Neurology 1978;28:439–46.
110. Ruegg UT, Nicolas-Métral V, Challet C, et al. Pharmacological control of cellular calcium handling in dystrophic skeletal muscle. Neuromuscul Disord 2002; 12(Suppl 1):S155–61.
111. Valentine BA, Cooper BJ, Gallagher EA. Intracellular calcium in canine muscle biopsies. J Comp Pathol 1989;100:223–30.
112. Stowell KM. Malignant hyperthermia: a pharmacogenetic disorder. Pharmacogenomics 2008;9:1657–72.
113. Mezin P, Payen JF, Bosson JL, et al. Histological support for the difference between malignant hyperthermia susceptible (MHS), equivocal (MHE) and negative (MHN) muscle biopsies. Br J Anaesth 1997;79:327–31.
114. O'Brien PJ, Cribb PH, White RJ, et al. Canine malignant hyperthermia: diagnosis of susceptibility in a breeding colony. Can Vet J 1983;24:172–7.
115. Gurnaney H, Brown A, Litman RS. Malignant hyperthermia and muscular dystrophies. Anesth Analg 2009;109:1043–8.

116. Ouyang L. Health care utilization and expenditures for children and young adults with muscular dystrophy in a privately insured population. J Child Neurol 2008;23:883–8.
117. The cost of muscular dystrophy. Report by Access Economics Pty Limited for the Muscular Dystrophy Association. Canberra, Melbourne, and Sydney (Australia), October 17, 2007.
118. Morley JE, Baumgartner RN, Roubenoff R, et al. Sarcopenia. J Lab Clin Med 2001;137:231–43.
119. Janssen I, Shepard DS, Katzmarzyk R, et al. The healthcare costs of sarcopenia in the United States. J Am Geriatr Soc 2004;52:80–5.
120. Bradley L, Yaworsky PJ, Walsh FS. Myostatin as a therapeutic target for musculoskeletal disease. Cell Mol Life Sci 2008;65:2119–24.
121. Patel K, Amthor H. The function of myostatin and strategies of myostatin blockade—new hope for therapies aimed at promoting growth of skeletal muscle. Neuromuscul Disord 2005;15:117–26.
122. Schuelke M, Wagner KR, Stolz LE, et al. Myostatin mutation associated with gross muscle hypertrophy in a child. N Engl J Med 2004;350:2682–8.
123. McPherron AC, Lee SJ. Double muscling in cattle due to mutations in the myostatin gene. Proc Natl Acad Sci U S A 1997;94(12):457–61.
124. Clop A, Marcq F, Takeda H, et al. A mutation creating a potential illegitimate microRNA target site in the myostatin gene affects muscularity in sheep. Nat Genet 2006;38:813–8.
125. Mosher DS, Quignon P, Bustamante CD, et al. A mutation in the myostatin gene increases muscle mass and enhances racing performance in heterozygote dogs. PLoS Genet 2007;3:779–86.
126. Wagner KR, McPherron AC, Winik N, et al. Loss of myostatin attenuates severity of muscular dystrophy in mdx mice. Ann Neurol 2002;52:832–6.
127. Wagner KR, Liu X, Chang X, et al. Muscle regeneration in the prolonged absence of myostatin. Proc Natl Acad Sci U S A 2005;102:2519–24.
128. Mendias CL, Marcin JE, Calerdon DR, et al. Contractile properties of EDL and soleus muscles of myostatin-deficient mice. J Appl Physiol 2006;101:898–905.
129. Parsons SA, Millay DP, Sargent MA, et al. Age-dependent effect of myostatin blockade on disease severity in a murine model of limb-girdle muscular dystrophy. Am J Pathol 2006;168:1975–85.
130. Li ZF, Shelton GD, Engvall E. Elimination of myostatin does not combat muscular dystrophy in dy mice but increases postnatal lethality. Am J Pathol 2005;166:491–7.
131. Mendias CL, Bakhurin KI, Faulkner JA. Tendons of myostatin-deficient mice are small, brittle, and hypocellular. Proc Natl Acad Sci U S A 2008;105:388–93.
132. Lin JH. Applications and limitations of genetically modified mouse models in drug discovery and development. Curr Drug Metab 2008;9:419–38.
133. Schneider MR, Wolf E, Braun J, et al. Canine embryo-derived stem cells and models for human diseases. Hum Mol Genet 2007;17(R1):R42–7.
134. Tsai KL, Clark LA, Murphy KE. Understanding hereditary diseases using the dog and human as companion model systems. Mamm Genome 2007;18:444–51.
135. Lindblad-Toh K, Wade CM, Mikkelsen TS, et al. Genome sequence, comparative analysis and haplotype structure of the domestic dog. Nature 2005;438:803–19.
136. Hong SG, Kim MK, Jang G, et al. Generation of red fluorescent protein transgenic dogs. Genesis 2009;47:314–22.
137. Yushkevich PA, Piven J, Hazlett HC, et al. User-guided 3D active contour segmentation of anatomic structures: significantly improved efficiency and reliability. Neuroimage 2006;31:1116–28.

Exercise Testing in Metabolic Myopathies

Mark Tarnopolsky, MD, PhD, FRCPC[a,b,*]

KEYWORDS

- Mitochondrial disease • Fatty acid oxidation defects
- Glycogen storage disease • Rhabdomyolysis

OVERVIEW OF METABOLIC MYOPATHIES

Metabolic myopathies are a group of genetic disorders specifically affecting glucose/glycogen, lipid, and mitochondrial metabolism. The main metabolic myopathies that are evaluated in this article are the mitochondrial myopathies, fatty acid oxidation defects (FAOD), and glycogen storage disease (GSD). Traditionally, defects in the enzyme myoadenylate deaminase (AMPD1) were considered to be a common metabolic myopathy; however, it is unlikely that AMPD1 deficiency is a true metabolic myopathy given the high prevalence in the general population (2%), that otherwise asymptomatic people (even athletes) can have this mutation with no exercise intolerance, and that high-intensity exercise does not alter energy status in skeletal muscle of patients homozygous for the common AMPD1 mutation.[1] A summary of some of the more common metabolic myopathies is presented in **Table 1**.

There are also medications that can interfere with intermediary metabolism and unmask or exacerbate an underlying genetic metabolic myopathy. The most common example of this phenomenon is 3-hydroxy-3-methylglutaryl-coenzyme A (HMG-CoA) reductase inhibitor (statins) medications leading to rhabdomyolysis and occurring in about 0.1% of all patients taking statins.[2–4] The cause of statin-associated myopathies is unclear; however, the depletion of coenzyme Q10 may be a more relevant mechanism in the rare cases when a patient with a genetic metabolic myopathy is prescribed a statin.[3] It is also known that patients taking statin medications are more susceptible to exercise-induced muscle damage with an increased serum creatine kinase level (hyperCKemia),[5] and this must be considered in the evaluation of a patient with exercise-induced muscle cramps/myalgias and hyperCKemia. Statin myopathies are classified as toxic myopathies and are not considered further in this article, which focuses on the usefulness of exercise in the evaluation of genetic metabolic myopathies.

[a] Department of Pediatrics, McMaster University, HSC – 2H26, Hamilton, ON L8N 3Z5, Canada
[b] Department of Medicine, McMaster University, HSC – 2H26, Hamilton, ON L8N 3Z5, Canada
* Department of Pediatrics, McMaster University, HSC – 2H26, Hamilton, ON L8N 3Z5, Canada.
E-mail address: tarnopol@mcmaster.ca

Phys Med Rehabil Clin N Am 23 (2012) 173–186
doi:10.1016/j.pmr.2011.11.011
1047-9651/12/$ – see front matter © 2012 Elsevier Inc. All rights reserved.

Table 1	
Genetic metabolic myopathies affecting skeletal muscle	
Mitochondrial myopathy	MELAS syndrome, complex IV deficiency, cytochrome b mutations, complex I deficiency, Kearn-Syre syndrome, chronic progressive external ophthalmoplegia
Fat oxidation defect	CPT2 deficiency, trifunctional protein deficiency, VLCAD deficiency, glutaric aciduria type 2
GSD	Myophosphorylase deficiency (McArdle disease), PFK deficiency (Tarui disease), phosphorylase b kinase deficiency, lactate dehydrogenase deficiency

Abbreviations: CPT2, carnitine palmitoyltransferase 2; MELAS, mitochondrial encephalomyopathy, lactic acidosis and strokelike episodes; PFK, phosphofructokinase; VLCAD, very-long-chain acyl-CoA dehydrogenase.

THE METABOLIC RESPONSES TO EXERCISE

The specific metabolic fuel supplied to muscle is a function of the intensity and duration of exercise. At the onset of muscle contraction, there is the hydrolysis of adenosine triphosphate (ATP) to drive the various ATPases in muscle (myosin ATPase, calcium ATPase, Na^+/K^+ ATPase). The alteration in cellular energy charge leads initially to the activation of the anaerobic pathways through a variety of mechanisms via mediators such as inorganic phosphate, protons, adenosine monophosphate (AMP), and calcium. Instantaneously, the accumulation of adenosine diphosphate (ADP) in muscle results in ATP generation through the adenylate kinase and AMP deaminase system, with flux through this pathway ultimately leading to the production of ammonia and uric acid (**Box 1**). Within the first couple of seconds of contraction, there is also rephosphorylation of ADP to ATP through phosphocreatine stores catalyzed by the enzyme creatine kinase. The energy-buffering action of phosphocreatine is a function of muscle phosphocreatine stores, which can usually provide energy for close to 10 seconds of sustained muscle contraction. Within the first seconds of

---

Box 1
The anaerobic energy pathways in skeletal muscle

1. Adenylate kinase/myoadenylate deaminase

   a. ATP>(*ATPase*)>ADP+ADP>(*AK*)>ATP+AMP>(*AMPD1*)>IMP+NH_3>>(*XO*)>uric acid

2. Phosphocreatine/creatine temporal energy buffering

   a. ATP>(*ATPase*)>ADP+PCr+H^+>(*cCK*)>Cr+ATP

3. Anaerobic glycogenolysis/glycolysis

   a. Glycogen>(*myophosphorylase*)>glucose-6-phosphate (see glycolysis)

   b. Glucose>(*hexokinase*)>glucose-6-phosphate+ATP>fructose-6-phosphate+ADP>(*PFK*)> fructose1,6-bisphosphate>glyceraldehyde-3-phosphate+NAD> 1,3-bisphosphoglycerate+NADH+H^++ADP>3-phosphoglycerate+ATP≫ phosphoenylpyruvate+ADP>pyruvate+ATP+NADH+H^+>(*LDH*)>lactate+NADH

Note: the key enzymes are in italics.
Abbreviations: AK, adenylate kinase; AMPD1, myoadenylate deaminase; ATP, adenosine triphosphate; cCK, cytosolic creatine kinase; LDH, lactate dehydrogenase; NAD, nicotinamide adenine dinucleotide; PFK, phosphofructokinase; XO, xanthine oxidase.

contraction, there is also the activation of glycogenolysis by phosphorylation of myo-phosphorylase (activated form) and glycolysis through phosphofructokinase (PFK) activation by allosteric regulation. In anaerobic conditions, the glycolytic pathway leads to the accumulation of lactate and protons that can eventually inhibit muscle contraction and limit the duration of activities supported solely by anaerobic glycolysis/glycogenolysis (see **Box 1**).

Even with lower intensity activity, the first seconds to minutes of muscle contraction are relatively anaerobic; however, as capillaries dilate and deliver more oxygen to the working muscle there is a progressive increase in delivery of oxygen and activation of oxidative metabolism. The creatine kinase system leads to an increase in ADP in the mitochondrial matrix that further activates mitochondrial respiration (a form of state 3 respiration). The contraction-induced increase in intracellular calcium activates the tricarboxylic acid cycle; the increase in AMP also leads to activation of AMP-dependent kinase (AMPK), which phosphorylates several rate-limiting enzymes involved in the regulation of aerobic metabolism.

The final common pathway for aerobic metabolism is the mitochondria, where reducing equivalents (NADH + H^+ and $FADH_2$) are delivered to complex I and II respectively, from the decarboxylation of amino acids, free fatty acids (FFAs), and carbohydrate (glucose). Most of the glucose for glycolysis comes from muscle glycogen; however, some is supplied from blood glucose derived from hepatic glycogenolysis or gluconeogenesis. FFAs are derived from adipocyte-derived triacylglycerol lipolysis (peripheral lipolysis) and from the intramuscular hydrolysis of intramyocellular lipids (IMCL). Several amino acids can be oxidized in exercising skeletal muscle; however, at most they contribute 5% to the total energy requirements and usually under conditions of glycogen depletion.[6] In addition, there are no known disorders of amino acid metabolism that lead to an exercise-induced metabolic myopathy, with most leading to central nervous system disorders with developmental delay, regression, and seizures.

Exercise intensity during endurance exercise is measured as oxygen consumption (Vo_2). At the cellular level, Vo_2 is a function of cardiac output (heart rate [HR] × stroke volume) and the peripheral oxygen extraction by the tissues (arterial–venous oxygen content of blood). Vo_2 is measured during exercise testing at the whole body level using a metabolic cart that consists of oxygen and carbon dioxide sensors and a pneumotachometer to measure ventilation. Vo_2 reflects the total oxygen consumption over unit time calculated from the difference between room oxygen (20.93%) and expired gas as a percentage, multiplied by the minute ventilation in liters per minute. Carbon dioxide sensors are also included in the metabolic cart to measure the volume of carbon dioxide production (Vco_2); the ratio of the Vco_2/Vo_2 is called the respiratory exchange ratio (RER), which reflects the type of fuel being consumed during steady state exercise (**Fig. 1**). During the maximal Vo_2 (Vo_{2max}) exercise test, the intensity (load) and/or speed (in the case of a treadmill) are progressively increased until the patient reaches maximal capacity and Vo_2 plateaus. During this progression, there is a gradual increase in reliance on anaerobic energy systems, with an exponential increase in respiration and lactate production (anaerobic/lactate threshold); the RER will exceed unity and is usually more than 1.12 at Vo_{2max}.

At low exercise intensities ($\sim$35% Vo_{2max}), energy supply is derived from peripheral lipolysis, IMCL hydrolysis, and plasma glucose, with minimal contribution from muscle glycogen (see **Fig. 1**). At an exercise intensity of $\sim$65% of Vo_{2max}, there is proportionately greater contribution from IMCL and glycogen, and at 85% of Vo_{2max} there is a proportionately greater contribution to the energy supply from intramuscular glycogen stores. For top sport runners, most of the energy supply to run a marathon

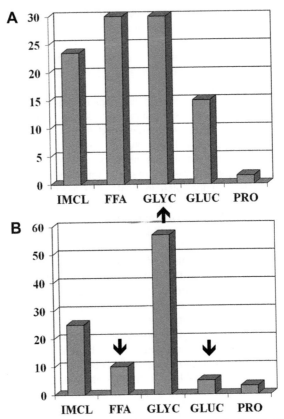

Fig. 1. Energy pathways during exercise. (*A*) Percentage contribution for the fuel sources to total energy during exercise at 35% of maximal oxygen uptake (Vo_{2max}); (*B*) percentage contribution for the fuel sources to total energy during exercise at 65% of Vo_{2max}. GLUC, blood glucose; GLYC, muscle glycogen; IMCL, intramyocellular lipids (triacylglycerol); PRO, protein/amino acids.

comes from muscle glycogenolysis.[7] During fixed lower intensity exercise for a long duration (ie, 2-hour cycle at 65% of Vo_{2max}), there is also a progressive increase in the contribution from FFAs (IMCL and plasma FFA) as muscle glycogen stores begin to deplete (see **Fig. 1**).

GLYCOGEN STORAGE DISEASE

Glycogen storage disorders refer to the inborn errors of metabolism that block the breakdown of tissue glycogen (glycogenolysis) and/or glycolysis. Although glycogen is important to muscle metabolism, it is also important in the liver, and some of the GSDs are liver specific (ie, glucose-6-phosphatase deficiency, GSD type 1; hepatic phosphorylase deficiency GSD type 6). Although the liver-specific GSDs lead to metabolic derangement, including hypoglycemia and lactic acidosis, the clinical features are severe and these patients do not present with a metabolic myopathy and with exercise intolerance. In addition, Pompe disease (GSD type 2, α-glucosidase deficiency) results in intralysosomal glycogen storage, which causes a fixed myopathy, but the intralysosomal glycogen is not used metabolically and patients do not present with a metabolic myopathy picture.

McArdle disease is the most common of the metabolic GSDs and is caused by a mutation in myophosphorylase blocking muscle glycogenolysis. GSD type 7 (PFK deficiency, Tarui disease) is less common than McArdle disease but is probably the second most common GSD affecting muscle. There are several other enzyme deficiencies in the glycolytic and glycogenolytic pathway that can lead to exercise-induced cramps, myalgias, and exercise intolerance; including phosphorylase b kinase deficiency, phosphoglycerate kinase and phosphoglycerate mutase deficiency, as well as lactate dehydrogenase deficiency. In general, all of the GSDs that affect muscle glycogenolysis or glycolysis have similar symptoms consisting of muscle cramps, premature fatigue, and occasionally rhabdomyolysis with myoglobinuria usually with higher intensity exercise. Given that anaerobic glycolysis/glycogenolysis is essential in the transition from rest to exercise when the muscle is anaerobic or in conditions of high-intensity exercise, these symptoms usually develop with high-intensity exercise, early after the onset of exercise, or during a stepwise increase in exercise intensity such as going for a bike ride and then suddenly having to go up a hill. Suspicion for these disorders comes from the pattern of exercise that induces the symptoms. In general, patients with McArdle disease have a second-wind phenomenon in which, after symptom onset and a period of rest or lowered exercise intensity, there is a feeling of lowered rating of perceived exertion as blood-borne fuels are delivered to the muscle to bypass the defects. Furthermore, patients with McArdle disease usually show improved exercise tolerance shortly (~ 20 min) after consuming glucose or sucrose (glucose-fructose).[8,9] In contrast, patients with glycolytic defects usually do not have a second wind, and may find that exercise tolerance is better after a prolonged fast.[10]

The diagnosis of the muscle metabolic GSDs is made from forearm exercise testing (discussed later), plasma creatine kinase (CK) levels, muscle biopsy, enzyme assays, and genetic testing. Plasma CK levels are almost universally increased in McArdle disease, but are seen in many muscle disorders (high sensitivity but low specificity). The muscle biopsy often shows a nonspecific increase in non–membrane-bound glycogen, and specific enzyme activities (PFK and phosphorylase) can be assayed from histologic sections and show the specific deficiency. The mainstay of therapy for McArdle disease is regular exercise training,[11] preexercise carbohydrate administration,[8,9] with possible benefit from creatine monohydrate supplementation.[12]

FATTY ACID OXIDATION DEFECT

The oxidation of FFAs in skeletal muscle is a complex process. FFAs are bound to albumin in the plasma and are transported across the muscle membrane by 1 of 3 different fatty acid transport proteins where they are reesterified into triglycerides and stored as IMCL lipid during the fed state or enter the mitochondria for β-oxidation. The long-chain FFAs (oleate, stearate, palmitate) are the FFAs predominately oxidized during exercise and these long-chain FFAs are transported into the mitochondria through the carnitine palmitoyltransferase (CPT) 1-carnitine acyl-transferase-CPT2 system. Medium-chain and short-chain fats are quantitatively less important during exercise and can enter the mitochondria without the CPT system. Once in the matrix of the mitochondria, the acyl-CoA moiety enters the 4 enzyme steps of β-oxidation, in which the acyl-CoA is converted to an n-2 acyl-CoA plus acetyl-CoA in a 4-step process involving dehydrogenation, hydration, dehydrogenation, and thiolysis. With each turn of β-oxidation, 1 mol of $FADH_2$ and 1 mol of $NADH + H^+$ is formed and they enter the electron transport chain of the mitochondria (discussed later). Very-long-chain acyl-CoA dehydrogenase (VLCAD) is the enzyme responsible for the first step of long-chain β-oxidation and trifunctional protein (TFP) combines catalytic activity of the long-chain–specific isoforms of the 3 final enzymes in β-oxidation. VLCAD and TFP deficiency are common β-oxidation defects, second in incidence only to defects in CPT2.

In general, patients with FAODs do well with brief high-intensity bouts of contraction, with activities such as weight training, peak strength activities, and sprinting being well tolerated; however, symptoms can occur if the patient is fasted or has a superimposed illness, and they can become more prominent with longer duration of activity. In general, therapy consists of avoidance of exercise during fasting or concurrent illness and consumption of a high-carbohydrate diet.[13] The plasma CK levels are usually normal between events, but increase during acute rhabdomyolysis. During a metabolic crisis leading to rhabdomyolysis, there is often an abnormal serum acylcarnitine profile and dicarboxylic aciduria (in the β-oxidation defects).[2,14] In general, the GSDs produce more of a muscle cramping sensation, whereas the FAODs produce myalgia sensations during exercise but can produce cramps on occasion.

MITOCHONDRIAL MYOPATHIES

The mitochondria are organelles that carry out the final common pathways for aerobic metabolism. Mitochondria are composed of approximately 1500 proteins, with the core function being the electron transport chain, which consists of 5 enzyme complexes. Reducing equivalents from the decarboxylation of fat, protein, and carbohydrates are used to reduce NAD^+ and FAD^+, which are delivered as $NADH + H^+$ and $FADH_2$ to complexes I and II, respectively, of the electron transport chain. The electrons from complex I and II reduce coenzyme Q10 and the electron flow through complex III is eventually passed on to cytochrome c and to complex IV (cytochrome c oxidase) where oxygen is reduced to water. The potential energy from the reducing equivalents is used to pump protons from the matrix of the mitochondria to the intramembrane space to build up the proton motive force. The protons then flow through ATP synthase (complex V) where ADP is rephosphorylated to ATP. Because the mitochondria represent the final common pathway for aerobic energy metabolism and also represent the terminal oxygen acceptor, many patients have endurance exercise intolerance and a low Vo_{2max}. The diagnosis of mitochondrial cytopathies is complex and involves clinical features, plasma analysis (alanine, lactate, CK), urine testing (organic acids such as 3-methylglutaconic acid), muscle biopsy, genetic analysis, and magnetic resonance (MR) spectroscopy; readers are referred to more comprehensive reviews in this regard.[2,15,16] For a more comprehensive review of many aspects of the metabolic myopathies, the reader is referred to a recent update.[2]

EXERCISE TESTING IN METABOLIC MYOPATHIES

In general, exercise testing is similar to any other test in that it has varying levels of sensitivity and specificity for ruling in (specific test) or ruling out (sensitive test) a given disorder. These testing characteristics are particularly important in patients with highly probable metabolic myopathies and those with highly unlikely metabolic myopathies. The latter case represents a substantial number of people referred for exercise intolerance and, in patients with nonspecific fatigue, when it is sometimes as important to rule out a metabolic myopathy as it is to rule one in other situations. For example, the patient complaining of generalized fatigue with a completely normal Vo_{2max} and RER is unlikely to have a primary mitochondrial myopathy (a sensitive test being normal rules out the disease in question). Conversely, there are several disorders in which secondary mitochondrial dysfunction can lead to a false-positive test, and it is important to be aware of these conditions and consider this in the interpretation of an exercise test. For example, we have shown that a 30% reduction in mitochondrial enzyme activity occurs after 2 weeks of immobilization in completely healthy university students,[17] and other disorders, such as type 2 diabetes and obesity, can be associated with secondary mitochondrial dysfunction, as can prolonged bed rest and other chronic debilitating disorders leading to hypodynamia.

An extensive number of exercise tests have been described in the literature[15,18–24]; however, a consensus for exercise testing in metabolic myopathies has not been adopted universally adopted. The most important consideration is to establish exercise testing based on sound biological principles, with individual laboratories establishing their own norms using positive controls (patients with confirmed metabolic myopathies) and negative controls (completely healthy individuals without evidence of metabolic myopathy). In general, there are 2 main types of exercise tests that are used in a metabolic myopathy laboratory, including forearm exercise testing, which is usually higher intensity to evaluate possible GSDs, and aerobic exercise testing (cycling or walking protocol) to stress the aerobic pathways and evaluate suspected mitochondrial defects and FAODs. An example of the setup for exercise testing patients with suspected metabolic myopathies is given in **Fig. 2**.

FOREARM EXERCISE TESTING

The first description of forearm exercise testing was in the evaluation of McArdle disease.[25] This test is based on the premise that any block of glycogenolysis or glycolysis should lead to a blunted/nonexistent increase in lactate following anaerobic exercise and an exaggerated ammonia response (caused by increased flux through the adenylate kinase/AMPD1 system). The increased flux through adenylate kinase/AMPD1 ultimately leads to an increase in uric acid (termed myogenic hyperuricemia), which can lead to gout.[26] The original versions of the testing used a sphygmomanometer around the upper arm to render the muscle ischemic, and most exercise protocols are about 1 minute in duration; however reports of testing-induced rhabdomyolysis,[27] and theoretic concerns for this phenomenon, led to the development of nonischemic or semi-ischemic tests.[22,28,29] As we have argued before,[22] the term nonischemic is a misnomer. All the tests render the muscle partially anaerobic (otherwise the test would technically not work) and all people doing these tests should be cognizant of the potential to induce a contracture, and potentially a forearm compartment syndrome and/or rhabdomyolysis, and should stop the test if a painful contracture occurs.

The test begins with the insertion of a plastic catheter into an antecubital vein of the arm to be exercised and blood is drawn into prechilled tubes for the determination of ammonia (usually green top with heparin) and lactate (usually gray top with glycolysis inhibitor). In theory, preexercise glucose ($\sim$20 minutes before) can falsely raise the lactate level and lead to the generation of some exercise-induced lactate (the premise behind preexercise glucose); however, in our tests, the lactate response is still massively blunted and the ammonia is exaggerated in McArdle disease during forearm testing (Mocellin, MSc thesis, manuscript in preparation, 2011); the preexercise glucose/sucrose is more of a confounder (false-negative directional change) during aerobic testing.[22] In practice, if a patient has eaten before arriving at the clinic, we wait at least an hour before starting the test, but our routine is to tell patients to fast

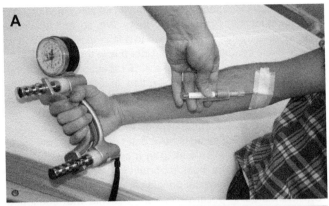

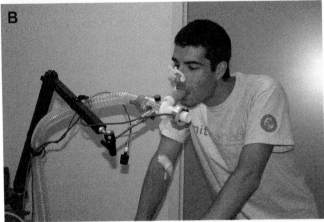

Fig. 2. Setup for metabolic myopathy testing. (*A*) Forearm exercise testing. A catheter (22 or 20 Ga) is placed in the antecubital vein with a Luer-Loc cap for sampling (a 3-way stopcock is also suitable). (*B*) Aerobic exercise testing. The catheter setup is identical to the forearm testing, and the participant cycles or walks on a treadmill (cycle shown here) with the established laboratory protocol.

for 2 hours before coming in. The participant then performs exercise for 30 to 60 seconds, with an intermittent contraction pattern (1:1 to 9:1 contraction/relaxation cycle) at 50% to 100% of maximal contraction (depending on the protocol).[22,28,29] In general, any of the many testing protocols can be used and it is likely that the specificity and sensitivity will be similar. We have the patient squeeze a Jamar dynamometer for 8 to 9 seconds and then relax for 1 to 2 seconds, and repeat this cycle for a minute (ie, six 9:1 rest/exercise squeezes = 60 seconds total) with verbal encouragement to work as hard as possible; the exercise force usually starts at about 90% of peak and decreases to about 35% of peak by the final cycle. We then draw blood into the tubes prepared the same way as described earlier at 1 minute and 3 minutes after exercise. It is critical that the blood tubes either be centrifuged and the plasma separated or transported to the laboratory on ice and run within 60 minutes of sampling (on ice). We do not recommend storage of the plasma, even in a freezer at −80°C, because the ammonia levels are spurious after only a week (lactate is unaffected for up to 6 months for research studies). We find that extending the postexercise sampling time beyond 3 minutes does not add to the sensitivity or specificity of the test.[22] In general, an increase in lactate of more than threefold compared with the baseline and an increase in ammonia of more than threefold are normal responses.[22] Patients with glycogenolytic/glycolytic defects usually have a minimal lactate response (<30% increase) and a normal to exaggerated (sometimes tenfold) ammonia response.

Although AMPD1 deficiency per se is not a cause of rhabdomyolysis, the measurement of ammonia has 2 other important uses in the testing. First, a patient with nonspecific fatigue or pain may not exert sufficient exercise intensity to activate the glycogenolytic or glycolytic pathway and, if both metabolites show a suboptimal response to the test, it is likely that there are local pain issues or supratentorial issues limiting force output. Alternatively, we have seen 1 patient with genetically confirmed McArdle disease who was also homozygous for the common AMPD1 mutation[30] and who had a suboptimal ammonia and lactate response to forearm exercise testing. This patient had a classic history of several bouts of rhabdomyolysis with high-intensity exercise, persistent hyperCKemia, a second-wind phenomenon, and a positive family history of similar symptoms in his brother, all of which led to further testing and the correct diagnosis.[30] Despite having molecular double trouble (ie, 2 mutations in the anaerobic pathways), he was no more symptomatic than his 2 brothers with McArdle disease and still plays competitive hockey with preexercise glucose, regular exercise after a warm-up, listening to his body, and taking creatine monohydrate supplements. A more common scenario in the neurology/metabolic clinic is a suboptimal test secondary to pain inhibition (myofascial pain) or supratentorial fatigue issues.

The sensitivity for McArdle disease or any of the glycolytic disorders is close to unity,[22] and a normal test rules out the glycogenolytic/glycolytic disorders; further testing is not needed unless there is compelling evidence to support the disorder (ie, multiple bouts of rhabdomyolysis induced by high-intensity exercise and a second wind [McArdle disease]). The specificity for the glycogenolytic and glycolytic disorders is high and an abnormal test warrants further testing. The only exception to the rules discussed earlier is phosphorylase b kinase deficiency, in which the response to the high-intensity forearm exercise test is reportedly normal and only apparent with aerobic testing.[31] The latter GSD is likely one of the mildest forms and there has even been some question as to whether or not it is a significant metabolic myopathy.[31] In the rare case when rhabdomyolysis occurs under high-intensity conditions, concern exists to rule out a metabolic myopathy, and the high-intensity forearm exercise test is normal, the advice would be to proceed to the aerobic testing to rule in or out an FAOD or mitochondrial disease. The very rare patient with phosphorylase b kinase deficiency would also be revealed with a suboptimal lactate response to exercise.

AEROBIC EXERCISE TESTING

The main value of this type of testing is to stress the aerobic energy systems in which FAODs and mitochondrial myopathies would be expected to show defects. The lactate response to phosphorylase b kinase and all other glycogenolytic and glycolytic defects would show a suboptimal lactate response; however, these disorders (except for phosphorylase b kinase deficiency) are usually suspected from the history and evaluated first with forearm exercise testing, so there would be no need to proceed to an aerobic test. There are occasions when a patient with McArdle disease notes symptoms during a more prolonged activity (eg, experienced rhabdomyolysis after a long walk and then climbing a hill) and it is possible that the history would suggest an FAOD or mitochondrial disease. Such a patient could first be investigated with aerobic testing (and identified from the suboptimal ammonia response).

In general, aerobic testing can be performed with either a cycle ergometer or a tread-mill, and the core samples include assessment of preexercise CK, lactate, ammonia, and postexercise (immediate or +1 minute) lactate, ammonia, and acylcarnitine. We do not measure CK after exercise because it takes many hours for an exercise-induced CK increase to occur.[32,33] For the reasons mentioned earlier, and because the RER would be falsely increased, the aerobic testing should occur at least 2 hours after eating. In general, we perform the tests in the morning after an overnight fast and provide a high-carbohydrate snack immediately after blood sampling. If patients have experienced fasting-induced rhabdomyolysis and/or fasting-induced pigmenturia or have a strong history of a likely FAOD, we do not recommend an overnight fast and allow them to have a snack 2 hours before the test and provide carbohydrates after the sampling.

Many different tests have been suggested for the diagnosis of possible mitochon-drial disorders and the reader is directed toward dedicated articles on the subject.[15,16] In general, a high resting lactate has moderate sensitivity (60%–70%) but good spec-ificity (>90%) in adults with suspected mitochondrial myopathy.[15,34–36] Exercise testing improves the sensitivity only marginally (postexercise lactate)[34–36]; however, a very high RER (>1.4), a low Vo_{2max}, and a high postexercise lactate strongly suggest further testing for a mitochondrial disease. There is an ongoing debate about the pros and cons of an absolute versus a relative exercise test.[15,35,36] The absolute testing is advocated because patients give a constant and identical workload for a set time and the response to the same workload is recorded (Vo_2, RER, HR, ventilation).[35,36] Advo-cates of the absolute testing protocol suggest that relative testing (ie, symptom-limited Vo_{2max}, or to 70% of Vo_{2max}) relies on a symptom-limited test, and motivation, pain, or other noncontrolled factors can limit the test. The advantages of a maximal test is that the Vo_{2max} can be determined and the metabolic stress is higher. Irrespec-tive of the testing mode that is chosen, it is important to establish normal values for controls (negative control) and to test patients with known disease (positive controls). Exercise testing in mitochondrial myopathies (using either method) has a sensitivity of between 0.63 and 0.75 and a specificity of 0.70 to 0.90 (see Ref.[15]).

Most cardiopulmonary testing laboratories (commonly available in most hospitals) use a symptom-limited Vo_{2max} test and it is easy for the nonmetabolic genetic exercise laboratory to use their testing to establish normal values for the variables mentioned earlier. We use a symptom-limited Vo_{2max} test in our laboratory with the blood measurements mentioned earlier. In cases of FAOD in which the resting acylcarnitine profile is normal, there can be an unmasking after exercise. A high resting response and/or an exaggerated lactate response to exercise in combination with a low Vo_{2max} and/or high RER can suggest a mitochondrial myopathy. However, high postexercise lactate is often seen in young healthy people who can push hard and drive the lactates high, which leads to an overlap with mitochondrial patients and limits the sensitivity of the test; however, extrapolating the postexercise lactate to peak power, or a dispro-portionate cardiovascular response at a given workload,[19] may help. In the rare case of a glycogenolytic or glycolytic defect that was not suspected and evaluated with the forearm testing, the lack of a lactate increase following exercise requires further eval-uation (assuming a true test, ie, ammonia increase and an HR close to the predicted maximum).

There are several additional tests that have been proposed to improve the diagnostic usefulness (sensitivity and specificity) of aerobic exercise testing in the mitochondrial myopathies, including near-infrared spectroscopy,[37] venous blood gas measurements,[18,20,38] MR spectroscopy,[24,39–41] and cardiac output measure-ments.[19] Near-infrared spectroscopy measures the myoglobin/hemoglobin content of muscle/blood over the working muscle (usually forearm aerobic protocols) and the classic mitochondrial pattern is a lack of or attenuated deoxygenation with exercise.[37] We find that this testing is tedious and not well suited to the clinic. It much easier to use routine venous blood gases to establish deoxygenation of the working forearm in response to exercise, as has been described by others.[20,28] The latter test just requires that the blood be taken in a blood gas syringe and immediately sent to the laboratory on ice. A complete lack or major attenuation of deoxygenation of hemoglobin in the draining vein following exercise is highly suspicious for mitochondrial myopathy, but a normal test does not rule it out.[28] There is an extensive body of literature using MR spectroscopy to evaluate mitochondrial function during exercise (eg, PCr/Pi ratio, acidosis),[39–41] but this is beyond the scope of this article; however, in general, the cost, time, effort, limited additional sensitivity or specificity,[39] and the confounding effect of physical inactivity (false-positive test)[42] make this an impractical and imprecise tool for the diagnosis of mitochondrial disease. In addition, it has been shown that the circulatory response to mitochondrial disease[19] and McArdle disease[43] is hyperkinetic (high cardiac output [stroke volume × HR]); however, cardiac

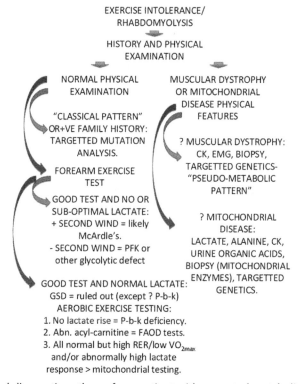

EXERCISE INTOLERANCE/
RHABDOMYOLYSIS

HISTORY AND PHYSICAL
EXAMINATION

NORMAL PHYSICAL
EXAMINATION

MUSCULAR DYSTROPHY
OR MITOCHONDRIAL
DISEASE PHYSICAL
FEATURES

"CLASSICAL PATTERN"
OR+VE FAMILY HISTORY:
TARGETTED MUTATION
ANALYSIS.

? MUSCULAR DYSTROPHY:
CK, EMG, BIOPSY,
TARGETTED GENETICS-
"PSEUDO-METABOLIC
PATTERN"

FOREARM EXERCISE
TEST

GOOD TEST AND NO OR
SUB-OPTIMAL LACTATE:
+ SECOND WIND = likely
McArdle's.
- SECOND WIND = PFK or
other glycolytic defect

? MITOCHONDRIAL
DISEASE:
LACTATE, ALANINE, CK,
URINE ORGANIC ACIDS,
BIOPSY (MITOCHONDRIAL
ENZYMES), TARGETTED
GENETICS.

GOOD TEST AND NORMAL LACTATE:
GSD = ruled out (except ? P-b-k)
AEROBIC EXERCISE TESTING:
1. No lactate rise = P-b-k deficiency.
2. Abn. acyl-carnitine = FAOD tests.
3. All normal but high RER/low VO_{2max}
and/or abnormally high lactate
response > mitochondrial testing.

Fig. 3. Proposed diagnostic pathway for a patient with suspected metabolic myopathy (ie, rhabdomyolysis, exercise intolerance, positive family history, and symptoms). If all of the testing is normal, we tell the patient that it is unlikely that the rhabdomyolysis was caused by an inborn error of metabolism, and request that, if it happens in the future, we are to be contacted and, during an acute event, that the following should be assesses: CK, creatinine, acylcarnitines, FFA, ketones, lactate, urinalysis (with myoglobin), liver function tests, thyroid stimulating hormone, viral serology, and hemolysis screen (for rare cases of sickle cell trait and also in PFK deficiency, although they would be diagnosed with the paradigm given). P-k-b, phosphorylase b kinase.

output measurements are not done routinely, but experienced clinicians may find that it adds to the diagnostic usefulness of testing in mitochondrial myopathy cases.[19]

SUMMARY

As with all of medicine, most diagnoses come from the history. A history of cramps/pigmenturia with higher intensity exercise may indicate a defect in glycolysis/glycogenolysis and a history of myalgias/cramps/pigmenturia with longer duration exercise or exercise in the fasted state or with a concomitant illness may indicate an FAOD or mitochondrial disease. Exercise testing may be helpful to rule in or rule out a given disease and prompt further testing. In general, patients with symptoms during higher intensity exercise should first undergo a forearm exercise test, which can be done in the office at the time of the initial consultation. Patients with exercise symptoms that suggest a mitochondrial myopathy or FAOD should be booked for a subsequent aerobic exercise test. Exercise testing is an extension of the history and examination and may add to the initial round of testing, but is not always necessary. For example, a patient with sensory neural hearing loss, type 2 diabetes, and strokelike episodes would be sent for MELAS (mitochondrial encephalomyopathy, lactic acidosis and strokelike episodes) 3243 testing followed by a muscle biopsy (if the genetic test for 3243, 3271, and 3291 was normal), even though exercise intolerance would undoubtedly be part of the history. Conversely, a patient with a history of pigmenturia with the flu as a child and exercise-induced rhabdomyolysis during a 3-hour hike would first be screened with an acylcarnitine profile (which may be increased even without provocation and sometimes can indicate the genetic defect: VLCAD, TFP, or CPT2). A practical approach to exercise testing in the patient with a suspected metabolic myopathy is presented in **Fig. 3**.

ACKNOWLEDGMENTS

Support for the testing laboratory came from Giant Tiger Stores. Tucker's Time Golf Tournament, the Costabile family, MitoCanada and Warren Lammert and Family have contributed to our work with mitochondrial myopathy patients.

REFERENCES

1. Tarnopolsky MA, Parise G, Gibala MJ, et al. Myoadenylate deaminase deficiency does not affect muscle anaplerosis during exhaustive exercise in humans. J Physiol 2001;533(Pt 3):881–9.
2. van Adel BA, Tarnopolsky MA. Metabolic myopathies: update 2009. J Clin Neuromuscul Dis 2009;10(3):97–121.
3. Vladutiu GD, Simmons Z, Isackson PJ, et al. Genetic risk factors associated with lipid-lowering drug-induced myopathies. Muscle Nerve 2006;34(2):153–62.
4. Baker SK, Tarnopolsky MA. Statin-associated neuromyotoxicity. Drugs Today (Barc) 2005;41(4):267–93.
5. Meador BM, Huey KA. Statin-associated myopathy and its exacerbation with exercise [review]. Muscle Nerve 2010;42(4):469–79.
6. Tarnopolsky M. Protein requirements for endurance athletes. Nutrition 2004; 20(7-8):662–8.
7. O'Brien MJ, Viguie CA, Mazzeo RS, et al. Carbohydrate dependence during marathon running. Med Sci Sports Exerc 1993;25(9):1009–17.
8. Vissing J, Haller RG. The effect of oral sucrose on exercise tolerance in patients with McArdle's disease. N Engl J Med 2003;349(26):2503–9.

9. Andersen ST, Haller RG, Vissing J. Effect of oral sucrose shortly before exercise on work capacity in McArdle disease. Arch Neurol 2008;65(6): 786–9.

10. Haller RG, Vissing J. No spontaneous second wind in muscle phosphofructokinase deficiency. Neurology 2004;62(1):82–6.

11. Haller RG, Wyrick P, Taivassalo T, et al. Aerobic conditioning: an effective therapy in McArdle's disease. Ann Neurol 2006;59(6):922–8.

12. Vorgerd M, Grehl T, Jager M, et al. Creatine therapy in myophosphorylase deficiency (McArdle disease): a placebo-controlled crossover trial. Arch Neurol 2000;57(7):956–63.

13. Orngreen MC, Ejstrup R, Vissing J. Effect of diet on exercise tolerance in carnitine palmitoyltransferase II deficiency. Neurology 2003;61(4):559–61.

14. Tein I. Metabolic myopathies. Semin Pediatr Neurol 1996;3(2):59–98.

15. Tarnopolsky M. Exercise testing as a diagnostic entity in mitochondrial myopathies. Mitochondrion 2004;4(5–6):529–42.

16. Tarnopolsky MA, Raha S. Mitochondrial myopathies: diagnosis, exercise intolerance, and treatment options. Med Sci Sports Exerc 2005;37(12):2086–93.

17. Abadi A, Glover EI, Isfort RJ, et al. Limb immobilization induces a coordinate down-regulation of mitochondrial and other metabolic pathways in men and women. PLoS One 2009;4(8):e6518.

18. Jensen TD, Kazemi-Esfarjani P, Skomorowska E, et al. A forearm exercise screening test for mitochondrial myopathy. Neurology 2002;58(10):1533–8.

19. Taivassalo T, Jensen TD, Kennaway N, et al. The spectrum of exercise tolerance in mitochondrial myopathies: a study of 40 patients. Brain 2003; 126(Pt 2):413–23.

20. Taivassalo T, Abbott A, Wyrick P, et al. Venous oxygen levels during aerobic forearm exercise: an index of impaired oxidative metabolism in mitochondrial myopathy. Ann Neurol 2002;51(1):38–44.

21. Vissing J, Haller RG. A diagnostic cycle test for McArdle's disease. Ann Neurol 2003;54(4):539–42.

22. Tarnopolsky M, Stevens L, MacDonald JR, et al. Diagnostic utility of a modified forearm ischemic exercise test and technical issues relevant to exercise testing. Muscle Nerve 2003;27(3):359–66.

23. Hanisch F, Eger K, Bork S, et al. Lactate production upon short-term non-ischemic forearm exercise in mitochondrial disorders and other myopathies. J Neurol 2006;253(6):735–40.

24. Argov Z, De Stefano N, Arnold DL. ADP recovery after a brief ischemic exercise in normal and diseased human muscle–a 31P MRS study. NMR Biomed 1996; 9(4):165–72.

25. McArdle B, Verel D. Responses to ischaemic work in the human forearm. Clin Sci (Lond) 1956;15(2):305–18.

26. Knochel JP. Myogenic hyperuricemia: what can we learn from metabolic myopathies? [letter]. Muscle Nerve 1996;19(4):535–6.

27. Meinck HM, Goebel HH, Rumpf KW, et al. The forearm ischaemic work test–hazardous to McArdle patients? J Neurol Neurosurg Psychiatry 1982;45(12): 1144–6.

28. Kazemi-Esfarjani P, Skomorowska E, Jensen TD, et al. A nonischemic forearm exercise test for McArdle disease. Ann Neurol 2002;52(2):153–9.

29. Hogrel JY, Laforet P, Ben Yaou R, et al. A non-ischemic forearm exercise test for the screening of patients with exercise intolerance. Neurology 2001;56(12): 1733–8.

30. Isackson PJ, Tarnopolsky M, Vladutiu GD. A novel mutation in the PYGM gene in a family with pseudo-dominant transmission of McArdle disease. Mol Genet Metab 2005;85(3):239–42.
31. Orngreen MC, Schelhaas HJ, Jeppesen TD, et al. Is muscle glycogenolysis impaired in X-linked phosphorylase b kinase deficiency? Neurology 2008; 70(20):1876–82.
32. Stupka N, Lowther S, Chorneyko K, et al. Gender differences in muscle inflammation after eccentric exercise. J Appl Physiol 2000;89(6):2325–32.
33. Stupka N, Tarnopolsky MA, Yardley N, et al. Cellular adaptation to repeated eccentric exercise-induced muscle damage. J Appl Physiol 2001;91(4):1669–78.
34. Jeppesen TD, Olsen D, Vissing J. Cycle ergometry is not a sensitive diagnostic test for mitochondrial myopathy. J Neurol 2003;250(3):293–9.
35. Finsterer J. The usefulness of lactate stress testing in the diagnosis of mitochondrial myopathy. Concerning the paper "Cycle ergometry is not a sensitive diagnostic test for mitochondrial myopathy" by Jeppesen et al. J Neurol 2005; 252(7):857–8.
36. Finsterer J, Milvay E. Stress lactate in mitochondrial myopathy under constant, unadjusted workload. Eur J Neurol 2004;11(12):811–6.
37. McCully K. Near infrared spectroscopy in the evaluation of skeletal muscle disease. Muscle Nerve 2002;25(5):629–31.
38. Hanisch F, Muller T, Muser A, et al. Lactate increase and oxygen desaturation in mitochondrial disorders–evaluation of two diagnostic screening protocols. J Neurol 2006;253(4):417–23.
39. Jeppesen TD, Quistorff B, Wibrand F, et al. 31P-MRS of skeletal muscle is not a sensitive diagnostic test for mitochondrial myopathy. J Neurol 2007;254(1): 29–37.
40. Argov Z, Arnold DL. MR spectroscopy and imaging in metabolic myopathies. Neurol Clin 2000;18(1):35–52.
41. Argov Z, Lofberg M, Arnold DL. Insights into muscle diseases gained by phosphorus magnetic resonance spectroscopy. Muscle Nerve 2000;23(9):1316–34.
42. Tartaglia MC, Chen JT, Caramanos Z, et al. Muscle phosphorus magnetic resonance spectroscopy oxidative indices correlate with physical activity. Muscle Nerve 2000;23(2):175–81.
43. Haller RG, Lewis SF, Cook JD, et al. Hyperkinetic circulation during exercise in neuromuscular disease. Neurology 1983;33(10):1283–7.

Nutrition Strategies to Improve Physical Capabilities in Duchenne Muscular Dystrophy

J. Davoodi, PhD[a,b], C.D. Markert, PhD[c], K.A. Voelker, PhD[a],
S.M. Hutson, PhD[a], Robert W. Grange, PhD[a,*]

KEYWORDS

• Duchenne muscular dystrophy • Nutrition • Physical activity
• Nutraceuticals

Duchenne muscular dystrophy (DMD) is a lethal, X-linked recessive, muscle-wasting disease[1] caused by mutations in the dystrophin gene, located on chromosome Xp21. Mutations of the dystrophin gene result in the absence of the dystrophin protein, which leads to an impaired linkage between the F-actin cytoskeleton and the extracellular matrix protein laminin 2 via the membrane-bound dystrophin-glycoprotein complex (DGC).[2,3]

In the absence of dystrophin, the mechanical links from the cytoskeleton of the muscle cell to the membrane and the components of the DGC are absent.[4] Progressive and ultimately fatal rounds of skeletal muscle degeneration and regeneration are hypothesized to result from either a fragile or weakened skeletal muscle membrane[5,6] or altered cell signaling.

Beyond these general hypotheses, the specific cellular mechanisms and the temporal progression of the dystrophic process are as yet unclear. There is no current cure for DMD, and palliative and prophylactic interventions to improve the quality of life of patients remain limited, with the exception of corticosteroids. Corticosteroids are effective at prolonging ambulation but have several undesirable side effects, including growth retardation, obesity, glucose intolerance, and bone demineralization.[7] Nevertheless, despite these side effects, a recent panel of experts recommended glucocorticoid therapy for all patients who have DMD. This recommendation suggests that until

[a] Department of Human Nutrition, Foods and Exercise, Virginia Tech, Blacksburg, VA 24061, USA
[b] Institute of Biochemistry and Biophysics, University of Tehran, Iran
[c] Wake Forest Institute for Regenerative Medicine, Winston-Salem, NC 27106, USA
* Corresponding author.
E-mail address: rgrange@vt.edu

Phys Med Rehabil Clin N Am 23 (2012) 187–199
doi:10.1016/j.pmr.2011.11.010
1047-9651/12/$ – see front matter © 2012 Elsevier Inc. All rights reserved.

a suitable corticosteroid substitute is available, any additional palliative and prophylactic treatment approaches will likely be in conjunction with corticosteroids.[8]

This article describes two potential nutritional interventions for the treatment of DMD, green tea extract (GTE) and the branched-chain amino acid (BCAA) leucine, and their positive effects on physical activity. Both GTE and leucine are suitable for human consumption; are easily tolerated with no side effects; and, with appropriate preclinical data, could be brought forward to clinical trials rapidly. In dystrophic mdx mice, both GTE[9] and leucine (Voelker KA, unpublished data, 2010) improve whole animal endurance and skeletal muscle function. Mechanistically both are mediated by signaling pathways to evoke these and other positive adaptations that attenuate the effects of dystrophic progression. To date, not all the specific pathways have been described.

CHARACTERISTICS OF DMD

The characteristics of DMD have been well described at the genetic, molecular, cellular, tissue, organ systems, and clinical levels (**Table 1**). Detailed descriptions are provided in several excellent reviews.[6,7,10–14]

Best Practices of Care

DMD is a complex disease to manage. Bushby and colleagues[7,10] recently published a detailed set of recommendations for the management of DMD. Among the many recommendations are those related to nutrition and exercise (physical activity). It is not the authors' intent here to discuss all the difficulties associated with nutrition (eg, swallowing problems) or exercise (eg, spinal deformities) but to focus on simple nutritional possibilities that may attenuate disease severity and progression.

Importance of Mobility

A goal for treatment of patients with DMD should be to improve quality of life,[7,10] one important aspect of which is mobility. Mobility is dependent on sufficient strength and endurance in skeletal muscles to move joints through a range of motion to accomplish a movement task. Some tasks may be occasional movements significant in everyday

Table 1 Characteristics of DMD	
Level of Pathology	Definitions and Descriptors at Various Levels of the Disease
Genetic	X-linked, hereditary or spontaneous
Cellular	Absence of the protein dystrophin, mechanical weakening of the sarcolemma, inappropriate calcium influx, recurrent muscle ischemia, aberrant cell signaling, increased oxidative stress, histologic z-disk disruption, central nucleation, fiber size heterogeneity, reduced expression and mislocalization of dystrophin-associated proteins
Tissue	Intramuscular accumulation of fibrous connective and fatty tissue, pseudohypertrophy
Organ systems	Musculoskeletal system, nervous system, digestive system, immune system, cardiorespiratory system
Clinical	Lethal, progressive, 1:3500 live male births, muscle wasting and weakness, susceptibility to fatigue, muscle pain, elevated serum creatine kinase, myoglobinuria, Gower sign, lordosis, progressive difficulty with ambulation, contractures, contraction-induced injury, secondary disuse atrophy, increased fat mass, side effects of medications, cardiorespiratory failure

life, such as reaching for a glass. Other movements may be repetitive and rhythmic, such as walking. Because ambulatory muscles, the diaphragm, and the heart are all adversely affected by dystrophin deficiency, mobility in individuals with DMD is severely compromised. Can nutritional therapies improve mobility?

WHY NUTRITIONAL AND PHYSICAL ACTIVITY THERAPIES?

The US government has established guidelines for a balanced diet to meet the energy demands and macronutrient and micronutrient requirements for health (http://health.gov/dietaryguidelines/2010.asp), which includes balancing calories with physical activity to manage weight. Similarly, guidelines have been established by the Centers for Disease Control and Prevention for a minimum participation in physical activity on a daily basis (http://www.cdc.gov/physicalactivity/everyone/guidelines/index.html). At the most basic level, nutrition represents energy intake and adequate vitamins and minerals; physical activity represents energy output. These requirements are no less, and likely more, important for individuals with DMD.

WHAT IS CURRENTLY KNOWN

There has been little research published on effective nutrition[7,8,10] or physical activity[15,16] for individuals with DMD. Although it is recognized that genetic and molecular biological approaches will ultimately reveal a cure for DMD, is it prudent to overlook potential simple approaches, such as diet and physical activity, as palliative and prophylactic treatments until the cure is found? Unfortunately, these treatments are simply not being investigated rigorously. Simply put, little is known about the nutritional needs of patients with DMD and little is known about the potential positive (or negative) adaptive responses of dystrophic muscles to physical activity.

Nutrition

Davidson and Truby[8] reported in their review that of approximately 1500 references they found on DMD, only 6 directly investigated the nutritional requirements of boys with DMD. Bushby and colleagues[10] cited a similar small number of references, although some differed from those cited by Davidson and Truby. The total number of nutritional investigations seems to be only about 10 to 12. Based on these studies, the recommendations for nutritional guidance could be dramatically improved.[8]

Physical Activity

The effects of physical activity to treat DMD have been investigated for several decades (eg, Refs.[17,18]), yet there are still no defined exercise prescriptions that include intensity, duration, and frequency.[15,16] A recent review by Markert and colleagues[16] suggested that appropriately prescribed physical activity might counter key dystrophic pathogenic mechanisms, including (1) mechanical weakening of the sarcolemma, (2) inappropriate calcium influx, (3) aberrant cell signaling, (4) increased oxidative stress, and (5) recurrent muscle ischemia.

Energy Balance

Although this article focuses on two specific nutritional interventions, monitoring the energy content of diet is also a cornerstone of health and is especially important to consider in disease states such as DMD, which affect multiple organ systems.[10] Excessive caloric intake leads to conditions of overweight or obesity, whereas inadequate caloric intake precedes weight loss. Boys treated with steroids gain nonfunctional mass (eg, fat, not muscle) because appetite is stimulated.[8] In boys with DMD whose mobility is compromised, this problem is exacerbated because they take in more energy but expend less.

Energy IN is determined by the amount consumed and the content of the diet in kilocalories. Energy OUT includes the sum of the resting metabolic rate, the thermic effect of food, the nonexercise energy expenditure, and exercise energy cost, also measured in kilocalories.[19] In addition, the disease and medications can contribute to energy status in patients with DMD.[8] When energy IN exceeds energy OUT, weight gain results. Systematic studies of energy expenditure in patients with DMD, using metabolic equivalents[20] (MET = 3.5 mL oxygen/kg body mass/min), have been suggested[16] to better prescribe physical activity and exercise guidelines. These studies would also help inform dietary guidelines for energy intake.

Pharmaceutical and Nutritional Interventions

Although the main impetuses to cure DMD are focused on genetic and molecular biological approaches, nutritional therapies could represent an appropriate and simple palliative approach.[21–23] For example, treatment with the amino acids glutamine[24,25] and arginine plus deflazacort[23] were reported to improve nitrogen retention and maintain protein balance in patients with DMD. However, at present there have been few detailed investigations of nutritional interventions in DMD. Radley and colleagues[26] succinctly provided a summary and analysis of several potential pharmaceutical and nutritional interventions as therapeutic agents in mdx mice and DMD. Among the potential nutritional interventions cited was GTE, which the investigators suggested was ready for clinical trial with the exception of the appropriate dose. In addition, several amino acids were also cited for possible use in treating DMD including taurine, glutamine, alanine, and arginine (alone or in various combinations). However, a caveat to the use of these amino acids was that they had yet to be formally evaluated. The potential benefits of leucine were not reported. The authors now summarize briefly the current literature on GTE, provide the likely signaling pathways of leucine to induce protein synthesis, and provide evidence of the benefits of leucine on strength in mdx mice and whole-body endurance.

GTE

GTE has been reported to ameliorate dystrophic pathology in mdx mice. Initial studies indicated that oxidative stress may contribute to muscular dystrophy symptoms,[27–32] and early administration of dietary GTE to young mdx mice (and their dams, before weaning) protected against muscle necrosis in the extensor digitorum longus (EDL) muscle.[33] Recognized for its antioxidative properties, GTE was investigated further as a possible protection against progression of muscular dystrophy. Administration early in the course of the disease was repeated in a study that compared GTE with its major component, epigallocatechin gallate (ECGC),[34] a polyphenol. This study also showed reduced necrosis in muscles from GTE-treated and ECGC-treated mice, and furthermore reported improved muscle strength and fatigue resistance in functional assays.

In another study,[9] voluntary exercise (wheel running) and GTE were investigated in 21-day-old mdx mice. Both conditions independently showed beneficial effects in assays of contractile properties, metabolic activity, lipid peroxidation, and antioxidant capacity. Synergistic effects of the combined treatments were also reported to benefit endurance capacity, although some other beneficial effects of GTE were mitigated by running. Mechanistic and time-course data[35] indicate that GTE potentially ameliorates pathology by acting on the nuclear factor κB pathway. Histologic assays of GTE-treated mdx muscle showed a reduced area of regenerating fibers, indicating a protective effect, and a fiber morphology more like that of non-diseased muscle. In summary, GTE and its polyphenolic constituents merit further study as possible regulators of oxidative stress and inflammation. Just as light swimming exercise may benefit aerobic and cardiorespiratory capacity, particularly of young ambulatory patients with DMD,[10] nutraceuticals such as BCAAs and GTE may provide benefit in additional biochemical and functional outcome measures (**Fig. 1**).

Leucine

Leucine is an essential BCAA with unique features. In addition to being a building block of proteins, it is an anabolic signal that induces protein synthesis.[36] In addition, it plays a role in glucose homeostasis.[37] Leucine also acts as a nitrogen donor for the synthesis of alanine and glutamine in the muscle.[38] Glutamate, which itself is the precursor of γ-aminobutyric acid (GABA), is produced from the transamination reaction of leucine and other BCAAs, and is a major excitatory neurotransmitter.[39]

Leucine also improves nitrogen retention by increasing muscle protein synthesis and decreasing myofibrillar breakdown in normal pigs.[40–43] Although both of these leucine-related effects would be relevant to reversal of the degradation processes in dystrophic muscle, it is not known whether dystrophic muscle will respond similarly. There is only one controlled clinical trial (conducted in 1984) that has investigated the therapeutic potential of leucine.[44] This study demonstrated a transient increase in muscle strength reported after the first month of a 12-month trial, but results were later confounded by the unusual rate of functional decline in the placebo group. More recently, D'Antona and colleagues[45] reported that supplementation with BCAAs promoted longevity as well as skeletal and cardiac muscle biogenesis in middle-aged mice, including enhanced physical endurance. Similarly, the authors' recent preliminary data demonstrating improved contractile and endurance performance in the mdx mouse indicate that leucine may be an effective nutritional therapy for DMD.

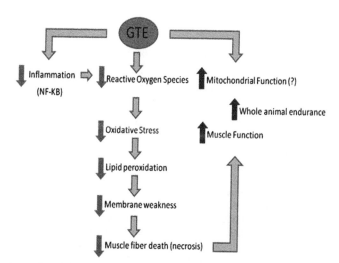

Fig. 1. Overview of positive physiologic effects of green tea extract (GTE) in mdx mice. The potential beneficial effects of GTE on mitochondrial function have not yet been determined mechanistically. NF, nuclear factor.

Mammalian target of rapamycin

Although it is well established that leucine can stimulate protein synthesis through the mammalian target of rapamycin (mTOR) signaling pathway,[36,46–51] the identity of sensor(s) for leucine is not known.[52] The strongest link between amino acids and mTOR complex 1 (mTORC1) is the Rag guanosine triphosphatases, which, in response to amino acids, bind to raptor (**Fig. 2**).[53,54] This interaction alters the intracellular location of the mTORC1 to a compartment where its activator Rheb is present. Activated mTORC1 phosphorylates substrates, of which ribosomal S6 protein kinase (S6K) and 4E-binding protein-1 (4EBP-1) are well known.

Phosphorylated S6K phosphorylates many substrates including S6 ribosomal protein, which is an essential component of the protein translation initiation machinery. On the other hand, 4EBP-1 phosphorylation causing its release from eukaryotic initiation factor 4E (eIF4E), allowing the initiation of CAP-dependent protein synthesis.[55,56] In addition to nutrients, mTORC1 is activated by growth factors, especially insulin.[57] Insulin binding activates Ras-Erk1/2 and phosphatidylinositol-3-kinase (PI3K)-AKT

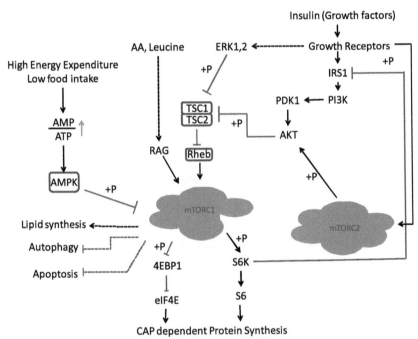

Fig. 2. Regulation of mammalian target of rapamycin complex (mTORC) signaling networks. Growth factors/mitogens (insulin, epidermal growth factor) and nutrients (eg, amino acids, energy) promote mTORC1 signaling via phosphorylation cascades that converge on tuberous sclerosis complex (TSC) and the mTORCs themselves. Insulin signals via its receptor (Insulin-R) to activate the phosphatidylinositol 3-kinase (PI3K)/Akt/TSC/Rheb pathway; amino acid sufficiency signals via hVps34 and the Rag and RalA guanosine triphosphatases; and energy sufficiency suppresses AMP-activated protein kinase (AMPK). Insulin/PI3K signaling likely promotes mTORC2 signaling via an unknown pathway. An mTORC1/S6 protein kinase (S6K)-mediated negative feedback loop signals via 2 pathways to suppress PI3K/mTORC2/Akt signaling. AA, amino acids; AMP, adenosine monophosphate; ATP, adenosine triphosphate; 4EBP-1, 4E-binding protein-1; eIF4E, eukaryotic initiation factor 4E; ERK, extracellular signal–regulated kinase; IRS1, Insulin Receptor Substrate 1; PDK1, Phosphoinositide Dependent Protein Kinase 1; S6, S6 Ribosomal Protein.

pathways, which merge at tuberous sclerosis complex 2 (TSC2).[52] The TSC1-TSC2 complex inactivates the mTORC1 complex through the hydrolysis of guanosine triphosphate, which is required for Rheb to activate mTORC1. Phosphorylation of TSC2 inhibits the activity of the TSC1-TSC2 complex, allowing the activation of Rheb and consequently mTORC1.[52] Activation of the PI3K pathway activates another TOR complex known as mTORC2. mTORC2 is believed to participate in cell growth and cytoskeletal organization.[58]

The mTORC1 and mTORC2 complexes consist of mTOR plus several proteins, some common to both complexes and others unique to each complex. These components play a role in substrate recognition, or act as positive and negative regulators of the TOR complexes.[59,60] Insulin can regulate mTORC2 by increasing phosphatidylinositol(3,4,5)P(3) (PIP3) through PI3K, which ultimately leads to the phosphorylation and activation of AKT.[52,61] mTORC1 and mTORC2 phosphorylate different substrates and respond differently to rapamycin. Short-term treatment of cells with rapamycin inhibits mTORC1 with no effect on mTORC2, whereas prolonged treatment causes the inhibition of the mTORC2 complex perhaps through sequestration of the cellular pool of mTOR in a complex with rapamycin-FKBP12.[62] Increasing evidence suggests that the two complexes directly or indirectly interact with each other. Activation of mTORC1 activates S6K, which in turn phosphorylates IRS1, downregulating insulin response.[63,64] Decreased insulin response reduces the PI3K-AKT pathway activity, which would negatively affect mTORC2.[65] In addition, active S6K phosphorylates Rictor, negatively affecting mTORC2 activity.[66] It was shown that mTORC1 phosphorylates the growth factor receptor-bound protein 10 (Grb10) resulting in its stability, and leading to a feedback inhibition of the PI3K and extracellular signal-regulated, mitogen-activated protein kinase (ERK-MAPK) pathways.[67,68] The presence of these cross talks and negative feedback loops ensures controlled cell growth. Therefore, understanding the pathways and identifying molecules involved in the cross talk between mTORC1 and mTORC2 will enable these pathways to be exploited in various pathologic conditions ranging from muscular atrophy to cancer and diabetes.

Amelioration of mdx pathology by leucine

In animal models of other muscle-wasting disorders such as sepsis and cachexia, supplementation with leucine helped maintain muscle mass.[55,69–74] The mdx mouse is a widely used preclinical model of DMD, because muscles of these mice, like boys with DMD, lack the protein dystrophin. Preliminary data from a pilot study conducted in the Grange Laboratory suggest that both running endurance and muscle strength in mdx mice are dramatically improved after 4 weeks of treatment with leucine-supplemented water. As shown in **Fig. 3**, the mean distance run was significantly higher in weeks 2 to 4 in mdx mice supplemented with leucine. Cages were equipped with a running wheel automated to measure voluntary wheel-running time. At the end of 4 weeks, muscle parameters such as stress-generating capacity were measured in vitro. Stress-generating capacity for EDL muscles was increased at all electrical stimulation frequencies (**Fig. 4**, $P<.05$). What is remarkable is that EDL muscle mass was not different between the mdx (9.4 ± 0.8 mg) and mdx-leucine groups (10.2 ± 1.4 mg), nor was fiber size (data not shown), indicating that hypertrophy did not account for the increased stress production. Furthermore, there was no change in fiber number, number of centralized nuclei, or myosin heavy chain distribution (data not shown). Collectively, these data suggest that even if skeletal muscle in leucine-treated mdx mice does not hypertrophy, it still improves endurance capacity and the ability to produce force.

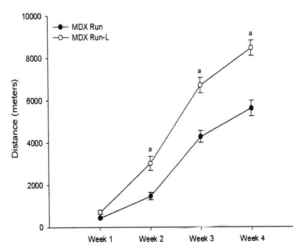

Fig. 3. Weekly running distance for the MDX Run Leucine (MDX Run-L) group was greater at weeks 2, 3, and 4 (*P*<.05). Leucine treatment clearly improved whole animal endurance, suggesting potential changes in muscle metabolism and the cardiovascular system.

Evaluation of Nutraceuticals and Nutritional Interventions

Experimental designs focused on elucidating the role of nutrition in the treatment of DMD may benefit from (1) incorporating previously defined standard operating procedures (SOPs) for preclinical experiments,[13] and (2) approaching nutrition research questions with the same mechanistic framework[16] used to define the role of exercise in the treatment of DMD. In brief, when designing experiments and selecting outcome measures in studies on both exercise and nutrition, DMD researchers should consider the reliability of the measures, their validity, how they represent DMD pathophysiology,

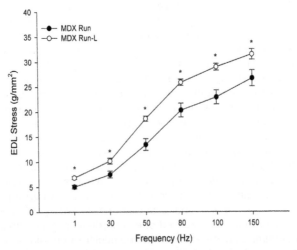

Fig. 4. Stress-frequency curve of MDX Run and MDX Run-L extensor digitorum longus (EDL) muscles. All tests were performed in vitro, in an oxygenated bath. *MDX Run-L group was significantly greater than the MDX Run group. Values are reported as mean ± SEM, *P*<.05.

Table 2
Examples of experimental designs to test nutritional interventions

Study	Mechanism	Intervention	Evaluation Method	Outcome Measure
De Luca et al,[75] 2003	Inappropriate Ca^{2+} ion influx	Dietary taurine	Electrophysiology	Chloride conductance
Evans et al,[35] 2010	Aberrant cell signaling; inflammation	Dietary green tea extract	Histology	Macrophage infiltration

and whether the measures facilitate translation of results from animal models to the human condition.[13] Blinded assessment of outcome measures is another consideration, as is using data to generate hypotheses and plan future statistical analyses. Established SOPs for many relevant outcome measures are readily available (http://www.treat-nmd.eu/research/preclinical/dmd-sops/). In addition, selection of appropriate outcome measures may be more straightforward if the measures target specific mechanisms of DMD pathophysiology.

In brief, if sarcolemmal weakening and damage is the mechanism of disease, and an exercise or nutrition intervention is hypothesized to ameliorate the damage, then outcome measures based on methods such as Evans blue dye injection, Procion orange injection, the creatine kinase assay, current clamp, voltage clamp, histology, immunohistochemistry, force production measures, and intracellular Ca^{2+} indicators, are indicated.[16] Interventional studies in mdx mice provide examples of experimental designs for the evaluation of nutrition in muscular dystrophy,[35,75] as shown in **Table 2**.

RECOMMENDATIONS

1. There is an immediate need to gather sufficient preclinical evidence to move forward to clinical trials.
2. As with studies of physical activity in muscular dystrophy, future studies of nutritional interventions, in both animals and humans, need to use standardized, reliable, systematic methods to assess outcomes. This approach allows for cross-study comparison.
3. Granting agencies play a key role in determining whether studies of nutrition-related topics in DMD are prioritized and funded. Targeted requests for proposals, and identification of grant reviewers who have specific expertise in evaluating the potential therapeutic benefits of nutritional interventions, may reinvigorate this area of research.
4. Whatever nutritional and/or physical intervention is studied, there will be a requisite need to assess combined therapy, particularly with prednisolone or deflazacort (or new corticosteroid derivatives as they are developed).

SUMMARY

There is a dearth of knowledge regarding effective interventions based on nutrition and physical activity for enhancement of physical capabilities in DMD.[10,16] As a result, guidelines for each are limited. However, concerted efforts by funding agencies and the DMD research community have the potential to overcome these limitations by expanding the available data base. Promising nutritional interventions, such as GTE and leucine, may find their path to the clinic expedited in the context of reprioritized policy and funding.

REFERENCES

1. Durbeej M, Campbell KP. Muscular dystrophies involving the dystrophin-glycoprotein complex: an overview of current mouse models. Curr Opin Genet Dev 2002;12(3):349–61.
2. Blake DJ, Weir A, Newey SE, et al. Function and genetics of dystrophin and dystrophin-related proteins in muscle. Physiol Rev 2002;82(2):291–329.
3. Davies KE, Nowak KJ. Molecular mechanisms of muscular dystrophies: old and new players. Nat Rev Mol Cell Biol 2006;7(10):762–73.
4. Ervasti JM, Ohlendieck K, Kahl SD, et al. Deficiency of a glycoprotein component of the dystrophin complex in dystrophic muscle. Nature 1990;345(6273):315–9.
5. Petrof BJ, Shrager JB, Stedman HH, et al. Dystrophin protects the sarcolemma from stresses developed during muscle contraction. Proc Natl Acad Sci U S A 1993;90(8):3710–4.
6. Petrof BJ. The molecular basis of activity-induced muscle injury in Duchenne muscular dystrophy. Mol Cell Biochem 1998;179(1-2):111–23.
7. Bushby K, Finkel R, Birnkrant DJ, et al. Diagnosis and management of Duchenne muscular dystrophy, part 1: diagnosis, and pharmacological and psychosocial management. Lancet Neurol 2010;9(1):77–93.
8. Davidson ZE, Truby H. A review of nutrition in Duchenne muscular dystrophy. J Hum Nutr Diet 2009;22(5):383–93.
9. Call JA, Voelker KA, Wolff AV, et al. Endurance capacity in maturing mdx mice is markedly enhanced by combined voluntary wheel running and green tea extract. J Appl Physiol 2008;105(3):923–32.
10. Bushby K, Finkel R, Birnkrant DJ, et al. Diagnosis and management of Duchenne muscular dystrophy, part 2: implementation of multidisciplinary care. Lancet Neurol 2010;9(2):177–89.
11. Ervasti JM, Sonnemann KJ. Biology of the striated muscle dystrophin-glycoprotein complex. Int Rev Cytol 2008;265:191–225.
12. Petrof BJ. Molecular pathophysiology of myofiber injury in deficiencies of the dystrophin-glycoprotein complex. Am J Phys Med Rehabil 2002;81(Suppl 11): S162–74.
13. Willmann R, De Luca A, Benatar M, et al. Enhancing translation: Guidelines for standard pre-clinical experiments in mdx mice. Neuromuscul Disord 2011. [Epub ahead of print].
14. Willmann R, Possekel S, Dubach-Powell J, et al. Mammalian animal models for Duchenne muscular dystrophy. Neuromuscul Disord 2009;19(4):241–9.
15. Grange RW, Call JA. Recommendations to define exercise prescription for Duchenne muscular dystrophy. Exerc Sport Sci Rev 2007;35(1):12–7.
16. Markert CD, Ambrosio F, Call JA, et al. Exercise and Duchenne muscular dystrophy: toward evidence-based exercise prescription. Muscle Nerve 2011; 43(4):464–78.
17. Hudgson P, Gardner-Medwin D, Pennington RJ, et al. Studies of the carrier state in the Duchenne type of muscular dystrophy. I. Effect of exercise on serum creatine kinase activity. J Neurol Neurosurg Psychiatry 1967;30(5):416–9.
18. Sockolov R, Irwin B, Dressendorfer RH, et al. Exercise performance in 6-to-11-year-old boys with Duchenne muscular dystrophy. Arch Phys Med Rehabil 1977;58(5):195–201.

19. Levine JA. Measurement of energy expenditure. Public Health Nutr 2005;8(7A): 1123–32.
20. American College of Sports Medicine Position Stand. The recommended quantity and quality of exercise for developing and maintaining cardiorespiratory and muscular fitness, and flexibility in healthy adults. Med Sci Sports Exerc 1998; 30(6):975–91.
21. Passaquin AC, Renard M, Kay L, et al. Creatine supplementation reduces skeletal muscle degeneration and enhances mitochondrial function in mdx mice. Neuromuscul Disord 2002;12(2):174–82.
22. Ruegg UT, Nicolas-Metral V, Challet C, et al. Pharmacological control of cellular calcium handling in dystrophic skeletal muscle. Neuromuscul Disord 2002; 12(Suppl 1):S155–61.
23. Archer JD, Vargas CC, Anderson JE. Persistent and improved functional gain in mdx dystrophic mice after treatment with L-arginine and deflazacort. FASEB J 2006;20(6):738–40.
24. Hankard RG, Hammond D, Haymond MW, et al. Oral glutamine slows down whole body protein breakdown in Duchenne muscular dystrophy. Pediatr Res 1998;43(2):222–6.
25. Mok E, Eleouet-Da Violante C, Daubrosse C, et al. Oral glutamine and amino acid supplementation inhibit whole-body protein degradation in children with Duchenne muscular dystrophy. Am J Clin Nutr 2006;83(4):823–8.
26. Radley HG, De Luca A, Lynch GS, et al. Duchenne muscular dystrophy: focus on pharmaceutical and nutritional interventions. Int J Biochem Cell Biol 2007;39(3): 469–77.
27. Bornman L, Rossouw H, Gericke GS, et al. Effects of iron deprivation on the pathology and stress protein expression in murine X-linked muscular dystrophy. Biochem Pharmacol 1998;56(6):751–7.
28. Disatnik MH, Chamberlain JS, Rando TA. Dystrophin mutations predict cellular susceptibility to oxidative stress. Muscle Nerve 2000;23(5):784–92.
29. Disatnik MH, Dhawan J, Yu Y, et al. Evidence of oxidative stress in mdx mouse muscle: studies of the pre-necrotic state. J Neurol Sci 1998;161(1):77–84.
30. Murphy ME, Kehrer JP. Free radicals: a potential pathogenic mechanism in inherited muscular dystrophy. Life Sci 1986;39(24):2271–8.
31. Ragusa RJ, Chow CK, Porter JD. Oxidative stress as a potential pathogenic mechanism in an animal model of Duchenne muscular dystrophy. Neuromuscul Disord 1997;7(6-7):379–86.
32. Rando TA, Disatnik MH, Yu Y, et al. Muscle cells from mdx mice have an increased susceptibility to oxidative stress. Neuromuscul Disord 1998;8(1): 14–21.
33. Buetler TM, Renard M, Offord EA, et al. Green tea extract decreases muscle necrosis in mdx mice and protects against reactive oxygen species. Am J Clin Nutr 2002;75(4):749–53.
34. Dorchies OM, Wagner S, Vuadens O, et al. Green tea extract and its major polyphenol (-)-epigallocatechin gallate improve muscle function in a mouse model for Duchenne muscular dystrophy. Am J Physiol Cell Physiol 2006;290(2):C616–25.
35. Evans NP, Call JA, Bassaganya-Riera J, et al. Green tea extract decreases muscle pathology and NF-kappaB immunostaining in regenerating muscle fibers of mdx mice. Clin Nutr 2010;29(3):391–8.
36. Anthony JC, Anthony TG, Kimball SR, et al. Orally administered leucine stimulates protein synthesis in skeletal muscle of postabsorptive rats in association with increase eIF4F formation. J Nutr 2000;130:139–45.

37. Nair KS, Woolf PD, Welle SL, et al. Leucine, glucose, and energy metabolism after 3 days of fasting in healthy human subjects. Am J Clin Nutr 1987;46(4):557–62.

38. Norton LE, Layman DK. Leucine regulates translation initiation of protein synthesis in skeletal muscle after exercise. J Nutr 2006;136(2):533S–7S.

39. Lieth E, LaNoue KF, Berkich DA, et al. Nitrogen shuttling between neurons and glial cells during glutamate synthesis. J Neurochem 2001;76(6):1712–23.

40. Sugawara T, Ito Y, Nishizawa N, et al. Regulation of muscle protein degradation, not synthesis, by dietary leucine in rats fed a protein-deficient diet. Amino Acids 2009;37(4):609–16.

41. Escobar J, Frank JW, Suryawan A, et al. Regulation of cardiac and skeletal muscle protein synthesis by individual branched-chain amino acids in neonatal pigs. Am J Physiol Endocrinol Metab 2006;290:612–21.

42. Escobar J, Frank JW, Suryawan A, et al. Physiological rise in plasma leucine stimulates muscle protein synthesis in neonatal pigs by enhancing translation initiation factor activation. Am J Physiol Endocrinol Metab 2005;288(5): E914–21.

43. Escobar J, Frank JW, Suryawan A, et al. Amino acid availability and age affect the leucine stimulation of protein synthesis and eIF4F formation in muscle. Am J Physiol Endocrinol Metab 2007;293(6):E1615–21.

44. Mendell JR, Griggs RC, Moxley RT 3rd, et al. Clinical investigation in Duchenne muscular dystrophy: IV. Double-blind controlled trial of leucine. Muscle Nerve 1984;7(7):535–41.

45. D'Antona G, Ragni M, Cardile A, et al. Branched-chain amino acid supplementation promotes survival and supports cardiac and skeletal muscle mitochondrial biogenesis in middle-aged mice. Cell Metab 2010;12(4):362–72.

46. Anthony JC, Yoshizawa F, Anthony TG, et al. Leucine stimulates translation initiation in skeletal muscle of postabsorptive rats via a rapamycin-sensitive pathway. J Nutr 2000;130(10):2413–9.

47. Buse MG, Reid SS. Leucine. A possible regulator of protein turnover in muscle. J Clin Invest 1975;56:1250–61.

48. Busquets S, Alvarez B, Lopez-Soriano FJ, et al. Branched-chain amino acids: a role in skeletal muscle proteolysis in catabolic states? J Cell Physiol 2002; 191(3):283–9.

49. Fulks RM, Li JB, Goldberg AL. Effects of insulin, glucose, and amino acids on protein turnover in rat diaphragm. J Biol Chem 1975;250(1):290–8.

50. Hong SO, Layman DK. Effects of leucine on in vitro protein synthesis and degradation in rat skeletal muscles. J Nutr 1984;114:1204–12.

51. Nakashima K, Ishida A, Yamazaki M, et al. Leucine suppresses myofibrillar proteolysis by down-regulating ubiquitin-proteasome pathway in chick skeletal muscles. Biochem Biophys Res Commun 2005;336(2):660–6.

52. Zoncu R, Efeyan A, Sabatini DM. mTOR: from growth signal integration to cancer, diabetes and ageing. Nat Rev Mol Cell Biol 2011;12(1):21–35.

53. Kim E, Goraksha-Hicks P, Li L, et al. Regulation of TORC1 by Rag GTPases in nutrient response. Nat Cell Biol 2008;10(8):935–45.

54. Sancak Y, Peterson TR, Shaul YD, et al. The Rag GTPases bind raptor and mediate amino acid signaling to mTORC1. Science 2008;320(5882):1496–501.

55. Armengol G, Rojo F, Castellvi J, et al. 4E-binding protein 1: a key molecular "funnel factor" in human cancer with clinical implications. Cancer Res 2007;67(16): 7551–5.

56. Avruch J, Long X, Ortiz-Vega S, et al. Amino acid regulation of TOR complex 1. Am J Physiol Endocrinol Metab 2009;296(4):E592–602.

57. Scott PH, Brunn GJ, Kohn AD, et al. Evidence of insulin-stimulated phosphorylation and activation of the mammalian target of rapamycin mediated by a protein kinase B signaling pathway. Proc Natl Acad Sci U S A 1998;95(13):7772–7.

58. Sparks CA, Guertin DA. Targeting mTOR: prospects for mTOR complex 2 inhibitors in cancer therapy. Oncogene 2010;29(26):3733–44.

59. Loewith R, Jacinto E, Wullschleger S, et al. Two TOR complexes, only one of which is rapamycin sensitive, have distinct roles in cell growth control. Mol Cell 2002;10(3):457–68.

60. Peterson TR, Laplante M, Thoreen CC, et al. DEPTOR is an mTOR inhibitor frequently overexpressed in multiple myeloma cells and required for their survival. Cell 2009;137(5):873–86.

61. Gan X, Wang J, Su B, et al. Evidence for direct activation of mTORC2 kinase activity by phosphatidylinositol 3,4,5-trisphosphate. J Biol Chem 2011;286(13): 10998–1002.

62. Sarbassov DD, Ali SM, Sengupta S, et al. Prolonged rapamycin treatment inhibits mTORC2 assembly and Akt/PKB. Mol Cell 2006;22(2):159–68.

63. Tremblay F, Brule S, Um SH, et al. Identification of IRS-1 Ser-1101 as a target of S6K1 in nutrient- and obesity-induced insulin resistance. Proc Natl Acad Sci U S A 2007;104:14056–61.

64. Um SH, D'Alessio D, Thomas G. Nutrient overload, insulin resistance, and ribosomal protein S6 kinase 1, S6K1. Cell Metab 2006;3:393–402.

65. Dobashi Y, Watanabe Y, Miwa C, et al. Mammalian target of rapamycin: a central node of complex signaling cascades. Int J Clin Exp Pathol 2011; 4(5):476–95.

66. Dibble CC, Asara JM, Manning BD. Characterization of Rictor phosphorylation sites reveals direct regulation of mTOR complex 2 by S6K1. Mol Cell Biol 2009; 29(21):5657–70.

67. Hsu PP, Kang SA, Rameseder J, et al. The mTOR-regulated phosphoproteome reveals a mechanism of mTORC1-mediated inhibition of growth factor signaling. Science 2011;332(6035):1317–22.

68. Yu Y, Yoon SO, Poulogiannis G, et al. Phosphoproteomic analysis identifies Grb10 as an mTORC1 substrate that negatively regulates insulin signaling. Science 2011;332(6035):1322–6.

69. Ventrucci G, Mello MA, Gomes-Marcondes MC. Effect of a leucine-supplemented diet on body composition changes in pregnant rats bearing Walker 256 tumor. Braz J Med Biol Res 2001;34(3):333–8.

70. Gomes-Marcondes MC, Ventrucci G, Toledo MT, et al. A leucine-supplemented diet improved protein content of skeletal muscle in young tumor-bearing rats. Braz J Med Biol Res 2003;36(11):1589–94.

71. Siddiqui R, Pandya D, Harvey K, et al. Nutrition modulation of cachexia/proteolysis. Nutr Clin Pract 2006;21(2):155–67.

72. Ventrucci G, Mello MA, Gomes-Marcondes MC, et al. Leucine-rich diet alters the eukaryotic translation initiation factors expression in skeletal muscle of tumour-bearing rats. BMC Cancer 2007;7:42.

73. De Bandt JP, Cynober L. Therapeutic use of branched-chain amino acids in burn, trauma, and sepsis. J Nutr 2006;136(Suppl 1):308S–13S.

74. Vary TC, Lynch CJ. Nutrient signaling components controlling protein synthesis in striated muscle. J Nutr 2007;137(8):1835–43.

75. De Luca A, Pierno S, Liantonio A, et al. Enhanced dystrophic progression in mdx mice by exercise and beneficial effects of taurine and insulin-like growth factor-1. J Pharmacol Exp Ther 2003;304(1):453–63.

Aging of Human Muscle: Understanding Sarcopenia at the Single Muscle Cell Level

Walter R. Frontera, MD, PhD[a,b,*], Ana Rodriguez Zayas, PhD[b], Natividad Rodriguez, MT[b]

KEYWORDS

- Aging • Sarcopenia • Skeletal muscle fiber
- Muscle atrophy • Contractility

Sarcopenia (*sarx* = flesh and *penia* = loss), the loss of muscle mass, has become a major subject of scientific research as well as a public health problem of significant dimensions. Although an operational definition that is universally acceptable is not available, researchers agree that the incidence of sarcopenia increases with advanced adult age in both sexes but particularly in men. Further, preliminary studies suggest that the costs associated with sarcopenia in the United States may exceed $20 billion.[1] Thus, understanding sarcopenia and developing therapeutic and rehabilitative interventions to slow down its progress or partially reverse its effects is an important scientific and health care policy goal.

The loss of muscle mass seen in older men and women has significant physiologic, functional, and health consequences. Muscle weakness, a decrease in muscle power, a reduction in walking ability, and an increase in hospitalizations are all associated with sarcopenia.[2] Of importance is that several additional physiologic changes are associated with aging and sarcopenia influencing muscle function, even though these changes do not occur inside the muscle fibers and are not known to alter the basic structure and function of myofilament proteins. Examples of these changes are an increased accumulation of adipose tissue around and between muscle fibers and a decrease in the anabolic influence of the endocrine system. Further examples are

[a] Department of Physical Medicine and Rehabilitation, University of Puerto Rico School of Medicine, San Juan, PR 00936, USA
[b] Department of Physiology, University of Puerto Rico School of Medicine, PO Box 365067, San Juan, PR, USA
* Corresponding author. Department of Physical Medicine and Rehabilitation, University of Puerto Rico School of Medicine, San Juan, PR 00936.
E-mail address: walter.frontera@upr.edu

Phys Med Rehabil Clin N Am 23 (2012) 201–207
doi:10.1016/j.pmr.2011.11.012
1047-9651/12/$ – see front matter © 2012 Elsevier Inc. All rights reserved.

age-related changes in the nervous system such as the loss of motor neurons, the remodeling of motor units through collateral reinnervation, and the impairment of neuromuscular activation manifested as a decreased maximal firing rate of motor units.

The study of skeletal muscle function in humans (patients or healthy volunteers) has advanced significantly in the last 3 decades. However, many of tests of skeletal muscle function, particularly those used in the clinical environment, reflect the integrated actions of several physiologic systems. Although the integrated response measured as muscle strength or power is of clinical interest, the specific contribution of each of the systems is very difficult to isolate using these tests. For example, in vivo measurements of muscle strength and power reflect the integrated action of muscle fibers, tendons, the neuromuscular junctions, peripheral axons, and the activating central nervous system. Clinical testing protocols may identify the presence of weakness and dysfunction, but cannot identify the specific level at which the impairment is happening and cannot explain the underlying cellular mechanism.

The first experiments with normal single human muscle fibers were published in 1975.[3] Since that time several researchers have used various experimental techniques to isolate and activate segments of single human muscle fibers obtained with the percutaneous muscle biopsy needle (**Fig. 1**). These techniques have been applied to research in healthy volunteers, elite athletes, patients with various diseases of the neuromuscular system, and patients with spinal cord injuries, among others. The first application of this technique to the aging (sarcopenia) problem was published in 1997.[4] This approach allows the investigator to examine the performance of the actin-myosin cross-bridges and muscle regulatory proteins in the absence of the influence of the nervous or endocrine systems. Further, because the technique includes the biochemical identification of the type of myosin heavy chain expressed in individual fibers, it is possible to study muscle-fiber physiology without the confounding effect of the heterogeneity of fiber type that is typical of the intact human neuromuscular system. Fibers are made permeable and then segments are activated maximally with high calcium concentrations. Due to the permeability of fibers, there is no (or very little) sarcolemma or sarcoplasmic reticulum that could interfere with the movements of calcium ion. Thus, the level of activation (or voluntary drive) is eliminated as a confounder. Finally, the absence of the tendon and mechanical leverage system permits the measurement of force generation directly from the fiber and its myofilament structure and not at a distance from the site of force generation.

The single muscle fiber technique allows the measurement and/or calculation of several important morphologic/physiologic, mechanical (**Fig. 2**), and biochemical variables (**Table 1**).

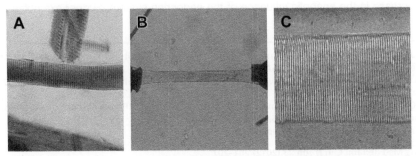

Fig. 1. (A) Dissected single human muscle fiber, (B) human muscle fiber attached to force transducer and servomotor, and (C) preserved sarcomere pattern at higher magnification.

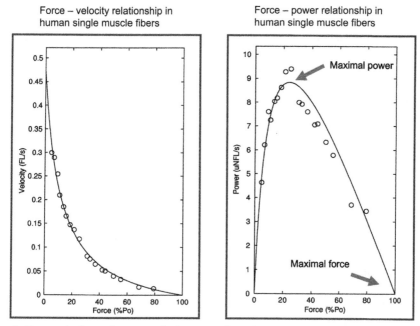

Force – velocity relationship in human single muscle fibers

Force – power relationship in human single muscle fibers

Fig. 2. Force-velocity and power-velocity curves from human single muscle fiber segments.

WHOLE-MUSCLE WEAKNESS

The presence of muscle weakness is a frequent clinical observation among elderly men and women. Muscle weakness contributes to the loss of functional capacity and independence, and is associated with a higher mortality in this population. Cross-sectional studies show a significant difference in muscle strength between young and old men and women in several muscle groups of both upper and lower limbs. This observation has been confirmed in longitudinal studies showing a larger annual decrement in strength (1.0%–1.5%) when compared with cross-sectional observations.[5,6] The loss of muscle strength with age is a highly variable process, as expected. For example, longitudinal studies of relatively healthy volunteers also show that women do not lose strength of the upper limbs over a 10-year period. Further, a relatively large percentage of men and women maintain the strength of the lower limbs over the same period of time. The reason for these observations is

Table 1		
Variables obtained from experiments with single muscle fibers		
Morphologic	**Physiologic/Mechanical**	**Biochemical**
Sarcomere length	Force	Myosin heavy chain expression
Depth	Shortening velocity	Myosin light chain expression
Length	Power	Regulatory proteins (ie, tropomyosin)
Cross-sectional area	Force-velocity curves	Structural protein (ie, titin)
Diameter	Power-velocity curves	
	Elasticity, stiffness	
	Specific force (force/size)	

not clear, although it is likely that the level of physical and/or occupational activity plays a role in the preservation of strength in some individuals.

Because of the significant correlation between muscle size and strength, it has been assumed that weakness is mainly due to the loss of muscle mass (or volume), that is, sarcopenia. However, the association between size and force is far from perfect, as illustrated in **Fig. 3**, and it is now known that factors other than size influence muscle strength (and weakness), even in the isolated fiber preparation. Experiments with single muscle fibers have allowed researchers to study muscle-fiber quality (defined as muscle force adjusted for muscle size) and have showed clearly that sarcopenia contributes to, but is not the only explanation of, muscle weakness. In other words, aging and sarcopenia are accompanied by reductions in muscle-fiber quality.[7] It appears that several changes at the cellular and molecular levels contribute to impaired muscle protein function.

WEAKNESS OF SINGLE MUSCLE FIBERS

Cross-sectional studies of single muscle fibers obtained from healthy, community-dwelling men and women[4,7] show a reduction in muscle-fiber quality in fibers express-ing type I or IIA myosin heavy chain (**Fig. 4**). This difference is more noticeable in both fiber types in men, and some of the changes observed in women did not reach statis-tical significance. It is interesting that when some of the same volunteers were tested approximately 10 years after baseline (the longitudinal phase of the study), muscle-fiber size and quality showed no significant changes over time and the only mechan-ical characteristic that showed a significant reduction was single muscle-fiber peak power.[8] One interpretation of these findings is that those fibers that survived and were not lost to the biological effects of aging compensated for those that were lost with the passage of time, maintaining their normal size and ability to generate force. This compensatory strategy has been observed in other populations such as post-polio survivors.

In addition to the ability to generate force, another important contractile property, maximum unloaded shortening velocity, is influenced by age and gender. For example it has been reported, although with some differential effects depending on the study, that among men and women shortening velocity was reduced with age in fibers expressing type I or type IIA myosin heavy chain isoforms.[9,10] Older women showed a slower shortening velocity than older men in both fiber types. A more recent compar-ison between older men and women of several contractile properties of single muscle

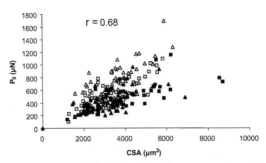

Fig. 3. Scatter plot of fiber cross-sectional area (CSA) and maximal force (P_0) for single muscle fibers from young (*open squares*, type I; *open triangles*, type IIa) and older men (*closed squares*, type I; *closed triangles*, type IIa).

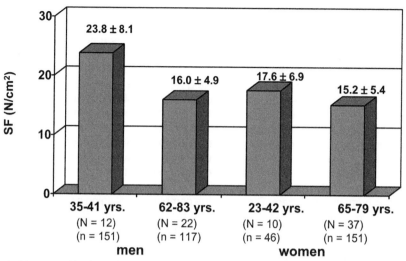

Fig. 4. Mean specific force (SF) of type IIA fibers (n = 465) from vastus lateralis muscle in young and older men (N = 34) and women (N = 47). Values are expressed as mean ± SD. N, number of subjects; n, number of fibers.

fibers, however, showed no significant differences at the level of single fibers that could explain differences at the whole-muscle level in strength and power.[11]

Finally, studies with human single fibers show that aging is associated with changes in fiber elasticity in both type I and IIA fibers.[12] A greater instantaneous stiffness per force unit was measured in fibers from older men. These findings at the cellular level may explain why the whole muscle-tendon unit of older men has been found to be stiffer. This increase in stiffness may be due to an increase in the number and proportion of actin-myosin cross-bridges in a low force state or alterations in the compliance of structures in series in muscle fibers. It is interesting that in these experiments the commonly seen increase in force after a quick stretch is preserved in older men. Thus, it could be speculated that the relative preservation of eccentric strength in the elderly may have a cellular basis.

PHYSIOLOGIC, CELLULAR, AND MOLECULAR CONTRIBUTORS TO SARCOPENIA AND WEAKNESS

From a physiologic point of view, muscle-fiber weakness can be explained by the interaction of several age-related alterations. The loss of anabolic stimuli is a characteristic of aging, partly due to the decline in the concentration of testosterone and other anabolic hormones. Moreover, both epidemiologic and clinical studies suggest that the elderly have a subclinical level of inflammation that may increase muscle catabolism. For example, higher concentrations of the messenger RNA and protein of inflammatory markers such as tumor necrosis factor α have been reported in frail elderly subjects.[13] This subclinical inflammation appears to be amenable to rehabilitation because it is partially reversed with exercise training. Research in the last decade[14] demonstrates a reduction in number and activation of satellite cells in older volunteers. The loss of satellite cells appears to be more significant in the population of cells associated with type IIA fibers. It is reasonable to suggest that this decline may result in the loss of the regenerative capacity of muscle fibers and an inability to compensate for the loss of fibers known to occur with aging. A final mechanism contributing to muscle loss in older men and women is the reported increase in the levels of myostatin in this population. Because myostatin is a negative regulator of muscle mass, an increase in circulating levels may lead to muscle atrophy. It is likely that no single mechanism can explain muscle dysfunction in the elderly, and that all of the above contribute to some degree to the development of sarcopenia.

Some research studies have looked at potential molecular contributors to sarcopenia and muscle dysfunction in the elderly. The concentration of myosin, the most important motor protein, has been shown to be reduced in fibers from elderly subjects expressing type I or IIA myosin heavy chain isoforms. This finding may suggest that old muscle fibers have fewer cross-bridges per muscle fiber area,[15] and therefore a lower capacity to generate force per area of contractile tissue. It must be noted that immobilization, commonly present in this population, further reduces the concentration of myosin in human single fibers. Therefore, the combination of aging and immobilization may have very deleterious effects on muscle function. Because the level of physical activity declines with adult age, the functional and clinical consequences of this synergistic effect should be obvious to the reader.[16] Another important change at the molecular level is the chemical alteration of the myosin molecule. It is possible that posttranslational chemical modifications such as protein methylation, glycosylation, and/or oxidation alter the function of the myosin filament.[17] In fact it has been shown that the velocity of filament sliding measured in vitro is impaired, although the immediate consequences for human muscle function of this observation have not been studied. Finally, at least 2 recent studies have demonstrated that sarcopenia is associated with a typical genetic pattern that includes the upregulation of a set of genes and the simultaneous downregulation of another set of genes.[18] This genetic signature is accompanied by a protein profile that appears to distinguish old and young skeletal muscle.[19] The specific contribution of this genetic signature to sarcopenia and the various expressions of muscle dysfunction in the elderly remains to be determined.

COUNTERMEASURES

It is not the purpose of this article to discuss in detail the possible benefits of various countermeasures that have been devised to slow down or reverse sarcopenia. Nevertheless, it is important to keep in mind that some of these have been shown to be effective and that it may be possible to reverse, at least partially, age-related muscle loss and dysfunction. The only strategy that has been shown to be safe and effective is some form of resistance (strength or power) exercise training; this is true even in very old individuals. Positive changes can be induced by exercise training at the whole-muscle and single-fiber levels. Some research indicates that dietary supplementation, particularly in the form of protein, may add to the benefits of exercise training. Finally, some studies have evaluated the potential benefits of hormonal strategies, particularly testosterone and growth hormone. Although some, but not all, short-term studies may suggest a positive benefit, it remains to be determined whether such an intervention is effective and/or safe in the long term.

REFERENCES

1. Janssen I, Shepard DS, Katzmatzyk PT, et al. The healthcare costs of sarcopenia in the United States. J Am Geriatr Soc 2004;52:80–5.
2. Cawthon PM, Fox KM, Gandra SR, et al. For the Health, Aging and Body Composition Study. Do muscle mass, muscle density, strength, and physical function

similarly influence risk of hospitalization in older adults? J Am Geriatr Soc 2009; 57:1411–9.

3. Wood DS, Zollman J, Reuben JP, et al. Human skeletal muscle: properties of the "chemically skinned" fiber. Science 1975;187:1075–6.

4. Larsson L, Li X, Frontera WR. Effects of ageing on shortening velocity and myosin isoform composition in single skeletal muscle cells from man. Am J Physiol (Cell Physiol) 1997;272:C638–49.

5. Frontera WR, Hughes VA, Fielding RA, et al. Aging of skeletal muscle: a 12 yr longitudinal study. J Appl Physiol 2000;88:1321–6.

6. Hughes VA, Frontera WR, Wood M, et al. Longitudinal muscle strength changes in older adults: influence of muscle mass, physical activity and health. J Gerontol A Biol Sci Med Sci 2001;56:B209–17.

7. Frontera WR, Krivickas L, Suh D, et al. Skeletal muscle fiber quality in older men and women. Am J Physiol 2000;279:C611–8.

8. Frontera WR, Reid KF, Phillips EM, et al. Muscle fiber size and function in elderly humans: a longitudinal study. J Appl Physiol 2008;105:637–42. PMC2519941.

9. Krivickas L, Suh D, Wilkins J, et al. Age and sex related differences in maximum shortening velocity of skeletal muscle fibers. Am J Phys Med Rehabil 2001;80: 447–55.

10. Yu F, Hedström M, Cristea A, et al. Effects of aging and gender on contractile properties in human skeletal muscle and single fibres. Acta Physiol 2007;190: 229–41.

11. Krivickas LS, Fielding RA, Murray A, et al. Sex differences in single muscle power in older adults. Med Sci Sports Exerc 2006;38:57–63.

12. Ochala J, Frontera WR, Krivickas LS. Single skeletal muscle fiber elastic and contractile characteristics in young and older men. J Gerontol A Biol Sci Med Sci 2007;62:375–81.

13. Greiwe JS, Cheng B, Rubin DC, et al. resistance exercise decreases skeletal muscle tumor necrosis factor α in frail elderly humans. FASEB J 2001;15:475–82.

14. Kadi F, Ponsot E. The biology of satellite cells and telomeres in human skeletal muscle: effect of aging and physical activity. Scand J Med Sci Sports 2010;20: 39–48.

15. D'Antona G, Pellegrino MA, Adami R, et al. The effect of ageing and immobilization on structure and function of human skeletal muscle fibres. J Physiol 2003; 552:499–511.

16. Kortebein P, Ferrando A, Lombeida J, et al. Effect of 10 days of bed rest on skeletal muscle in healthy older adults. JAMA 2007;297:1772–4.

17. Clarke S. Aging as war between chemical and biochemical processes: Protein methylation and the recognition of age-damaged proteins for repair. Ageing Res Rev 2003;2:263–85.

18. Giresi PG, Stevenson EJ, Theilhaber J, et al. Identification of a molecular signature of sarcopenia. Physiol Genomics 2005;21:253–63.

19. Gelfi C, Vigano A, Ripamonti M, et al. The human muscle proteome in aging. J Proteome Res 2006;5:1344–53.

Index

Note: Page numbers of article titles are in **boldface** type.

A

Aerobic exercise testing
  in metabolic myopathies, 181–184
Arm
  function of
    surgical restoration of
      in tetraplegia
        neuromuscular assessments for, **33–50**. *See also* Tetraplegia, arm and hand
          function in, surgical restoration of, neuromuscular assessments for

B

Becker muscular dystrophy (BMD)
  muscle hypertrophy in, 150–152
Biomarker(s)
  MRI as
    in DMD, 7–8
BMD. *See* Becker muscular dystrophy (BMD)

C

Cine sequence-based feature tracking (FT), 125
Connective tissue remodeling
  in decreasing muscle stiffness, 54–55
Contractile activity
  in muscle length adjustment, 52–53
Contracture(s)
  muscle hypertrophy in muscular dystrophy and, 156–161

D

DENSE. *See* Fast cine displacement-encoded (DENSE)
DEXA. *See also* Dual-energy x-ray absorptiometry (DEXA)
DMD. *See* Duchenne muscular dystrophy (DMD)
Dog(s)
  neuromuscular disorders in, 79–80
  respiratory assessment in, 82–91
    described, 82
    invasive respiratory impedance, 83
    plethysmography chambers, 83
    pneumotachometer, 83
    RIP, 83, 85–86
    transdiaphragmatic pressure, 86–91
  XXMTM in, 80–82

Phys Med Rehabil Clin N Am 23 (2012) 209–220
doi:10.1016/S1047-9651(11)00125-2
1047-9651/12/$ – see front matter © 2012 Elsevier Inc. All rights reserved.

pmr.theclinics.com

Dual-energy x-ray absorptiometry (DEXA)
    described, 67
    in neuromuscular disease progression treatment and monitoring, **67–73**
        advantages of, 68–69
        clinical applications of, 71–72
        described, 70
        disadvantages of, 69
    regional
        in neuromuscular disease progression treatment and monitoring
            described, 68
Duchenne muscular dystrophy (DMD)
    cardiac MRI in, 129–130
    characteristics of, 188–189
    clinical course of, 2
    described, 2, 187–188
    diagnosis of, 2
    management of, 188
        current, 2–3
        GTE in, 190–191
        leucine in, 191–193
    mobility in, 188–189
    muscle hypertrophy in, 150–152
    physical activity in, 189
    physical capabilities in
        nutraceuticals and
            evaluation of, 194–195
        nutrition strategies to improve, **187–199**
          energy balance and, 189–190
          evaluation of, 194–195
          pharmaceutical interventions with, 190
          recommendations related to, 195
    postural instability and contractures in, 156–158
    skeletal muscle MRI in, **1–10**. See also Magnetic resonance imaging (MRI), skeletal muscle, in DMD

E

Echogenicity measurements
    in neuromuscular ultrasonography, 138–141
Edema
    skeletal muscle
        in muscular dystrophy, **107–122**. See also Muscular dystrophy, muscle change in
Elbow extension
    reconstruction of
        in tetraplegia, 35–36, 40
Electromyography (EMG)
    described, 23–24
    in neuromuscular function assessment, **23–29**
        in fatigue threshold identification, 25–27
        responses to isometric and dynamic submaximal to maximal muscle actions, 25
Electromyography (EMG) amplitude
    in fatigue threshold identification, 25–27

Electromyography (EMG) frequency
    in fatigue threshold identification, 27
EMG. *See* Electromyography (EMG)
Energy balance
    physical activity and nutrition in
        in DMD, 189–190
Evoked phrenic motor unit pressure
    in inspiratory muscle weakness assessment, 77
Exercise
    metabolic response to, 174–176
    muscle changes in muscular dystrophy related to, 116–118
Exercise testing
    in metabolic myopathies, **173–186**. *See also* Metabolic myopathies, exercise testing in
Expiratory muscle
    dysfunction of
        assessment of
            clinical end points for clinical translation of animal model research in, 78–82
Extrinsic finger flexors
    tendon lengthening of, 42

F

Fast cine displacement-encoded (DENSE), 125
Fat-suppression sequences
    in DMD, 4–5
Fatigability
    mental
        in neuromuscular disease, 19–20
    physical
        central *vs.* peripheral
            in neuromuscular disease, 19
Fatigue
    defined, 11–12
    inspiratory muscle
        assessment of
            clinical end points for clinical translation of animal model research in, 77–78
    in neuromuscular diseases
        assessment of, **11–22**
            in laboratory setting, 15–16
            questionnaires in, 12–15
            systemic approach to, 12–16
    physical
        origin of
            central *vs.* peripheral, 16–20
                twitch interpolation and TMS in differentiation of, 18–19
Fatigue Severity Scale (FSS)
    in fatigue assessment in neuromuscular diseases, 13–14
Fatigue threshold
    EMG in identification of, 25–27
Fatty acid oxidation defect
    exercise testing in, 177–178
Feline hypertrophic muscular dystrophy (FHMD), 153

Feline (*continued*)
  postural instability and contractures in, 159
FHMD. *See* Feline hypertrophic muscular dystrophy (FHMD)
Forearm exercise testing
  in metabolic myopathies, 179–181
Forearm pronation
  reconstruction of
    in tetraplegia, 37, 41
Frequency
  in EMG signal, 24
FSS. *See* Fatigue Severity Scale (FSS)
FT. *See* Cine sequence-based feature tracking (FT)

  G

Gadolinium enhancement
  in DMD, 3
  late
    of heart
      in muscular dystrophy, 129
Glycogen storage diseases (GSDs)
  exercise testing in, 176–177
Golden Retriever muscular dystrophy (GRMD)
  muscle hypertrophy in, 154–156
  postural instability and contractures in, 159–161
Green tea extract (GTE)
  in DMD, 190–191
Grip function
  reconstruction of
    in tetraplegia, 37
GRMD. *See* Golden Retriever muscular dystrophy (GRMD)
GSDs. *See* Glycogen storage diseases (GSDs)
GTE. *See* Green tea extract (GTE)

  H

Hand
  function of
    surgical restoration of
      in tetraplegia
        neuromuscular assessments for, **33–50**. *See also* Tetraplegia, arm and hand
          function in, surgical restoration of, neuromuscular assessments for
Hand opening
  reconstruction of
    in tetraplegia, 39, 42, 44
Harmonic phase tagging (HARP), 125
HARP. *See* Harmonic phase tagging (HARP)
Heart
  disorders of
    strain as early indicator of, 126–127
  MRI of
    in muscular dystrophy, **123–132**. *See also* Muscular dystrophy, cardiac MRI in

Homocysteine. *See also* Hypohomocysteinemia
   described, 59
   metabolism of, 60
   synthesis of, 60
Hypertrophy
   muscle
      in muscular dystrophy, **149–172**. *See also* Muscular dystrophy, muscle hypertrophy in
Hypohomocysteinemia, **59–66**. *See also* Homocysteine
   clinical ramifications of, 61–62
   discussion of, 62–64

I

Impedance leads
   implanted
      in respiratory assessment in dogs, 83
Infectious neuropathy
   quantitative ultrasonography in, 143–144
Inspiratory muscle
   fatigue of
      assessment of
         clinical end points for clinical translation of animal model research in, 77–78
   weakness of
      assessment of
         clinical end points for clinical translation of animal model research in, 76–77
Intrinsic muscles
   reconstruction of
      in tetraplegia, 37, 39, 43
Invasive respiratory impedance
   in respiratory assessment in dogs, 83

K

Key pinch
   reconstruction of
      in tetraplegia, 37, 41–42

L

Late gadolinium enhancement (LGE)
   of heart
      in muscular dystrophy, 129
Leucine
   in DMD, 191–193
LGE. *See* Late gadolinium enhancement (LGE)
Littler release, 42

M

Magnetic resonance imaging (MRI)
   cardiac
      in muscular dystrophy, **123–132**. *See also* Muscular dystrophy, cardiac MRI in
   muscle biopsy *vs.*
      in DMD, 7

Magnetic (*continued*)
  skeletal muscle
    described, 2
    in DMD, **1–10**
      as biomarker for clinical trials, 7–8
      correlation with functional outcome measures, 8
      fat-suppression sequences, 4–5
      findings from, 3
      T1-weighted imaging, 3–4
      T2-weighted imaging, 4
      three-point Dixon technique, 5–6
      treatment response, 8
      uses of, 3–6
Magnetic resonance spectroscopy (MRS)
  skeletal muscle
    described, 2
    in DMD, 6
Mammalian target of rapamycin (mTOR), 192–193
Maximal inspiratory pressure (MIP)
  in inspiratory muscle weakness assessment, 76
mdx mouse
  muscle hypertrophy in, 152–153
  postural instability and contractures in, 158–159
Mechanomyography (MMG)
  in neuromuscular function assessment, **29–31**
    in clinical populations, 28
    for continuous muscle actions, 28–29
    responses to isometric and dynamic submaximal and maximal muscle actions, 28
Medical Rehabilitation Research Infrastructure Network (MMRIN), 95–96
Metabolic myopathies. *See also specific types, e.g.,*. Glycogen storage diseases (GSDs)
  exercise testing in, **173–186**
    aerobic, 181–184
    described, 178–179
    forearm, 179–181
  overview of, 173–174
  types of, 173
MFI. *See* Multidimensional Fatigue Inventory (MFI)
MIP. *See* Maximal inspiratory pressure (MIP)
Mitochondrial myopathies
  exercise testing in, 178
MMG. *See* Mechanomyography (MMG)
MMRIN. *See* Medical Rehabilitation Research Infrastructure Network (MMRIN)
MRI. *See* Magnetic resonance imaging (MRI)
MRS. *See* Magnetic resonance spectroscopy (MRS)
mTOR. *See* Mammalian target of rapamycin (mTOR)
Multidimensional Fatigue Inventory (MFI)
  in fatigue assessment in neuromuscular diseases, 14
Muscle
  actions of
    continuous
      MMG in, 28–29

aging of, **201–207**
    countermeasures to, 206
    physiologic, cellular, and molecular contributors to, 205–206
    study of, 202
    weakness of single muscle fibers, 204–205
    whole-muscle weakness, 203–204
  imaging of, 2
  measurements of
    quantification of, **133–148**. *See also* Ultrasonography, neuromuscular
  skeletal
    properties of, 51
  stiffness of
    connective tissue remodeling effects on, 54–55
  weakness of
    physiologic, cellular, and molecular contributors to, 205–206
Muscle biopsy
  MRI *vs.*
    in DMD, 7
Muscle cell
  sarcopenia at level of, **201–207**. *See also* Sarcopenia, at muscle cell level
Muscle fibers
  weakness of, 204–205
Muscle hypertrophy
  in muscular dystrophy, **149–172**. *See also* Muscular dystrophy, muscle hypertrophy in
Muscle length
  adaptation of, 52
  adjustment of
    contractile activity in, 52–53
  stretching effects on
    active, **51–57**
    passive, **51–57**
      described, 53–54
Muscle mass
  loss of, 201–202
Muscular dystrophy. *See also specific types, e.g.,* Duchenne muscular dystrophy (DMD)
  cardiac MRI in, **123–132**
    analysis methods, 125
    described, 123–125
    full picture in, 130
    strain related to heart problems, 126–128
    T2 measurement in, 128–129
  muscle change in
    analysis technique considerations, 118–119
    correlation of inflammation to MRI findings in, 116
    exercise and, 116–118
    future directions in, 119
    patterns of, 111–113
    progression of
      imaging in assessment of, 108–111
    quantitative assessment of, 114–116
    semiquantitative assessment of, 114

Muscular (*continued*)
    muscle hypertrophy in, **149–172**
        BMD, 152–153
        DMD, 152–153
        FHMD, 153
        GRMD, 154–156
        mdx mouse and, 152–153
        mechanisms contributing to, 162–163
        postural instability and contractures, 156–161
        variable muscle involvement and, 150–156
    myostatin inhibition in, 163–165
    skeletal muscle edema in, **107–122**. *See also* Muscular dystrophy, muscle change in
    types of, 107–108
Myopathy(ies)
    metabolic
        exercise testing in, **173–186**. *See also* Metabolic myopathies, exercise testing in
    mitochondrial
        exercise testing in, 178
Myostatin
    inhibition of
        in muscle disease, 163–165

N

Nasal sniff pressure
    in inspiratory muscle weakness assessment, 77
National Skeletal Muscle Research Center (NSMRC), 96–97
    opportunities for rehabilitation researchers, 102
    sharing of expertise with rehabilitation community, 102–104
Nerve(s)
    measurements of
        quantification of, **133–148**. *See also* Ultrasonography, neuromuscular
Nerve transfers
    in tetraplegia, 44–47
Neuromuscular diseases. *See also specific diseases*
    central and peripheral physical fatigability in, 19
    in dogs
        described, 79–80
    fatigue in
        assessment of, **11–22**
        mental, 19–20
    myostatin inhibition in, 163–165
    progression of
        DEXA in treatment and monitoring of, **67–73**. *See also* Dual-energy x-ray
            absorptiometry (DEXA), in neuromuscular disease progression treatment and
            monitoring
    treatment of
        establishing clinical end points for clinical translation of animal model research in,
            75–94. *See also* Respiratory function, in large animals, establishing clinical end
            points for clinical translation
Neuromuscular function
    assessment of

EMG in, **23–29**. *See also* Electromyography (EMG), in neuromuscular function assessment

MMG in, **29–31**. *See also* Mechanomyography (MMG), in neuromuscular function assessment

Neuromuscular research

core descriptions, 97–102

administration core, 101

biomechanics core, 98

histology core, 97–98

imaging core, 98–100

muscle metabolism core, 100–101

new opportunities in, **95–105**

support of

novel paradigms in, **95–105**

Neuromuscular ultrasonography, **133–148**. *See also* Ultrasonography, neuromuscular

Neuropathy(ies)

infectious

quantitative ultrasonography in, 143–144

NSMRC. *See* National Skeletal Muscle Research Center (NSMRC)

Nutraceuticals

in improving physical capabilities in DMD

evaluation of, 194–195

Nutrition

in improving physical capabilities in DMD, **187–199**. *See also* Duchenne muscular dystrophy (DMD), physical capabilities in, nutrition strategies to improve

P

Peripheral neuropathology

hypohomocysteinemia and, **59–66**. *See also* Hypohomocysteinemia

PFS. *See* Piper Fatigue Scale (PFS)

Physical activity

in DMD, 189

Piper Fatigue Scale (PFS)

in neuromuscular diseases, 14–15

Plethysmography chambers

in respiratory assessment in dogs, 83

Pneumotachometer

in respiratory assessment in dogs, 83

Postural instability

muscle hypertrophy in muscular dystrophy and, 156–161

Power grip

reconstruction of

in tetraplegia, 37, 42

R

Range of motion

in neuromuscular assessment for surgical restoration of arm and hand function in tetraplegia, 34

Rehabilitation researchers

NSMRC opportunities for, 102

Respiratory function
    assessment of
        in neuromuscular disease patients, 75–76
    in dogs
        assessment of, 82–91. *See also* Dog(s), respiratory assessment in
    in large animals
        establishing clinical end points for clinical translation, **75–94**
            expiratory muscle dysfunction, 78–82
            inspiratory muscle fatigue, 77–78
            inspiratory muscle weakness, 76–77
            respiratory assessment, 75–76
Respiratory impedance plethysmography (RIP)
    in respiratory assessment in dogs, 83, 85–86
RIP. *See* Respiratory impedance plethysmography (RIP)

S

Sarcopenia
    defined, 201
    at muscle cell level, **201–207**
        countermeasures to, 206
        physiologic, cellular, and molecular contributors to, 205–206
Sensibility testing
    in neuromuscular assessment for surgical restoration of arm and hand function in
        tetraplegia, 34–35
Skeletal muscle
    properties of, 51
Skeletal muscle edema
    in muscular dystrophy, **107–122**. *See also* Muscular dystrophy, muscle change in
Spasticity
    procedures for
        in tetraplegia, 42–43
Spinal cord injury
    prevalence of, 33
Strain
    as early indicator of heart problems, 126–127
        across longitudinal course, 127
        complexity of interpreting metrics related to, 127
        as treatment index, 128
Stretching
    muscle length effects of, **51–57**. *See also* Muscle length, stretching effects on

T

T1-weighted imaging
    in DMD, 3–4
T2-weighted imaging
    in DMD, 4
    of heart
        in muscular dystrophy, 128–129

Tetraplegia
    arm and hand function in
        surgical restoration of
            combined procedures, 43–44
            elbow extension, 35–36, 40
            forearm pronation, 37, 41
            grip function, 37
            hand opening, 39, 42, 44
            immediate activation of tendon transfers, 44
            intrinsic muscles, 37, 39, 43
            key pinch, 37, 41–42
            nerve transfers, 44–47
            neuromuscular assessments for, **33–50**
                joint range of motion in, 34
                muscle testing in, 34
                sensibility testing in, 34–35
            new developments in, 43–47
            planning of, 35–43
            power grip, 37, 42
            for spasticity, 42–43
            wrist extension, 37
Three-point Dixon technique
    in DMD, 5–6
Time
    in EMG signal, 24
TMS. *See* Transcranial magnetic stimulation (TMS)
Transcranial magnetic stimulation (TMS)
    in central *vs.* peripheral fatigability differentiation, 18–19
Transdiaphragmatic pressure
    in inspiratory muscle weakness assessment, 77
    in respiratory assessment in dogs, 86–91
Twitch interpolation
    in central *vs.* peripheral fatigability differentiation, 18–19

U

Ultrasonography
    muscle
        in muscle disease assessment, 2
    neuromuscular, **133–148**
        echogenicity measurements in, 138–141
        in infectious neuropathy, 143–144
        muscle dynamics in, 141–142
        quantification of, 142–144
        size measurements in, 134–138

V

VAS. *See* Visual Analog Scale (VAS)
Visual Analog Scale (VAS)
    in fatigue assessment in neuromuscular diseases, 12–13

W

Whole-muscle weakness, 203–204
Wrist extension
    reconstruction of
        in tetraplegia, 37

X

X-linked myotubular myopathy (XXMTM)
    animal models of, 78–79
    described, 78
    in dogs, 80–82
XXMTM. *See* X-linked myotubular myopathy (XXMTM)

Moving?

Make sure your subscription moves with you!

To notify us of your new address, find your **Clinics Account Number** (located on your mailing label above your name), and contact customer service at:

Email: journalscustomerservice-usa@elsevier.com

800-654-2452 (subscribers in the U.S. & Canada)
314-447-8871 (subscribers outside of the U.S. & Canada)

Fax number: 314-447-8029

Elsevier Health Sciences Division
Subscription Customer Service
3251 Riverport Lane
Maryland Heights, MO 63043

*To ensure uninterrupted delivery of your subscription, please notify us at least 4 weeks in advance of move.